Anesthesia and Intensive Care for Patients with Liver Disease

Anesthesia and Intensive Care for Patients with Liver Disease

edited by
Gilbert R. Park, M.D., M.B.Ch.B., F.R.C.A.

Director of Intensive Care and Consultant in Anaesthesia
The John Farman Intensive Care Unit
Addenbrooke's Hospital, Cambridge

and
Yoogoo Kang, M.D.

Professor of Anesthesiology, University of Pittsburgh School of Medicine, and Director, Hepatic Transplantation Anesthesiology, Presbyterian University Hospital, Pittsburgh

with a Foreword by
Sir Roy Calne, F.R.S.

Professor of Surgery, University of Cambridge Clinical School, Cambridge

Butterworth–Heinemann
Boston   London   Oxford   Singapore   Sydney   Toronto   Wellington

Library of Congress Cataloging-in-Publication Data

Anesthesia and intensive care for patients with liver disease / edited
    by Gilbert R. Park and Yoo Goo Kang ; with foreword by Sir Roy
    Calne.
        p.   cm.
    Includes bibliographical references and index.
    ISBN 0-7506-9554-4 (alk. paper)
        1. Liver—Diseases—Complications. 2. Anesthesia—Complications.
    3. Liver—Surgery—Complications. I. Park, G.R. (Gilbert R.)
    II. Kang, Yoo Goo.
        [DNLM: 1. Liver Diseases—physiopathology. 2. Liver—drug
    effects. 3. Anesthesia—adverse effects. 4. Anesthesia.
    5. Preoperative Care. WI 700 1994]
    RD87.3.L53A54 1994
    617.5'56—dc20
    DNLM/DLC
    for Library of Congress   94-11812
                                                                          CIP

British Library Cataloguing-in-Publication Data
A catalogue record for this book is available from the British
Library

Butterworth-Heinemann
313 Washington Stereet
Newton, MA 02158

10 9 8 7 6 5 4 3 2 1

Printed in the United States of America

Contents

Contributors

Graeme Alexander, MRCP
Lecturer in Medicine, University of Cambridge; Consultant in Hepatology, Department of Medicine, Addenbrooke's Hospital, Cambridge

John C. Berridge, MB, ChB, MRCP, FRCA
Senior Lecturer in Anaesthesia, University of Leeds; Consultant in Anaesthetics and Intensive Care, The General Infirmary at Leeds, Leeds

Julian Bion, MB, BS, MRCP, FRCA, MD
Senior Lecturer in Intensive Care Medicine, University Department of Anaesthesia and Intensive Care, University of Birmingham; Consultant in Intensive Care, University Department of Anaesthetics and Intensive Care, The Queen Elizabeth Hospital, Birmingham

D. Ryan Cook, MD
Professor of Anesthesiology, University of Pittsburgh School of Medicine; Director, Department of Anesthesiology, Children's Hospital of Pittsburgh, Pittsburgh, Pennsylvania

Mervyn H. Davies, MB, ChB, MRCP
Research Fellow, The Liver and Hepatobiliary Unit, The Queen Elizabeth Hospital, Birmingham

Peter J. Davis, MD
Associate Professor of Anesthesia and Pediatrics, University of Pittsburgh School of Medicine; Associate Director, Department of Anesthesia, Children's Hospital of Pittsburgh, Pittsburgh, Pennsylvania

Andre M. De Wolf, MD
Associate Professor of Anesthesiology, University of Pittsburgh School of Medi-

cine; Department of Anesthesiology, Presbyterian University Hospital, Pittsburgh, Pennsylvania

Vincents J. Dindzans, MD
Division of Gastroenterology, University of Pittsburgh School of Medicine, Pittsburgh, Pennsylvania

A. C. Elston, FFARCSI
Research Registrar, The John Farman Intensive Care Unit, Addenbrooke's Hospital, Cambridge

Simon Gelman, MD, PhD
Leroy D. Vandam/Benjamin G. Covino Professor of Anaesthesia, Harvard Medical School; Chairman, Department of Anesthesia, Brigham and Women's Hospital, Boston, Massachusetts

K. E. J. Gunning, MB, BS, FRCS, FRCA
Consultant in Anaesthesia and Intensive Care, The John Farman Intensive Care Unit, Addenbrooke's Hospital, Cambridge

S. Kim Jacobson, MB, ChB, MRCP, MRCPath
Senior Registrar, Clinical Microbiology and Public Health Laboratory, Addenbrooke's Hospital, Cambridge

Yoogoo Kang, MD
Director, Hepatic Transplantation Anesthesiology, Department of Anesthesiology, Presbyterian University Hospital, Pittsburgh, Pennsylvania

John R. Klinck, MD, FRCA, FRCPC
Consultant in Anaesthesia and Intensive Care, Department of Anaesthesia, Addenbrooke's Hospital, Cambridge

Graham Neale, MA, BSc, MB, FRCP
Honorary Clinical Scientist, MRC Dunn Clinical Nutrition Centre; Consultant Physician, Department of Gastroenterology and Clinical Nutrition, Addenbrooke's Hospital, Cambridge

James M. Neuberger, DM, FRCS
Senior Lecturer in Medicine, University of Birmingham Medical School; Consultant Physician, The Liver and Hepatobiliary Unit, Department of Medicine, The Queen Elizabeth Hospital, Birmingham

Gilbert R. Park, MD, MBChB, FRCA
Director of Intensive Care and Consultant in Anaesthesia, The John Farman Intensive Care Unit, Addenbrooke's Hospital, Cambridge

Dale A. Parks, PhD
Associate Professor of Anesthesiology, Physiology and Biophysics, and Pediatrics, University of Alabama at Birmingham School of Medicine, Birmingham

Mordechai Rabinovitz, MD
Assistant Professor of Medicine, University of Pittsburgh School of Medicine; Division of Gastroenterology and Hepatology, University of Pittsburgh Medical Center, Pittsburgh, Pennsylvania

Steven R. Rettke, MD
Assistant Professor of Anesthesiology, Mayo Medical School; Chair, Division of Rochester Methodist Hospital North Anesthesia, Department of Anesthesiology, Mayo Clinic, Rochester, Minnesota

Paul G. Roe, BSc, MBBS, FRCA
Consultant in Anaesthesia and Intensive Care, The John Farman Intensive Care Unit, Addenbrooke's Hospital, Cambridge

Robert R. Schade, MD
Associate Professor of Medicine, Division of Gastroenterology, University of Pittsburgh Medical Center, Pittsburgh, Pennsylvania

Dagmar Schaps, Prof. Dr. Med.
Professor of Anaesthesia and Supervisor, Department of Anaesthesiology, Medizinische Hochschule Hannover, Hannover, Germany

Raymond D. Seifert, DO
Former Assistant Professor of Anesthesiology/Critical Care Medicine, University of Pittsburgh School of Medicine, Pittsburgh, Pennsylvania

Maire P. Shelly, FRCA
Consultant in Anaesthesia and Intensive Care, Intensive Care Unit, University Hospital of South Manchester, Manchester

David H. Van Thiel, MD
Medical Director of Transplantation, Oklahoma Transplant Institute, Baptist Medical Center of Oklahoma, Oklahoma City

Rosalind Ward, FRCA
Consultant Anaesthetist, Department of Anaesthesia, East Birmingham Hospital, Birmingham

Roderic E. Warren, MB, BChir, FRCPath.
Honorary Senior Lecturer, Department of Infection, University of Birmingham; Director, Public Health Laboratory, The Royal Shrewsbury Hospital, Shrewsbury

Foreword

This is an important new volume on anesthesia and perioperative care in patients with liver disease. It is edited by Dr. Park and Dr. Kang, pioneers in anesthesia and intensive care for liver transplantation, who have wide experience in this field. The editors have brought together a group of experts in different aspects of liver disease and anesthesia, and this text includes research that has been performed in patients in the anhepatic state. This has added important new knowledge to metabolism and interaction of drugs and complements a large body of information that has been gained over the years from patients with severe liver dysfunction, both acute and chronic.

Liver transplantation has become a success story, in terms of therapy, providing a good chance not only of survival but also excellent rehabilitation except when the original disease was malignant or viral. Unfortunately, these last two conditions are prone to recur and these two areas are, of course, important fields for further investigation. I am sure this up-to-date volume will be of great interest to anybody caring for patients who are in a vulnerable state due to impaired liver function.

Sir Roy Calne, FRS
Professor of Surgery, University of Cambridge
Clinical School, Cambridge, England

Preface

Liver disease is complex and usually brings about changes in many other organ systems. These changes have tended to limit surgical operations to the minimum possible in the past. Many recent advances in surgical and anesthetic techniques, blood transfusion, microbiology, immunology, and nutrition have now made longer and more invasive operations possible. Furthermore, liver disease may develop after nonhepatic surgery if complications arise that cause multiorgan dysfunction. The increased frequency with which liver disease is now being seen by clinicians concerned with the care of patients after operative has prompted this book. We believe the time is now right for a book that covers the many problems that liver disease causes in this group of patients.

Many specialties are involved in the care of patients after surgery. No longer is it just the anesthesiologist and surgeon, but physicians, microbiologists, nutritionists, and many others. We have tried to incorporate as wide a group as possible of contributors. The only criterion for inclusion as an author is active involvement with patients of this type.

Surgery is a continuum. It starts with assessment before operation by the physician, surgeon, and anesthesiologist and continues through the operation into the postoperative period. This book addresses the various difficulties that may be faced in the same order, although some may occur at any stage and their placement is arbitrary.

We are grateful to our many colleagues in the clinics, operating room, laboratories, and intensive care units who have helped us with this book.

G.R.P.
Y.K.

ONE

Assessment

Chapter 1

Normal Liver Function and the Hepatic Circulation

Dale A. Parks and Simon Gelman

Introduction

The liver lies in the right upper quadrant of the abdominal cavity and is attached to the diaphragm. It is the largest gland in the body, weighing approximately 1.5 kg. This represents 2% of the body weight in an adult and 5% in a neonate. The liver is divided into four lobes. Its circulation is supplied by the portal vein and hepatic artery and drains into the hepatic veins, which subsequently empty into the inferior vena cava. Bile drains into the right and left hepatic ducts. The liver is covered by a thin connective tissue capsule, called Glisson's capsule, which serves as a supportive framework for the hepatic parenchyma, vessels, and nerves.

The splanchnic vasculature receives, at rest, approximately 25–30% of the cardiac output (about 1500–1800 mL/min in a 70-kg adult). The arterial supply of the splanchnic organs originates primarily from three branches of the abdominal aorta: the celiac, superior mesenteric, and inferior mesenteric arteries. The superior mesenteric artery supplies most of the small intestine, the proximal colon, and the pancreas, while the inferior mesentric artery supplies the distal colon and the rectum. It is the celiac artery that supplies the liver, pancreas, stomach, and duodenum.

Anatomy

Extrahepatic Anatomy

Hepatic Artery

Anatomic variations in the hepatic artery are very common, with the usual pattern being present in only about 50% of individuals. In a typical person, the celiac axis arises from the anterior surface of the abdominal aorta immediately below the aortic hiatus of the diaphragm. After a very short course of only about 1 cm, the celiac artery trifurcates into the splenic, common hepatic, and left gastric arteries. The splenic artery is the largest of the branches. After running a tortuous course along the upper border of the pancreas, it provides branches to the pancreas, stomach, and spleen. The smallest branch of the celiac axis is the left gastric artery. This vessel runs cephalad and anterior to reach the stomach near the esophagogastric junction. The left gastric artery contributes most of the blood supply to the anterior and posterior walls of the stomach as well as sending several small branches to the esophagus and cardiac regions. The common hepatic artery arises from the right side of the celiac artery, passing along the upper border of the pancreas. It passes cephalad and posterior to the duodenum, usually giving off the gastroduodenal artery as its first branch. The common hepatic artery then ascends toward the liver, giving rise to the right gastric artery. After this point, it is referred to as the proper hepatic artery. In the lesser omentum, the proper hepatic artery runs medial to the common bile duct and anterior to the portal vein. It normally proceeds upward parallel to both these structures and, as it nears the liver, divides to form the right and left hepatic branches at the porta hepatis. The right hepatic artery passes behind the common hepatic duct and, in the triangle between the common hepatic duct, cystic duct, and the visceral surface of the liver (triangle of Calot), it commonly gives off the cystic artery. The cystic artery supplies the gallbladder before finally dividing terminally to supply the parenchyma of the right lobe of the liver. The left hepatic artery gives off branches to the caudate and quadrate hepatic lobes before ending as the arterial supply of the left lobe of the liver.

Portal Vein

The portal vein is the terminal vessel that collects and returns the whole of the effluent of the splanchnic vasculature to the liver. This relatively short vessel, approximately 5 cm, is formed behind the head of the pancreas by the union of the splenic and superior mesenteric veins. The portal vein also drains the inferior mesenteric vein, which enters, although variably, the terminal portion of the splenic vein. In addition, the portal vein receives tributaries from the stomach and the upper portion of the pancreas and duodenum. The veins and entry are highly variable, but commonly include the right and left gastric veins and less often a cystic vein. The portal vein runs posterior to the first part of the duodenum and enters the lesser omentum before ascending into the porta hepatis where it divides into right and left terminal branches.

Hepatic Veins

The blood in the sinusoids, derived from both the arterial and portal circulations, is collected into three major hepatic veins. The right hepatic vein is the largest of these and lies between the anterior and posterior segments of the right lobe. It drains the entire posterior portion of the right lobe and a variable portion of the anterior superior segment. The right

hepatic vein is actually a bundle of several veins that converge into a single, occasionally double, opening into the anterior wall of the inferior vena cava. The left hepatic vein lies between the medial and lateral segments of the left lobe and drains the lateral portion of the left lobe. The middle hepatic vein lies in the lobar fissure and drains the medial segment of the left lobe and a variable portion of the right lobe. Most often, the left and middle hepatic veins join so that only two major hepatic veins empty into the vena cava.

Intrahepatic Anatomy

The microcirculation of the liver has recently been described in detail by Campra and Reynolds.[1] Briefly, major trunks of the portal vein ramify and eventually penetrate the liver substance. Interlobular or conducting veins give rise to smaller axial and marginal distributing veins before branching extensively and eventually becoming continuous with the sinusoids. Hepatic arteries run with branches of the portal vein before branching to form arterioles, terminal arterioles, precapillaries, and capillaries. These terminal branches of the hepatic artery can subsequently form into:

1. a general plexus supplying the portal tract other than bile ducts;
2. the peribiliary plexus, a network of capillaries surrounding the bile ducts;
3. arterial capillaries that empty directly into the sinusoid.

Both afferent and efferent hepatic vessels are richly innervated. McCuskey has described smooth muscle sphincters at the bifurcation of the arterioles.[2] Sphincters have been described at the junction of the sinusoid with the portal venules (inlet sphincters) and with the terminal hepatic veins (outlet sphincters). These sphincters may play a major role in the regulation of hepatic blood flow through both intrinsic and extrinsic regulatory mechanisms.

Hepatic Sinusoids

Blood is carried by the terminal portal venules into the hepatic sinusoids. The hepatic sinusoid is structurally unique among the microvasculature, consisting of three major cell types: endothelial cells,

Kupffer cells, and fat-storing cells, also referred to as Ito cells, perisinusoidal cells, lipocytes, or stellate cells. The endothelial cells or Kupffer cells are in direct contact with the bloodstream and are located "littoral," or "on the shore," whereas the fat-storing cells and parenchymal cells (hepatocytes) are in contact with the plasma only in the space of Disse.[3]

In the early 1970s, electron microscopic studies revealed that hepatic endothelial cells are unique with highly characteristic ultrastructural features.[4] The endothelial cells, which constitute approximately 44% of all cells in the liver, possess a cell body with a nucleus and thin extended processes containing multiple fenestrae or pores arranged in clusters termed "sieve-plates." The fenestrations are quite large, with diameters ranging from 100–500 nm in many species, and have no diaphragm to close the fenestrae.[5] Unlike normal vascular endothelium, liver endothelial cells, at least in humans and the rat, are devoid of an underlying basement membrane. The porous nature of the sinusoidal wall allows almost unrestricted communication of the blood plasma between the vascular space and the space of Disse. Interestingly, the endothelial cells also contain features indicative of a well-developed endocytic capability such as membrane invaginations, lysosome-like vacuoles, and numerous vesicles.[3] In spite of the significant numbers of vesicles, their role in macromolecular transport is considered to be insignificant compared with that occurring through the massive endothelial gaps.

Kupffer cells also contribute to the sinusoidal wall, consisting of about 33% of all cells in the liver. These cells are distinguished from other hepatic cells on the basis of morphologic, cytochemical, biochemical, and functional criteria. Kupffer cells are highly phagocytic and constitute 80–90% of the fixed macrophages of the reticuloendothelial (RE) system. Kupffer cells are attached to the endothelial cells of the cytoplasmic processes. Within the acinus, Kupffer cell morphology and cellular density appear to be heterogeneous. Approximately 43% of the Kupffer cells are preferentially located in the periportal region of the hepatic acinus.[6] These cells appear to be larger, contain larger and more heterogeneous lysosomes, and have higher lysosomal enzyme activities than in midacinic and perivenous regions. This preferential location is consistent with the primary function of Kupffer cells, that is, the endocytosis of large quantities of particulate material entering the sinusoid.

The remaining cell type that constitutes the sinusoid is the "pit" cell. These cells are in contact with both the sinusoidal lumen and the hepatocytes. On the basis of the high content of intracytoplasmic granules, it is postulated that pit cells have a neuroendocrine function or "natural killer cell" function.

Terminal Hepatic Venules

Most of the sinusoids empty into terminal hepatic venules (central veins). The terminal hepatic venules connect at right angles with sublobular veins, which in turn empty into collecting hepatic veins and eventually drain into three major hepatic veins.

Microcirculatory Unit: The Liver Acinus

The gastrointestinal tract and other visceral vascular beds are arranged in parallel with the venous blood draining into the portal vein. This is a low-pressure (6–10 mmHg), low-resistance circuit that provides 70–75% of the blood supply to the liver. The remaining 25–30% of the blood supply is derived from the high-pressure, high-resistance circuitry of the hepatic artery. The high-pressure hepatic and low-pressure portal afferent systems meet within the sinusoidal bed of the structural and functional unit of the hepatic parenchyma, the simple liver acinus. Here, the pressure is estimated to be 2–4 mmHg above that of the inferior vena caval pressure. The simple acinus consists of a three-dimensional, microscopic mass of irregular size and shape arranged around a small, triangular, vascular axis consisting of a terminal hepatic arteriole, a terminal portal venule, a bile ductule, lymph vessels, and nerves.[7]

The terminal hepatic venule, and the glomus of sinusoids that branch off from it, join with a terminal hepatic arteriole before entering the sinusoidal inlet to perfuse the liver acinus. Blood flows from the acinar core and exits the liver acinus by two or more hepatic venules (central veins in lobular terminology). The unidirectional perfusion of the hepatic acinus allows arbitrary divisions into three zones.[7] Cells in zone 1 are in close proximity to the arterioles and are bathed in blood with a composition closer to that of the hepatic arterial blood than to that of the portal venous blood. Cells of zone 3 (perivenular) are on the periphery of the acinus and are perfused with blood modified by the uptake and secretion of solutes of cells from zones 1 and 2. In between zones 1 and 3 is an intermediate area referred to as zone 2. Cells in zone 3 are the most sensitive and those in zone 1 the least sensitive to damage resulting from anoxia, ischemia, congestion, and nutritional deficiency. In addition to differences in the microenvironment surrounding the hepatocytes, there are zonal morphological and biochemical differences among the hepatocytes which optimize the cells to their particular physiologic function. The more aerobic hepatocytes of zone 1 are preferentially equipped with enzymes required for oxidative energy metabolism, β-oxidation, amino acid catabolism, gluconeogenesis, and ureagenesis from amino acids. Zone 1 is also preferentially equipped with oxidant protective enzymes (antioxidants). Zone 3 is relatively hypoxic as the hepatocytes are equipped for less oxygen-dependent processes such as glycolysis, liponeogenesis, and biotransformation.[8]

Hepatocellular Function

The unique interposition of the liver between the digestive tract and the systemic circulation assists the liver in handling the large amount of nutrients, amino acids, carbohydrates, lipids, and even pollutants presented to it. One of the primary functions of the liver is the metabolism of carbohydrates, protein, lipids, porphyrins, and bile acids. In addition, the vast majority of serum proteins are synthesized within the liver, with two notable exceptions in the adult: gamma globulin and hemoglobin. The infant retains the ability to synthesize hemoglobin. The liver is a major site for storage of iron, glycogen, lipids, and vitamins. The liver also plays a critical role in the excretion of toxic metabolic products such as bilirubin, ammonia, and urea. In addition, the liver is instrumental in the detoxification of xenobiotics, foreign materials such as drugs, and environmental toxins. Finally, the liver serves as a significant reservoir for blood during episodes of decreased arterial blood pressure and/or circulatory blood volume.

Hemodynamics and Oxygenation

The liver is supplied by a varying mixture of oxygenated hepatic arterial and partially deoxygenated portal venous blood. As a result, the hepatic artery delivers approximately 25–30% of total hepatic blood flow and approximately 45–50% of hepatic oxygen supply, whereas the portal vein provides 70–75% of total hepatic blood supply and only 55% of hepatic oxygen supply. Under normal conditions, extraction of oxygen by the liver is less than 40% of oxygen delivered, with oxygen uptake estimated at 4–6 mL/min/100 g liver.[1] The primary mechanism for meeting oxygen demand is increased oxygen extraction. The afferent and efferent vessels within each hepatic unit are symmetrical and all sinusoidal inlets and all sinusoidal outlets are adjacent.[9] Because blood flow in adjacent sinusoids is concurrent (unidirectional), there is no opportunity for intrahepatic short-circuiting of oxygen. Therefore, oxygen extraction in the liver is potentially more efficient than that in most other organs and is the primary mechanism by which increased hepatic oxygen requirements are satisfied.

Regulation of Hepatic Blood Flow

Total blood flow, as well as distribution between the hepatic arterial and portal venous vascular beds, is determined primarily by:

1. hepatic arterial vascular resistance
2. intrahepatic portal venous vascular resistance
3. portal venous blood flow, which is determined by vascular resistance in the preportal splanchnic organs.[10]

Intrinsic Regulation

Hepatic Arterial–Portal Venous Interactions

The reciprocal interaction between the hepatic artery and the portal vein has been extensively studied since its description by Burtin-Opitz over 80 years ago.[11] The principal purpose of this reciprocal relationship is the attenuation of potentially large transient fluctuations in total hepatic blood flow and oxygen delivery that would otherwise occur as a result of changes in portal blood flow. A decrease in portal venous blood flow is usually accompanied by an increase in hepatic arterial blood flow.[12–14] Since the liver cannot control portal venous flow, and hepatic clearance of a number of endogenous and exogenous compounds is known to be flow dependent,[13–15] prevention of transient shifts in hepatic blood flow resulting from a decrease in portal blood flow could be of major homeostatic importance.[14] Compensation by the hepatic artery for changes in portal blood flow, at least to some extent, adjusts total hepatic blood flow to minimize alterations in hepatic clearance of endogenous substances.[13,14] This increase in hepatic arterial blood flow could also help maintain oxygen supply to the liver.[12,16,17] This control, the so-called hepatic arterial buffer response, functions to regulate blood flow per se and does not respond to altered oxygen content of the blood, altered metabolic activity, or altered oxygen uptake or biliary secretion. This situation is much different from that for most arteries in the body, which are highly responsive to the metabolic status of tissues they supply. Several mechanisms have been proposed to account for the reciprocal relationship between portal venous and hepatic arterial blood flows, including intrinsic neural control, a myogenic mechanism, and a metabolic or dilator washout phenomenon. The dilator washout hypothesis postulates that a hepatic arterial vasodilator, namely adenosine, is produced within the liver.[13,14] When portal blood flow is decreased, adenosine accumulates, resulting in dilation of the hepatic arterial vasculature.[15] Although the mechanism controlling the arterial buffer response is unclear, the presence and importance of the response are obvious.

Venous Pressure Elevation

The liver, by virtue of its unique microcirculation, is highly vulnerable to disturbances in hydrostatic pressure because no effective protein osmotic pressure is generated across the highly porous sinusoidal endothelium to oppose the hydrostatic pressure. Continued elevation of the venous pressure results in increased hepatic blood volume, increased fluid filtration, increased liver lymph flow, and formation of ascitic fluid.[5] To help offset the elevation in venous pressure, the precapillary sphincters and small arterioles constrict. This response is postulated to result from a myogenic mechanism

based on the observation that the vasodilator papaverine abolishes this effect. The mechanism remains undefined, however, because papaverine also increases oxygen delivery, which subsequently alters tissue levels of metabolites.

Pressure-Flow Autoregulation

Autoregulation is the tendency for local blood flow to be maintained despite alterations in perfusion pressure. There is some evidence that the hepatic artery, although apparently not the portal vein, exhibits autoregulatory ability. A reduction in hepatic artery pressure in innervated[18] or denervated[19] liver preparations results in a substantial reduction in hepatic artery resistance. Obliteration of this response by the vasodilator papaverine or by *Escherichia coli* endotoxin is consistent with a myogenic mechanism. However, the dependency of the response on both the duration and the extent of the arterial occlusion[10] suggests a progressive buildup of vasodilator metabolites and a metabolic mechanism.

Extrinsic Regulation of Hepatic Blood Flow

Neural Control

The hepatic plexus receives fibers from the celiac plexus, the vagi, and sometimes the right phrenic nerves to form a thick coat around the hepatic artery. The sympathetics and parasympathetics form two separate, but intercommunicating, plexuses. Stimulation of the hepatic periarterial sympathetic nerves increases hepatic arterial vascular resistance, followed by a brief period of hyperemia. Stimulation of the hepatic nerves increases vascular resistance in the portal vein, which is manifested by an increased portal pressure with no reduction in blood flow.[20] The hepatic artery exhibits autoregulatory escape in the cat, but not in the dog.[7] The portal bed does not exhibit autoregulatory escape in either the dog or the cat.

Respiratory Control

A cyclic pattern of alterations in blood flow appears to occur during spontaneous ventilation. Outflow of blood from the hepatic vein is maximal during expiration and decreases substantially during inspiration.[1] The alteration during inspiration has been attributed to the increased pressure on the sus-pending matrix of the liver, with a resulting partial collapse of the vasculature due to downward dis-placement by the diaphragm. Blood then accumu-lates behind the liver in the splanchnic vasculature, and splanchnic outflow decreases. At the same time, intrathoracic and caval vein pressure de-crease. This facilitates inferior vena caval blood flow from the kidneys and lower extremities. Op-posite effects occur during expiration, when the diaphragm is displaced upward, releasing the com-pression of the liver, decreasing hepatic venous pressure, and thereby facilitating an increase in splanchnic outflow. At the same time, intrathoracic and vena caval pressures increase, diminishing the pressure gradient for venous return and venous out-flow from the lower part of the body. It is clear that such an arrangement maintains the stability of ve-nous return through the inferior vena cava, which predominantly consists of blood flow from the lower part of the body during inspiration and from the splanchnic system during expiration.[21] Myo-genic mechanisms apparently modify, to a certain extent, such fluctuations in splanchnic blood flow.

Osmoreceptors

Changes in portal venous osmolality increase he-patic artery blood flow with little change in portal vascular resistance. It has been demonstrated that infusion of hypertonic solution results in a release of arginine vasopressin in direct proportion to the osmolality of the stimulus. Increased osmolality is a probable contributor to postprandial hepatic hyperemia.[10]

*Gastrointestinal (GI) and
Pancreatic Hormones*

It is improbable that any GI hormone, acting alone, is an important physiologic mediator of hepatic blood flow. Several GI hormones known to increase blood flow in the mesenteric circulation, including pentagastrin, cholecytokinin, secretin, and vasoac-tive intestinal polypeptide (VIP), produce only mild to moderate increases in portal blood flow.[1,10] Intra-venous glucagon increases total hepatic blood flow, presumably through a large increase in portal ve-nous flow as a result of vasodilation of the mesen-teric circulation.[22] There is also an accompanying

transient increase in hepatic arterial blood flow as a result of antagonism of hepatic arterial vasocon-striction by an unknown mechanism.[23]

Methods for Measurement of Hepatic Blood Flow

Essential to the understanding of the pathoetiology of organ dysfunction is the awareness of organ per-fusion. Since inadequate hepatic perfusion is com-mon to the etiology of many pathologic states, the need for a reliable technique to estimate hepatic blood flow is obvious. However, the relatively in-accessible dual blood supply of the liver coupled with the location of the hepatic veins deep in the he-patic parenchyma has made it difficult to devise methods for the determination of blood flow. The ideal method should be simple, safe, noninvasive, continuous, quantitative, accurate, reproducible, in-dependent of tissue metabolism and disease states, and inexpensive and have no effect on blood flow.[24,25] Methods for measurement of hepatic blood flow can generally be divided into two categories: direct and indirect methods.

Direct methods include timed collections of he-patic vein output, plethysmography, thermodilu-tion, and electronic or ultrasonic flow probes. These techniques are invasive and require visual-ization and manipulation of the liver and its ves-sels. A recently reported pulsed Doppler technique may have potential in clinical use.[26] In this report, the portal vein was visualized and the vessel diam-eter determined by sonography before the determi-nation of velocity of blood in the selected segment of the vessel. From the velocity and diameter of the vessel, blood flow per minute was calculated. In spite of the problems with variability of the critical measurements of portal vein diameter and the problems associated with measuring and interpret-ing Doppler signals, this relatively noninvasive technique may have tremendous value in its ability to measure dynamically portal blood flow. The use of most direct measurement techniques remains limited to animal investigations and a few selected surgical procedures.

Indirect methods for determination of hepatic blood flow are variably invasive and are more ap-plicable clinically. Indirect methods also have some inherent limitations, such as inability to discriminate between portal vein and hepatic artery blood flow and to respond to rapid changes in flow rate.

Clearance techniques, based on the use of a substance that is extracted by the hepatocytes (hepatocyte clearance) or by the Kupffer cells (reticuloendothelial clearance) present in the normal parenchyma of the liver are suitable for obtaining information on either hepatic blood flow or function.[27] The extent to which flow or function determines the rate of clearance depends on the biochemical efficiency of the liver for removal of the substance relative to flow. Substrates with efficient removal relative to flow can be used to estimate hepatic blood flow, whereas substrates with low efficiency of removal relative to flow are useful for estimation of hepatic function. If the rate of entry of a substance into an organ is constant, then the rate of removal (R) of that substance equals the product of blood flow (Q) and the difference in inflow (c_i) and outflow (c_o) concentrations:

$$R = Q(c_i - c_o) \qquad 1$$

The ratio of the rate of removal to the inflow concentration is the clearance (Cl) of the substance.

$$Cl = Q[(c_i - c_o)c_i] = Q \times ER \qquad 2$$

The quotient $[(c_i - c_o)/c_i]$ is referred to as the extraction fraction or extraction ratio (ER). Therefore,

$$Q = Cl/ER \qquad 3$$

The ER determines the degree to which the clearance of the substance approximates flow. If 100% of the test substance is cleared by the liver in a single pass through the liver, the $ER = 1.0$ and $Q = Cl$. Ethanol, propranolol, galactose, lidocaine, radiocolloids, and sorbitol[28,29] have high hepatic extraction ratios ($ER > 0.9$) and are eliminated in accordance with first-order kinetics, and pertubations in blood flow are accompanied by a proportional alteration in the rate of removal of the substance from the blood (blood flow dependent). In these situations, the substances are removed so efficiently in a single pass through the hepatic circulation that $c_o = 0$, and blood flow can be estimated without hepatic vein catheterization. As ER decreases, the relative importance of intrinsic metabolic capacity becomes increasingly prominent, and the clearance of the indicator is dramatically affected by disturbances in hepatic function (function dependent or intrinsic clearance). Correction for

this less efficient extraction, lower ER, requires correction by determination of the test substance in the hepatic vein (c_o) through catheterization. This procedure is invasive and somewhat variable, since it must be assumed that blood collected from the cannulated vessel is representative of the venous drainage of the entire liver.[30]

Hepatocyte Clearance Methods

Liver blood flow measurements based on hepatocyte uptake of a substance determined by concentration measurements in arterial and venous blood and subsequent calculation according to Fick's principle have been extensively used since their introduction by Bradley and coworkers in 1945. These methods are greatly influenced by both hepatic blood flow and efficiency of extraction by the hepatocytes. Clearance of blood-flow–dependent substances estimates "nutrient" or "effective" hepatic blood flow (EHBF) as opposed to total hepatic blood flow, since clearance occurs only in metabolically active tissue. Hepatocellular diseases, such as cirrhosis and jaundice, may markedly decrease the efficiency of substrate clearance, thereby making total hepatic blood flow estimates unreliable. The validity of this method also depends on the assumption that the substance is cleared exclusively by the liver. Also, inaccuracies may result from the presence of intrahepatic shunts and extrahepatic portasystemic shunts associated with chronic liver disease and portal hypertension.[31,32]

Bromosulphalein (BSP) was the first test substance used for the estimation of hepatic blood flow.[31] The method involves an indirect application of the Fick's principle and requires catheterization of the hepatic vein and a constant infusion of BSP. The infusion rate of BSP is adjusted until the peripheral blood concentration of BSP is constant. When the infusion rate is in steady state with the dye clearance, the hepatic uptake of the dye equals the rate of infusion. Hepatic plasma flow can be calculated according to the following equation:

$$Q = BSP/(c_i - c_o) \qquad 4$$

Hepatic blood flow can be determined by correcting for hematocrit. This same principle has been applied to several other test substances. BSP is relatively inexpensive and readily quantitated. However, BSP is extracted by extrahepatic tissues (5–7%), is excreted by the kidneys, and is subjected to a certain amount of enterohepatic recirculation.[1] In patients with chronic liver disease, the ER falls precipitously and can reach as low as 5–15%, making the resulting calculations highly inaccurate.

Indocyanine green (ICG) has been used extensively to estimate hepatic blood flow. This method has several shortcomings:

1. in chronic liver disease, ER may be too low to provide a reliable measurement of hepatic plasma flow;
2. there have been several fatal anaphylactic reactions;[33]
3. the price of ICG is relatively high.

It is fairly well documented that hepatic clearance of ICG is of limited value for estimating absolute hepatic blood flow in patients with hepatic dysfunction.[31] Recent evidence with simultaneous measurements of ICG plasma clearance and hepatic blood flow by hepatic venous catheterizations suggests that neither the magnitude nor the direction of changes of hepatic blood flow can be determined from ICG clearance, even in healthy subjects.[34]

Galactose has many characteristics that make it a nearly ideal test substance for estimation of EHBF. Galactose is a simple monosaccharide that is converted to galactose 1-phosphate in the presence of galactokinase and ATP. Galactokinase is present in kidney, brain, gut, red blood cells (RBC), and muscle but in much lower concentrations than that found in the liver.[35] Galactokinase activity in RBC is second to that in the liver but appears to account for only 1–2% of the total elimination. The primary site of extrahepatic galactose elimination is urine, increasing linearly with concentration. In the concentration range used for EHBP determinations, urinary elimination is less than 1% of total elimination. In fact, the sum of galactose elimination in all extrahepatic sites is only 2%, certainly within the limits of Fick's criterion for use of a test substance for estimation of EHBF.[36] This method of determination of EHBF is safe, simple, and suitable for repeated measurements. It has tremendous potential for clinical measurements of EHBF in humans.

Sorbitol has been proposed as an alternative test substance to the more commonly used ICG for estimation of EHBF.[37] Hepatic elimination of sorbitol follows first-order kinetics with an *ER* approaching 1.0.[29] Extrahepatic, extrarenal elimination and enterohepatic recirculation appear to be negligible.

Significant differences between clearance of ICG and sorbitol have been reported in patients with advanced liver disease. It appears that clearance of sorbitol is maintained (*ER* > 0.40). It has been proposed that the high hepatic extraction, relative safety, and low price make this test substance far superior to ICG for estimation of EHBF.[29] Single-injection techniques, similar to those proposed for galactose clearance, have been developed, but must be conducted using very low plasma concentrations of sorbitol, which introduces a degree of uncertainty. The measurements of hepatic blood flow determining the clearance of a very low dose of ethanol infusion might find a place in clinical settings in the future.

Reticuloendothelial (RE) Clearance Methods

Reticuloendothelial clearance methods involve extracted or nonextracted radiotracers from which time-activity curves are determined by external counting or with a computerized gamma camera system to evaluate hepatic blood flow. These techniques have two major advantages over parenchymal (hepatocyte) cell clearance methods: extraction of radiolabeled colloids by RE cells does not appear to be influenced by the presence of hepatic disease[38] and the ratio of hepatic arterial and portal venous flows to total liver flow can be determined. In spite of these major advantages, widespread clinical application is limited because of inaccuracies related to dependency on several inherent assumptions:

1. the efficiency of extraction of the colloid is 100%;
2. extrahepatic uptake of colloids is negligible;
3. removal of the radiocolloids follows first-order kinetics;
4. the number of colloidal particles represents only a small fraction of the binding sites within the liver.

The assumption that extrahepatic extraction is negligible is problematic. The RE cells responsible for colloidal uptake are located primarily on the sinusoidal endothelium of the liver. Unfortunately RE clearance is influenced by extrahepatic extraction because RE cells are present in the spleen, bone marrow, and intestine. In the healthy human, extrahepatic extraction of colloid is relatively small (<10%). In a patient with chronic liver disease, the fractional clearance of colloid by the bone marrow becomes substantial. In addition, "intrahepatic" shunts may occur owing to pathologic modifications of the hepatic vasculature. Since intrahepatic shunts do not contain RE cells, a portion of the arterial blood supply to the liver would not be subjected to extraction by intrahepatic RE cells. In spite of the required approximations, results obtained using radiocolloidal extraction appear to be sufficiently accurate, reproducible, safe, and practical to be considered for clinical estimates of hepatic perfusion.[27]

Hydrogen Clearance Methods

Hydrogen gas clearance appears to have some promise in the clinical measurement of hepatic blood flow. This technique is based on the clearance of highly diffusible, biologically inert gas from a tissue. In practice, a low concentration (3%) of hydrogen gas is inhaled until the tissue becomes saturated with H_2. A platinum electrode, in contact with the surface of the tissue, generates a current proportional to the concentration of H_2 in the tissue. The rate of disappearance of H_2 from the tissue estimates blood flow. Several major methodologic problems have limited its application to the clinical measurement of hepatic blood flow. The technique, unfortunately, appears to measure blood flow only in the most superficial tissue layers, which are in contact with the platinum electrode. Comparison of the H_2 gas clearance method with ICG determinations suggests that only about 40% of the calculated blood flow by ICG is measured by H_2 clearance. Gouma and colleagues suggest that the apparent discrepancy between estimations is that H_2 gas clearance methods assess hepatic arterial perfusion rather than estimate total hepatic blood flow.[39] Other limitations of the technique are that the measurements are noncontinuous, relatively slow, and subject to alterations in local blood flow associated with contact of the electrode with the tissue. Although this method has potential for clinical applications, severe methodologic restrictions may limit its application.

Miscellaneous Techniques

A variety of other methods for determination of hepatic blood flow have been proposed and are well summarized in a recent article by Campra and Reynolds.[1] Briefly, these techniques include indicator dilution methods, electromagnetic flowmeters, inert gas washout, injection of lipiodol droplets, and ultrasonic pulsed Doppler flowmeters.

References

1. Campra, J.L. and Reynolds, T.B. (1988) Hepatic circulation. In *The Liver: Biology and Pathobiology,* 2nd edn., (Arias, I.M., Jakoby, W.B., Popper, H., Schachter, D., and Shafritz, D.A., eds.) New York: Raven Press, pp. 911–30.
2. McCuskey, S.R. (1971) Sphincters in the microvascular system. *Microvascular Research* 3:428–33.
3. Brouwer, A., Wisse, E., and Knook, D.L. (1988) Sinusoidal endothelial cells and perisinusoidal fat-storing cells. In *The Liver: Biology and Pathobiology,* 2nd edn., (Arias, I.M., Jakoby, W.B., Popper H., Schachter, D., and Shafritz, D.A., eds.) New York: Raven Press, pp. 665–82.
4. Widmann, J-J., Cotran, R.S. and Fahimi, H.D. (1972) Mononuclear phagocytes (Kupffer cells) and endothelial cells: Identification of two functional cell types in rat liver sinusoids by endogenous peroxidase activity. *Journal of Cellular Biology* 52:159–170.
5. Granger, D.N. and Barrowman, J.A. (1984) Gastrointestinal and liver edema. In *Edema,* (Staub, N.C. and Taylor, A.E., eds.) New York: Raven Press, pp. 615–56.
6. Jones, E.A. and Summerfield, J.A. (1988) Kupffer cells: In *The Liver: Biology and Pathobiology,* 2nd edn. (Arias, I.M., Jakoby, W.B., Popper, H., Schachter, D. and Shafritz, D.A., eds.) New York: Raven Press, pp. 683–704.
7. Rappaport, A.M. and Schneiderman, J.H. (1976) The function of the hepatic artery. *Review of Physiology Biochemistry and Pharmacology* 76:130–86.
8. Jungermann, K. and Katz, N. (1982) Functional hepatocellular heterogeneity. *Hepatology* 2:385–95.
9. Goresky, C.A. (1974) The lobular design of the liver: Its effect on uptake process. In *Regulation of Hepatic Metabolism,* (Lundquist, F. and Tygstrup, N., eds.) New York: Academic Press, pp. 808–19.
10. Richardson, P.D.I. (1982) Physiological regulation of the hepatic circulation. *Federation Proceedings* 41, 2111–6.
11. Burtin-Opitz, R. (1911) The vascularity of the liver: The influence of the portal blood flow upon the flow in the hepatic artery. *Quarterly Journal of Experimental Physiology* 4:93–102.
12. Gelman, S. and Ernst, E. (1977) The role of pH, P_{CO_2} and O_2 content of the portal blood in hepatic circulatory autoregulation. *American Journal of Physiology* 233: E255–62.
13. Lautt, W.W. (1977) Hepatic vasculature: A conceptual review. *Gastroenterology* 73:1163–69.

14. Lautt, W.W. (1983) Relationship between hepatic blood flow and overall metabolism: The hepatic arterial buffer response. *Federation Proceedings* 42:1662–66.

15. Lautt, W.W., Legare, D.J. and D'Almeida, M.S. (1985) Adenosine as putative regulator of hepatic arterial flow (the buffer response). *American Journal of Physiology* 248:H331–38.

16. Greenway, C.V. and Stark, R.D. (1971) Hepatic vascular bed. *Physiological Review* 51:23–65.

17. Gelman, S. (1975) The effect of enteral oxygen administration on the hepatic circulation during halothane anaesthesia: Experimental investigations. *British Journal of Anaesthesia* 47:1253–59.

18. Torrance, H.B. (1961) The control of the hepatic arterial circulation. *Journal of Physiology* (London) 158:39–49.

19. Hanson, K.M. and Johnson, P.C. (1966) Local control of hepatic arterial and portal venous flow in the dog. *American Journal of Physiology* 211:712–20.

20. Friedman, M.I. (1988) Hepatic nerve function. In: *The Liver: Biology and Pathobiology* 2nd edn. (Arias, I.M., Jakoby, W.B., Popper, H., Schachter, D. and Shafritz, D.A., eds.) New York: Raven Press, pp. 949–59.

21. Moreno, A.H. and Burchell, A.R. (1982) Respiratory regulation of splanchnic and systemic venous return in normal subjects and in patients with hepatic cirrhosis. *Surgery, Gynecology and Obstetrics* 154:257–67.

22. Granger, D.N., Richardson, P.D.I., Kvietys, P.R. and Mortillaro, J.A. (1980) Intestinal blood flow. *Gastroenterology* 78:837–63.

23. Gelman, S., Dillard E. and Parks, D.A. (1987) Glucagon increases hepatic oxygen supply-demand ratio in pigs. *American Journal of Physiology* 252:G648–53.

24. Granger, D.N. and Kvietys, P.R. (1985) Recent advances in measurement of gastrointestinal blood flow. *Gastroenterology* 88:1073–76.

25. Tepperman, B.L. and Jacobson, E.D. (1981) Measurement of gastrointestinal blood flow. *Annual Review of Physiology* 44:71–82.

26. Zoli, M., Marchesini, G., Cordiani, M.R., et al. (1986) Echo-Doppler measurement of splanchnic blood flow in control and cirrhotic subjects. *Journal of Clinical Ultrasound* 14:429–35.

27. Magrini, A., Izzo, G., Guerrisi, M., Favella, A., Picardi, R. and Valeri, L. (1985) A new approach to non-invasive quantitative study of hepatic haemodynamics using radiocolloids in vivo. *Clinical Physics and Physiological Measurements* 6:179–204.

28. Keiding, S. (1988) Galactose clearance measurements and liver blood flow. *Gastroenterology* 94:447–81.

29. Zeeh, J., Lang, H., Bosch, J., Pohl, S., Loesgen, H. and Eggers, R. (1988) Steady-state extrarenal sorbitol clearance as a measure of hepatic plasma flow. *Gastroenterology* 95:749–59.

30. Bradley, S.E., Ingelfinger, F.J., Bradley, G.P., et al. (1945) Estimation of hepatic blood flow in man. *Journal of Clinical Investigation* 24:890–97.

31. Bradley, E.L. (1974) Measurement of hepatic blood flow in man. *Surgery* 75:783–89.

32. McLean, A., du Souich, P. and Gibaldi, M. (1979) Noninvasive kinetic approach to the estimation of total hepatic blood flow and shunting in chronic liver disease. A hypothesis. *Clinical Pharmacology and Therapeutics* 25:161–66.

33. Carski, T.R. (1978) Adverse reactions after administration of indocyanine green. *Journal of the American Medical Association*. 240:635–36.

34. Kanstrup I-L. and Winkler, K. (1987) Indocyanine green plasma clearance as a measure of changes in hepatic blood flow. *Clinical Physiology* 7:51–54.

35. Cuatrecasas, P. and Segal, S. (1985) Mammalian galactokinase. *Journal of Biology and Chemistry* 240:2382.

36. Schirmer, W.J., Townsend, M.C., Schirmer, J.M., Hampton, W.W. and Fry, D.E. (1986) Galactose clearance as an estimate of effective hepatic blood flow: Validation and limitations. *Journal of Surgical Research* 41:543–56.

37. Molino, G.P., Cavanna, A., Avagnina, P., Ballare, M. and Torchio, M. (1987) Hepatic clearance of *D*-sorbitol. Noninvasive tests for evaluating functional liver plasma flow. *Digestive Diseases and Sciences* 32:753–58.

38. Shaldon, S., Chiandussi, L., Guevara, L., Caesar, J. and Sherlock, S. (1981) The estimation of hepatic blood flow and intrahepatic shunted blood flow by colloidal heat-denatured human serum albumin labeled with ^{131}I. *Journal of Clinical Investigation* 40:1346–54.

39. Gouma, D.J., Coelho, J.C.U., Schlegel, J., Fisher, J.D., Li, Y.F. and Moody, F.G. (1986) Estimation of hepatic blood flow by hydrogen gas clearance. *Surgery* 99, 439–45.

Chapter 2
Causes of Liver Disease

Mervyn H. Davies and James M. Neuberger

Introduction

This chapter briefly discusses the presentation, treatment, and investigation of various forms of liver disease that the anesthetist may encounter, either during surgery or in the intensive care unit. Patients in intensive care often have abnormal liver function tests in the absence of primary liver disease. In such patients, systemic infection is usually the cause; however, postoperative or posttraumatic state, circulatory failure, gastrointestinal failure, total parenteral nutrition, and cardiac failure may be contributory factors. A section on liver disease in pregnancy is included, since many women will require the attention of an anesthetist at the time of delivery.

Hepatic Cirrhosis

Cirrhosis is a syndrome with a number of different causes (Table 2-1). Essentially the clinicopathologic features are similar, irrespective of the cause. Cirrhosis is a diffuse process characterized by the loss of normal liver architecture, with fibrosis and nodule formation. Sinusoids no longer function effectively, so that metabolic exchange across basement membranes and hepatocytes is impaired. Cirrhosis can lead to both portal hypertension and progressive liver failure. Cirrhosis can be consid-

ered broadly in terms of biliary disease (for example, primary biliary cirrhosis or primary sclerosing cholangitis) in which jaundice is common or of parenchymal disease in which jaundice suggests advancing liver failure.

Cirrhosis may be suspected clinically because of findings such as spider nevi, palmar erythema, and clubbing. Other physical signs associated with late disease include leuconychia, sparse body hair,

Table 2-1. Causes of Hepatic Cirrhosis

Viral Hepatitis	Hepatitis B, B and D, and C
Metabolic Disease	Hemochromatosis
	Wilson's disease
	Alpha-1 antitrypsin deficiency
	Glycogen storage disease
	Galactosemia
	Tyrosinemia
Cholestasis	Primary biliary cirrhosis
	Secondary biliary cirrhosis
	Primary sclerosing cholangitis
Venous Outflow Obstruction	Budd Chiari syndrome
	Veno-occlusive disease
	Cardiac failure
Drugs and Toxins	Alcohol
	Amiodarone and many others
Autoimmune Cryptogenic	Chronic active hepatitis

caput medusae, and purpura. Biliary cirrhosis is typically associated with a large liver, while auto-immune chronic active hepatitis and alpha-1 anti-trypsin deficiency are associated with a small liver or with left lobe hypertrophy and right lobe atrophy.

Patients with decompensated cirrhosis suffer symptoms of severe fatigue and lethargy, which may be complicated by encephalopathy. Patients are weak and experience muscle wasting and weight loss. There may be profound electrolyte imbalance. Ascites and peripheral edema are frequent and may be unresponsive to diuretic therapy. Coagulopathy may result in spontaneous bleeding. Patients are at greatly increased risk of sepsis, especially from gram-negative organisms. Spontaneous bacterial peritonitis can develop without clinical signs in the abdomen.

If portal hypertension is present, the spleen is almost always palpable and enlarges progressively. The size of the liver correlates poorly with portal pressure. While portal hypertension contributes to the formation of ascites, the development of ascites is unusual without an element of liver cell dysfunction. The development of portal hypertension, whether caused by parenchymal liver disease or portal vein thrombosis, will lead to major changes in the pharmacokinetics of some drugs.[1-3] Systemic availability may be increased many fold because of spontaneous portosystemic shunting together with changes to sinusoidal fenestration and basement membrane thickening with collagenization of the space of Disse, which will diminish the extraction ratio of drugs as they traverse the liver. This reduces first-pass metabolism and, in the case of high extraction drugs, increases their bioavailability dramatically. Portal hypertension also results in the formation of esophageal and gastric varices, which may bleed catastrophically.

It is important to investigate the etiology of the underlying liver disease in patients who are found to be cirrhotic to exclude treatable causes. There is currently no convincing evidence in favor of prophylactic sclerotherapy before the first variceal bleed. Patients should be followed up to observe for signs of decompensation and to screen for early hepatocellular carcinoma (HCC).

Child's Classification

Child originally classified the severity of liver disease into three groups as a means of assessing risk before portocaval surgery.[4] This simple classification system has remained a consistent indicator of prognosis in the cirrhotic patient, although it has been amended by Pugh.[5] Individual measurements are allocated either 1, 2, or 3 points (Table 2-2) depending on the result. Points for the five variables are added to provide a score ranging from 5 to 15. Patients with a score of 5/6 are considered grade A, 7 to 9 points are grade B, and those with 10 points or more are graded C. In primary biliary cirrhosis (PBC) an increase in bilirubin occurs earlier than in other liver disease, so an allowance is made for this.

Primary Biliary Cirrhosis

Primary biliary cirrhosis (PBC) is a disease of unknown etiology characterized by progressive granulomatous destruction of intrahepatic bile ducts.[7,8] It usually affects middle-aged women. The reason for the 9:1 predominance of females is unknown. PBC has been reported from all parts of the world. It appears to have variable prevalence, which probably

Table 2-2. Pugh's Grading of the Severity of Liver Disease

	Points Scored for Increasing Abnormality		
Parameter	1	2	3
Bilirubin (μmol/l)	<35	35–51	>51
Albumin (g/l)	>35	28–35	<28
Ascites	Absent	Slight	Moderate
Encephalopathy*	Absent	Grades I and II	Grades III and IV
Prothrombin time (seconds, prolonged)	1–4	4–6	>6
For PBC			
Bilirubin (μmol/l)	17–68	68–170	>170

*Encephalopathy according to Trey[6]

reflects genetic or environmental factors but may reflect different diagnostic practice.

Clinical presentation usually occurs between the ages of 40 and 60 years. Most frequently it presents insidiously with symptoms of pruritis and malaise. Patients may first present to a dermatologist or even to a psychiatrist for investigation of pruritis.

Jaundice is not invariable but usually develops within 6 months to 5 years of the onset of pruritis. Fatigue is often prominent. The associated malabsorption of fat may cause steatorrhea and weight loss and is associated with impaired absorption of the fat-soluble vitamins A, D, E, and K.

Skin xanthomas may develop and serum cholesterol is usually elevated, sometimes massively. Bone disease can be disabling and is worse in the deeply cholestatic patient. It is caused by osteoporosis, which is accelerated by steroid therapy, and rarely by osteomalacia. Bleeding from esophageal varices may occur as a presenting event. Portal hypertension may be presinusoidal and so can develop in the absence of cirrhosis.

Associated autoimmune diseases occur, including connective tissue diseases such as mixed connective tissue disease, scleroderma, or CREST (*c*alcinosis, *R*eynaud's, *e*sophageal dysmotility, *s*clerodactyly, and *t*elangiectasia) syndrome. The sicca syndrome is a common association. Other associated diseases include autoimmune thyroiditis, celiac disease, and vitiligo.

As with other inflammatory cirrhotic processes affecting the liver, there is an increased incidence of primary hepatocellular carcinoma. There is also an increased prevalence of breast cancer in patients with PBC.

A diagnosis of PBC is usually suspected clinically and confirmed with laboratory investigations. Alkaline phosphatase is raised, with elevated serum IgM and positive antimitochondrial antibody (AMA). A number of antimitochondrial antibodies have been described.[9] The most specific is directed against the E2 component of the pyruvate dehydrogenase complex.

Primary biliary cirrhosis is characterized histologically (Figure 2–1) by inflammatory damage to interlobular bile ducts. Bile ducts may be destroyed, so that portal tracts are devoid of appropriately sized bile ducts (ductopenia). Ductular proliferation occurs. Histologic appearances are divided into four stages:

Stage I	florid bile duct lesions
Stage II	ductular proliferation
Stage III	septal fibrosis and bridging
Stage IV	cirrhosis

Endoscopic retrograde cholangiopancreatography (ERCP) excludes extrahepatic biliary disease in those studied; however, a normal ERCP is not a prerequisite for diagnosis.

Increased use of automated laboratory screening detects a number of asymptomatic patients. Despite

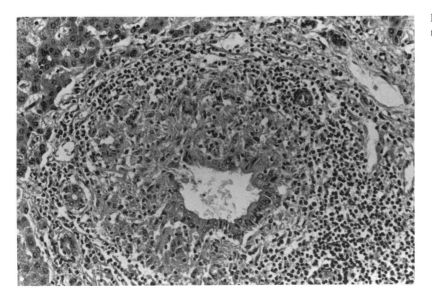

Figure 2-1. Histology in primary biliary cirrhosis (PBC).

the lack of symptoms and even in the presence of normal biochemical profile, patients with AMA in a titer ≥ 1/40 almost invariably have histological features of PBC. The course of asymptomatic cases is unpredictable, but most patients develop progressive disease.

Symptomatic patients presenting with jaundice have a median survival of around 7–10 years. While a number of complex prognostication indices have been developed, serum bilirubin provides the single best indicator of prognosis. When serum bilirubin has risen in excess of 150 μmol/L, expected survival is less than 2 years.

There are five considerations in the treatment of patients with PBC:

- Symptomatic therapy for pruritus
- Vitamin supplementation
- Treatment of associated disease, such as thyroxine
- Treatment of the disease itself
- Liver transplantation

Symptomatic treatment of PBC includes oral therapy with bile acid binding agents, such as cholestyramine, or choleretic agents, such as ursodeoxycholic acid. Antihistamines are of little value. The fat-soluble vitamins A, D, and K should be administered parenterally in cholestatic patients.

Treatment of the disease itself has been disappointing, and it is still without cure. Drug therapy tested includes corticosteroids; other immunosuppressants such as azathioprine, cyclosporin, and chlorambucil; antifibrotic agents; colchicine; and more recently the choleretic ursodeoxycholic acid.[10] Numerous controlled trials have been carried out and more are in progress. Liver transplantation is the only current treatment with a realistic chance of resumption of normal quality of life.

Primary Sclerosing Cholangitis

Primary sclerosing cholangitis (PSC) is a disease of unknown etiology characterized by chronic cholestasis due to an obliterative fibrosis of the biliary tract.[11–13] Males are affected twice as commonly as females. Most frequently patients present in adult life; however, disease occasionally occurs in childhood. Patients may present with symptoms attributable to cholestasis, such as pruritus and fatigue or jaundice. Weight loss and right upper quadrant pain may be present from the outset, in which case it is important to exclude a complicating cholangiocarcinoma, although weight loss may simply reflect fat malabsorption.

Increasing use of biochemical screening and recognition of the association between inflammatory bowel disease (IBD) and PSC has resulted in the diagnosis of increasing numbers of asymptomatic patients. Patients should have a rectal biopsy to determine whether associated ulcerative colitis is present.

Approximately half the patients with PSC have associated IBD. In the majority this is ulcerative colitis (UC); Crohn's disease is an infrequent association. The cause of the link with IBD is unknown, but it does not relate to disease severity or activity. Patients may present with liver disease several years after IBD becomes manifest. Conversely, patients may first present with PSC months or years after total colectomy for UC. Some evidence suggests familial occurrence of PSC and an association with HLA B8, DR3.[13]

Standard liver tests typically show evidence of cholestasis, with elevation of serum alkaline phosphatase. Serum bilirubin levels are variable and do not have the same prognostic value as in PBC. Antimitochondrial antibody is absent. Antineutrophil cytoplasmic antibodies (ANCA), with a characteristic perinuclear pattern of immunofluorescence, are not completely specific for PSC. Histologic features consist typically of portal infiltration, periductular inflammation and ductopenia (Figure 2-2). Ductal scars, surrounded by concentric rings of fibrosis, are classical of the disease.

ERCP is diagnostic (Figure 2-3), revealing stricturing, which may involve intrahepatic and/or extrahepatic bile ducts.

The routine monitoring of patients by ERCP is contraindicated because the investigation can be complicated by life-threatening suppurative cholangitis.

The course is variable, but many patients remain asymptomatic. The main complications are recurrent cholangitis, bleeding from esophageal or gastric varices, progression to cirrhosis, or development of cholangiocarcinoma.

The diagnosis of a complicating cholangiocarcinoma can be difficult but may be suggested by a rapid clinical deterioration. Investigation may include ultrasonography, computed tomography, MRI, cholangiography, aspiration cytology, wire-guided brush cytology, and measurement of carcinoembryonic antigen (CEA). Despite extensive

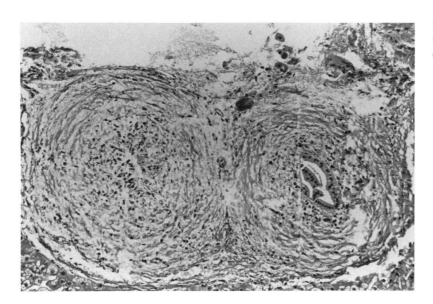

Figure 2-2. Histological features of primary sclerosing cholangitis (PSC).

investigations, the diagnosis is frequently made at laparotomy or autopsy.

Treatment is supportive. Although therapy such as ursodeoxycholic acid may provide biochemical improvement, there is no convincing evidence so far that it improves disease outcome. Therapy should be either aimed at relieving symptoms or prescribed as part of a controlled clinical trial. Ursodeoxycholic acid, bile acid binding agents, and antihistamines may be effective in controlling pruritus. Patients may have recurrent episodes of symptomatic cholangitis, in which case prophylactic antibiotics usually reduce the frequency of such episodes. Associated IBD should be treated along standard lines. A subgroup of patients have an overlap with autoimmune hepatitis, in which case a component of their disease may respond to corticosteroid therapy. Liver transplantation is indicated in some patients with advanced disease or symptoms of intolerable quality of life. The management of benign extrahepatic strictures in the setting of PSC is controversial. Surgical or endoscopic decompression carries major risks and some advocate transplantation in this group. Liver transplantation is not indicated if cholangiocarcinoma is present. PSC may recur after transplantation.[13a]

Chronic Hepatitis

Chronic hepatitis is defined as the presence of an inflammatory reaction within liver parenchyma persisting beyond 6 months. Histologically it is subdivided into three forms.

- *Chronic persistent hepatitis* is characterized by expansion of the portal zone, with the limiting plate remaining intact and no piecemeal necrosis.
- *Chronic lobular hepatitis* resembles acute viral hepatitis, with intralobular inflammation and necrosis. Piecemeal and bridging necrosis are absent.
- *Chronic active hepatitis* (CAH) is characterized by inflammation consisting mainly of lymphocytes and plasma cells expanding portal areas. The inflammatory infiltrate extends into the liver lobule, causing erosion of the limiting plate and piecemeal necrosis. Increasing severity is marked by fibrous septa surrounding groups of hepatocytes, or "rosettes."

Chronic persistent and chronic lobular hepatitis usually do not progress. Chronic active hepatitis may progress rapidly to cirrhosis if not treated.

The cause of chronic persistent hepatitis is frequently unknown. Diagnosis is usually made following the discovery of deranged liver tests. Viral hepatitis B and C should be excluded. Alcohol is another cause, since acute alcoholic hepatitis may not resolve completely following abstinence. Clinical features are generally mild and nonspecific, usually consisting of constitutional upset and fatigue. Physical examination is normal, although a liver edge may be palpable. There is modest elevation of

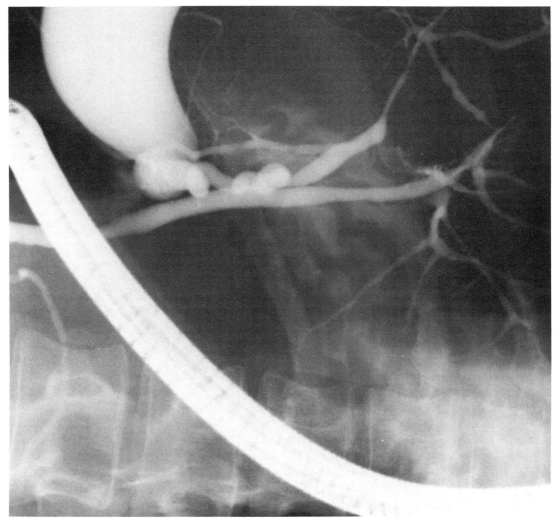

Figure 2-3. Endoscopic retrograde cholangiopancreatograph (ERCP) in primary sclerosing cholangitis (PSC).

serum transaminases and serum alkaline phosphatase is usually normal or minimally increased, as is serum bilirubin.

Chronic lobular hepatitis has many clinical and etiological factors in common with chronic persistent hepatitis. The prognosis is good if features of more aggressive hepatitis do not supervene.

Chronic active hepatitis may result from a range of etiological agents (Table 2-3).

Nonspecific symptoms of constitutional upset are usual and may be severe. Serum transaminases are elevated. Physical signs may include jaundice, spider nevi, and splenomegaly.

The cause of *autoimmune chronic active hepatitis* (AIH) is unknown. The disease predominantly affects the young. Fifty percent present before 20 years of age. A second peak occurs during middle age. Females predominate 4:1 in the younger group.

Presentation is often with jaundice, constitutional upset, and malaise. Secondary amenorrhea is frequent. Physical features typically include spider

Table 2-3. Etiology of Chronic Active Hepatitis

Viral Hepatitis	Hepatitis B, C, B and D
Other Viruses	Cytomegalovirus, rubella
Autoimmune	
Wilson's Disease	
Alpha-1 Antitrypsin Deficiency	
Drugs	
Alcohol	

nevi, skin striae, acne, and a small liver. Splenomegaly is frequent, which may be related to the immunologic nature of the disease, rather than portal hypertension. Jaundice is often a presenting feature but is also associated with disease exacerbations and may be intermittent.

AICAH is characterized by evidence of abnormal immunologic activity.[14–15] Serum gammaglobulins, especially IgG, may be grossly elevated and autoantibodies are usually present in the serum. Antinuclear factor is present in around 50% of patients. Smooth muscle antibody (anti-actin) is detected in 70%. Others include antibodies to soluble liver antigen and liver-kidney microsomal (LKM) antibodies. The latter are typically associated with hepatitis presenting in children or young adults. Mitochondrial antibody is present in around 30% of AICAH patients, but in low titer (< 1/40) and not the E2 subtype. Titers of autoantibodies vary with disease activity and usually disappear with remission of disease.

Untreated, the 5-year survival is around 50%.[16] Disease remission usually results from treatment with corticosteroids either alone or in combination with azathioprine. Symptoms and biochemical derangements usually resolve rapidly on starting therapy, so histology should ideally be obtained before therapy begins. If coagulopathy precludes a percutaneous biopsy, a transjugular liver biopsy should be considered.

A delay of 6 months frequently occurs between biochemical and histologic remission. Histologic remission is obtained in 80% after 3 years of therapy,[17] although some patients will fail to enter remission.

Treatment protocols vary. High-dose corticosteroid therapy is effective in inducing remission but is associated with a high incidence of toxicity, whereas combined therapy with corticosteriod and azathioprine permits a smaller dose of corticosteroid. Azathioprine used alone is not effective, although some studies suggest it may maintain remission once it is established. Therapeutic trials of cyclophosphamide and cyclosporin therapy have shown no clear evidence of additional benefit.

Patients should be maintained on the minimum effective dose of immunosuppressive therapy. In a few cases treatment can be successfully withdrawn, but it is mandatory to maintain careful follow-up because relapse is frequent and may be severe.

Some physicians advocate lifelong low-dose maintenance therapy.

Drugs

A number of drugs are associated with chronic active hepatitis. These include methyldopa, nitrofurantoin, and isoniazid. Clinical features mimic other forms of CAH, but rapid resolution usually follows withdrawal of the drug. Early diagnosis is important, since repeated drug challenge may produce fatal liver injury. Alcohol, another cause of chronic active hepatitis, is discussed later in this chapter.

Wilson's Disease

Wilson's disease[18,19] is a rare, autosomal recessive disease of copper metabolism, characterized by reduced biliary excretion of copper, increased urinary copper, reduced serum copper, and serum ceruloplasmin. The gene responsible for Wilson's disease is located on chromosome 13.[20] The function of the gene product and the precise mechanism of the metabolic abnormality is unknown, but it results in accumulation of copper and progressive injury of the liver, central nervous system, cornea, kidneys, and other organs.

Clinical presentation varies (Table 2-4), but characteristic patterns tend to occur at different ages. Hepatic syndromes are the most common form of presentation in children. Later in life neuropsychiatric manifestations are increasingly likely to occur, although the two forms may overlap.

Hepatic disease may present with either acute or chronic hepatitis, or cirrhosis may already have developed. Rarely, in children and young adults, Wilson's disease presents with fulminant hepatic failure, characterized by deep jaundice, ascites, and coagulopathy that progresses rapidly to hepatorenal failure and death.

Table 2-4. A Comparison of Clinical Features Occurring in Hepatic and Neuropsychiatric Presentations of Wilson's Disease

Hepatic Presentation	Neuropsychiatric Presentation
Acute hepatitis	Dystonia, dysarthria, dysphagia
Fulminant hepatic failure	Behavioral abnormalities
Chronic hepatitis	Depression
Cirrhosis	Psychosis

The deposition of copper in the cornea may result in Kayser Fleischer (KF) rings. Visualization of KF rings at the periphery of the cornea is assisted by examination with a slit lamp. KF rings are invariably present in those with neurologic disease but may be absent in cases presenting early. Very occasionally KF rings are present in other forms of chronic liver disease, such as PBC.[21]

Acute presentation is frequently associated with hemolysis and a low serum alkaline phosphatase. There may be jaundice, elevated transaminases, and hypergammaglobulinemia. Any young patient with liver disease accompanied by neurological dysfunction, hemolysis, or subnormal levels of serum alkaline phosphatase should be investigated for Wilson's disease.

A reduced serum ceruloplasmin (<200 mg/L) strongly suggests the diagnosis of Wilson's disease. In addition, hepatic copper content in excess of 250 µg/g dry liver or the presence of KF rings will confirm the diagnosis. Most symptomatic patients excrete in excess of 100 µg of copper in the urine over 24 hours. Occasionally liver biopsies from other chronic cholestatic diseases contain levels of copper similar to that in Wilson's disease.

The treatment of choice is penicillamine, which chelates copper, causing a large rise in urinary copper output. The importance of patient compliance should be emphasized because a lifelong commitment to therapy is required. Any secondary clinical or biochemical deterioration should arouse suspicion that therapy has been discontinued. Treatment with zinc or trientine is a safe and effective alternative.

Untreated, the disease is progressive. Prognosis is related to the extent of tissue damage before the onset of therapy. Fulminant presentation requires emergency liver transplantation, which will cure the disease.

Family screening is important to detect early and presymptomatic disease.

Iron Overload and Liver Damage

Fibrosis and hepatocyte damage are related to the absolute iron content, rather than its particular etiology. The severity of fibrosis is most marked in periportal areas, where iron is preferentially deposited. The damage to hepatocytes induced by iron is thought to result from lysosomal injury, resulting in the leak of enzymes into the cytosol and lipid peroxidation that produces functional disturbances in mitochondria and microsomes.

Genetic Hemochromatosis

Genetic hemochromatosis (GH)[22,23] is an autosomal recessive disease of disordered iron metabolism. The disease is related to excessive iron absorption and subsequent deposition of iron in various tissues. The primary abnormality is unknown, but an inappropriate rate of iron absorption dates from birth. There is genetic linkage with the histocompatibility antigen A3.[24] Females are relatively protected because menstrual blood loss eliminates some of the excess iron.

Alcohol excess is frequent in patients with clinically overt hemochromatosis, since alcohol appears to accelerate liver disease. Although liver disease may develop in nonalcohol abusers, it does so at a slower rate.

Genetic hemochromatosis (GH) results in a multisystem disease, since iron has a deleterious effect on the many different tissues in which it is deposited. Typically, it presents in a middle-aged man with symptoms of lethargy and fatigue, who complains of loss of libido and may be diabetic with hepatomegaly and arthropathy affecting the metacarpophalangeal joints of the hands. The liver is usually enlarged and may be painful. Cirrhosis may be present at the time of presentation. Splenomegaly is often present but not marked. A high rate of hepatic malignancy occurs in GH.

Endocrine manifestations include diabetes mellitus, hypopituitarism, and hypogonadotrophic testicular failure. Cardiac infiltration results in cardiomyopathy and arrhythmias. Arthropathy often resembles osteoarthrosis and is predominantly restricted to the hands and knees. Pseudogout may occur, which relates to deposition of calcium pyrophosphate.

Serum iron is often raised and transferrin saturation is grossly increased. Serum ferritin increases in proportion to the degree of iron excess. In GH, ferritin levels above 100 µmg/L are common. Liver biopsy permits a direct measurement of the hepatic iron concentration, and histologic examination determines the extent of siderosis and fibrosis and whether dysplastic changes are present. MRI scanning can detect iron overload and may be of value in assessing the response to therapy.

Prognosis is dependent on sex, time of diagnosis, and other cofactors such as alcohol ingestion. Patients diagnosed during the precirrhotic stage have an excellent prognosis if they comply with therapy. Even patients with established cirrhosis fare well from the point of view of hepatic function, although HCC may develop despite the removal of excess iron.

Treatment consists of venesection, since iron can be mobilized from tissue stores to replace blood loss. Five hundred milliliter of blood contains about 250 mg iron. Venesection may be needed weekly for up to 2 years. Reversal of the iron balance usually results in a renewed feeling of well-being, hepatosplenomegaly reverses, and liver tests improve. When tissue iron is normal, venesection should be performed every 3 months to prevent further iron accumulation.

Secondary Iron Overload

Various *hematologic disorders* are accompanied by secondary iron overload if they are associated with high rates of erythropoiesis or large transfusion requirements. These may be congenital such as thalassemia major, sickle cell disease, red cell dysplasia, and congenital sideroblastic anemia, or acquired, such as acquired refractory sideroblastic anemia and hypoplastic or myelodysplastic disorders. Excess iron is mainly deposited in parenchymal sites (hepatocytes, pancreas, and heart) in a similar fashion to genetic hemochromatosis. In the case of thalassemia major, hepatomegaly and fibrosis develop in the first decade. The second decade is marked by failure of growth and sexual development, together with cardiac dysfunction, which is the major cause of death.

Therapeutic maneuvers consist of dietary measures and the administration of subcutaneous desferrioxamine to chelate some of the excess iron. Supplementation with ascorbic acid increases urinary iron removal by desferrioxamine. Compliance with therapy in young patients is a major hurdle, since an effective orally active agent is not yet available.

Chronic alcoholic liver disease is associated with iron overload in around 30% of patients, but is usually mild to moderate and less than three times

the upper limit of normal. The patient may have hypogonadism, glucose intolerance, and elevated parameters of iron load such as ferritin, serum iron, and transferrin saturation. A diagnosis of genetic hemochromatosis may be considered, and in such a case it is important to measure hepatic iron content to confirm the diagnosis.

Porphyria cutanea tarda[25] is caused by deficient activity of the enzyme uroporphyrinogen decarboxylase. The excessive amount of porphyrins in the blood and skin accounts for the cutaneous photosensitivity. Clinical expression of the disease usually requires exogenous factors such as alcohol, estrogens, liver disease, or iron. The origin of the moderate iron overload is uncertain, but iron administration leads to disease exacerbations, whereas venesection reduces the clinical manifestations.

Toxic and Drug-Induced Liver Injury

Exposure to toxic xenobiotics, whether naturally occurring or synthetic, may mimic almost any liver disease. It is important to take note of deliberate and accidental exposure to potential hepatotoxins when considering the cause of liver disease, although it remains a diagnosis of exclusion.

The particular susceptibility of the liver to such damage presumably results from its primary role in the metabolism of many xenobiotics. Biotransformation reactions have been traditionally considered protective. There are a number of examples, however, in which such reactions produce active metabolites that require subsequent detoxification. The metabolism of paracetamol provides an example. Most is detoxified by conjugation with glucuronide or sulphate. A small proportion of the drug is metabolized by the cytochromes P450, producing a cytotoxic intermediary compound. Failure to detoxify this by glutathione conjugation results in liver cell necrosis. In paracetamol overdose, exhaustion of glutathione reserves predisposes to such injury.

Most toxic liver damage in the United Kingdom results from drug ingestion. Injury may be predictable, occurring in a dose-related fashion, such as following paracetamol overdose. In most other cases of drug-induced liver disease, injury is not predictable and results from idiosyncratic mechanisms, such as hypersensitivity or aberrant metabolic detoxification with resultant accumulation of hepatotoxic metabolites. This topic is discussed further in chapter 18.

Alcoholic Liver Disease

The prevalence of alcoholic liver disease (ALD) depends on cultural, social, religious, and economic factors.[26,27] Not all individuals who abuse alcohol develop liver disease. Those who develop ALD may be unreliable witnesses, which creates difficulty interpreting data concerning the dose of alcohol required to induce liver injury. Heavy drinking on a daily basis is more damaging than intermittent "binge" drinking. Women are more susceptible to alcohol toxicity. The enzymes responsible for alcohol metabolism are expressed polymorphically, with marked differences between individuals in the capacity to metabolize alcohol, which may account for some of the variable susceptibility to alcohol-induced liver disease. A number of studies have linked HLA type to susceptibility to ALD.[28,29]

The mechanisms of ethanol toxicity are unknown. Possible causes include acetaldehyde, the main product of alcohol metabolism, or changes in the intracellular redox potential precipitated by the marked increase in the NADH:NAD ratio.[30] Mallory's hyaline characterizes ALD, although it is nonspecific and occurs in a number of other conditions. Its role in disease pathogenesis is uncertain. Immunologic mechanisms may be important, since liver damage characterized by an active hepatitis may progress despite the patient's abstinence from alcohol, and immunosuppressive therapy with corticosteroids is beneficial in some subgroups of patients with alcoholic hepatitis.

Deposition of fat occurs after acute alcohol ingestion. It accumulates in zones 2 (mediolobular) and 3 (centrolobular) and is usually macrovesicular. Fatty infiltration reverses following alcohol withdrawal. A number of other causes of fatty liver are listed in Table 2-5.

Alcoholic hepatitis varies in its presentation from a mild anicteric illness with hepatomegaly to a rapidly progressive form of liver failure with jaundice, ascites, gastrointestinal bleeding, and hepatic coma. The majority of patients with mild or moderate alcoholic hepatitis present with nonspecific symptoms such as anorexia, lethargy, and malaise, but those with more aggressive disease will present with symptoms suggestive of hepatocellular failure,

Table 2-5. The Etiology of Fatty Liver

Nutritional	Metabolic Disease
Kwashiorkor	Diabetes mellitus
Gastrointestinal	Glycogenoses
Pancreatic disease	Hyperlipidemias
Obesity	Wilson's disease
Intestinal bypass	Tyrosinemia
Prolonged parenteral nutrition	
General	Drug Related
Viral infections	Alcohol
Cryptogenic	Corticosteroids
Fatty liver in pregnancy	Estrogens
	Amiodarone and others

such as jaundice, ascites, encephalopathy, or variceal hemorrhage. Patients with alcoholic hepatitis are more ill than those with simple fatty liver. Fever and leucocytosis are often present, even in the absence of bacterial sepsis. Patients may suffer a marked deterioration in clinical status when admitted to the hospital, and their poor nutritional status is made worse by anorexia and vomiting.

The combination of right upper quadrant pain, fever, leucocytosis, jaundice, and hepatomegaly may lead to the diagnosis of biliary tract disease. This erroneous diagnosis can have fatal consequences if the patient is subjected to a general anesthetic and laparotomy.

Fibrosis is the prelude to cirrhosis and is thought to relate predominantly to transformation of fat-storing Ito cells to fibroblasts, but the stimulus for such transformation is unknown. If alcoholic cirrhosis develops, it is characteristically micronodular. Fatty change and alcoholic hepatitis may coexist.

A patient may admit abusing alcohol, but otherwise diagnosis can prove difficult because patients may be extremely effective at concealing their abuse. The measurement of random ethanol levels in blood, urine, or breath may be indicated. A liver biopsy is useful both diagnostically and prognostically. Although biopsy features may be highly suggestive of ALD, there are no absolute diagnostic features. It is important to rule out other causes of liver disease. In particular, genetic hemochromatosis can be overlooked if iron deposition is considered to have occurred secondary to alcohol but, in fact, represents coexistent genetic hemochromatosis. Biochemical investigations typically show only a modest elevation of transaminases, even in severe acute alcoholic hepatitis. Serum aspartate transaminase (AST) tends to be more elevated than serum alanine transaminase (ALT), a ratio which may be used diagnostically.[31]

Prognosis is related to biopsy features and the patient's ability to abstain from alcohol. Even decompensated cirrhotics may improve with sustained abstinence. For those with acute alcoholic hepatitis and hepatorenal syndrome, mortality approaches 100%.

Neoplasms of the Liver

Advances in diagnostic medicine have led to increased interest in hepatic neoplasms, since some are diagnosed at a stage where surgical cure, by either resection or liver transplantation, is achievable. Unfortunately, the majority of tumors are still diagnosed at an advanced stage. Oncologists have developed a number of new chemotherapeutic agents and alternative modes of treatment, which may offer hope to those with unresectable tumors.

Most tumors in the liver are metastatic in origin. The microenvironment within the liver seems ideal for growth of populations of malignant cells that are spread hematogenously. Hepatic metastases may be asymptomatic; for example, metastatic melanoma is associated with such minimal tissue reaction that almost complete hepatic replacement can occur before symptoms develop, and liver tests may be normal. In contrast, metastases arising from the stomach or lung typically cause symptoms or jaundice with less than 60% of the original parenchyma replaced. Rarely, a patient may present with fulminant hepatic failure due to replacement of functioning hepatic parenchyma by a tumor, such as lymphoma.

Primary Malignant Tumors

Hepatocellular carcinoma (HCC) is a malignant epithelial cell tumor arising from the parenchymal liver cell. It is the most common primary malignancy of the liver. In the United Kingdom and Western populations it is relatively uncommon, but it is much more common in Africa and the Orient.[32]

Epidemiologic studies suggest an important role of hepatitis B virus (HBV) infection in HCC. In Taiwan up to 90% of patients with HCC are surface antigen (HBsAg) positive. In many populations the incidence of HCC tends to reflect proportionately the carriage rate for HBsAg. The importance of HBV is also suggested by familial clustering of cases and HBV carriage.

For many years the agent responsible for non-A, non-B hepatitis was assumed to be responsible for a large number of tumors in hepatitis-B–negative individuals. The recent discovery of hepatitis C virus (HCV) suggests there is a link between HCV and HCC, but it is uncertain whether malignant transformation is dependent on cirrhosis being present.

Other etiologic factors include chemical carcinogens. Epidemiologic studies have implicated aflatoxin, but direct evidence of its causal role is lacking. Synthetic carcinogens are thought to include chlorinated hydrocarbons and organochlorine pesticides. Oral contraceptive use in females is associated with benign tumors, focal nodular hyperplasia, and HCC. Androgenic steroids are also carcinogenic. There is a strong association between alcohol abuse and HCC, which may rely on the presence of cirrhosis, rather than a direct promotive effect of alcohol. The contrast medium thorotrast is the best documented hepatic carcinogen, predisposing to HCC, hepatic angiosarcoma, and cholangiocarcinoma.

Early diagnosis of HCC may result from routine screening of cirrhotic patients. The most cost-effective policy is to perform ultrasonography annually and serum alphafetoprotein (AFP) twice yearly in cirrhotic patients. HCC is highly likely if a space-occupying lesion is present and serum AFP exceeds 100 ng/dL or is rising rapidly. In such cases, histologic confirmation is not usually obtained, since biopsy may seed tumor cells along its track. Imaging techniques include radionuclide scanning, CT, MRI scanning, and CT scanning with lipiodol contrast (Figure 2-4). The latter is the most sensitive technique and can detect HCC of less than 1 cm. Lipiodol is an oily contrast medium that is cleared by hepatocytes but not by HCC. A CT scan repeated 2–4 weeks after injection of lipiodol will detect HCC which appears dense on the tomogram.

Small lesions in cirrhosis may be cured by liver transplantation, which removes the potential for premalignant foci elsewhere in the liver to develop following resection. The number of tumors amenable to transplantation, however, is few. Other options include arterial embolization,[33] chemotherapy,[34] and injection with absolute alcohol.[35]

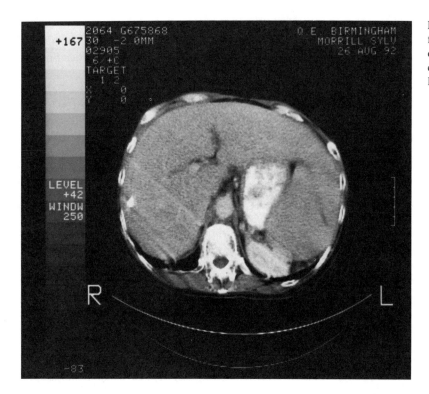

Figure 2-4. A CT scan performed three weeks after lipiodol injection reveals a 1.1 cm lesion in the right lobe of liver. R=right; L=Left.

Benign Infiltrative Disease of the Liver

There are several forms of systemic amyloidosis,[36] and any of these can affect the liver. The degree of amyloid infiltration varies greatly. Clinical manifestations are related to the degree of hepatic involvement. Hepatomegaly may occur and can be massive. In rare cases, disease is complicated by jaundice, portal hypertension, and liver failure. Rarely, a severe form of intrahepatic cholestasis may be precipitated, which is associated with a poor prognosis.

Diagnosis may be suspected on clinical grounds (e.g., a smoothly enlarged liver in association with known involvement of other organs or an associated primary disease). Liver biopsy, which is associated with a higher risk of bleeding, provides histologic diagnosis. Prognosis depends on causation and degree of involvement of other organs, since death is not caused by liver failure. Treatment is generally supportive, except in the case of familial Mediterranean fever in which colchicine is of value.[37]

Other infiltrative conditions that affect the liver include lipid storage diseases, glycogenoses, and other metabolic diseases that predominantly present in childhood.

Granulomatous Liver Disease

Granulomas are seen in a number of liver diseases. They consist of epithelioid cells with surrounding lymphocytes and are situated most frequently in the periportal regions. They may have giant cells, central caseation, and necrosis. Granulomas cause little functional hepatic disturbance.

Granulomas may be found in around 5% of liver biopsies. Despite extensive investigation, their cause may remain obscure. The two conditions most closely associated with granulomatous disease are tuberculosis and sarcoidosis, which account for a high proportion of cases. Rarer infectious causes include brucellosis, histoplasmosis, syphilis, leprosy, AIDS, cytomegalovirus, infectious mononucleosis, and schistosomiasis. Drugs that may induce granulomatous change include sulphonamides, carbamazepine, allopurinol, and quinine.

"Granulomatous hepatitis"[38] is a separate clinical entity associated with prolonged fever and constitutional upset. Occasionally lymphoma is found to be the cause, but in other cases the cause is not found despite extensive investigation. Liver tests are persistently abnormal, typically with moderate elevation of serum alkaline phosphatase and slight increases in serum transaminases. A trial of anti-tuberculous chemotherapy may be prescribed but, if unsuccessful, corticosteroids may be substituted when an infectious cause has been excluded.

Sarcoidosis is a multisystem disease of unknown etiology.[39] Hepatic involvement occurs frequently, as shown by noncaseating granulomas on liver biopsy. Hepatic disease is usually asymptomatic and trivial, although severe manifestations can develop. A vanishing bile duct syndrome may develop, which may be immune mediated. Some cases develop noncirrhotic portal hypertension, which is attributed to portal granulomas, and this occurs more commonly in those of African descent. Some patients with sarcoidosis are cirrhotic, but the link between the two is not clear and may occur by coincidence.

Viral Hepatitis

Five specific hepatitis viruses are recognized. A number of other viruses affect the liver secondarily. Acute hepatitis of any etiology is frequently associated with constitutional and gastrointestinal symptoms, lethargy, malaise, nausea, anorexia, and aching abdominal pains.

Hepatitis A and E are spread through the feco-oral route and cause self-limited disease. Hepatitis B, C, and D are spread parenterally and infection is frequently chronic. Other causes of hepatitis may be assumed to be viral in origin and are designated non-A, non-B, and non-C. It is likely that a number of hepatitis viruses are yet to be identified.

The pathologic reaction to acute infection with any of these agents is similar. Acute inflammatory changes are present that affect the entire liver. Hepatocyte necrosis is associated with infiltration of leucocytes and histiocytes. Portal tracts have increased cellularity. Bile duct proliferation is usual, but bile duct damage is rare. Occasionally necrosis may be confluent (submassive) and affect substantial groups of adjacent liver cells. In massive necrosis the whole acinus is involved.

Hepatitis A

Hepatitis A (HAV) is due to a 27 nm RNA picorna virus. Only a single serotype has been identified.

The disease occurs sporadically or in epidemic form and is spread by the fecal-oral route. Infection occurs most frequently in childhood. Spread is related to overcrowding and poor sanitation.

The illness is usually mild and may be subclinical, especially in childhood. The disease tends to be more serious and prolonged in adults and very rarely causes fulminant hepatic failure. However, overall mortality is less than one per 1000.[40] Chronicity does not develop, although occasionally the disease takes a biphasic form. Complete resolution of hepatitis and eradication of the virus is the rule. Diagnosis is confirmed serologically by the presence of serum IgM anti-HAV.

Cholestatic hepatitis A affects adults and is characterized by prolonged jaundice and pruritus.[41] The duration of cholestasis can be reduced by a course of corticosteroids, which may be indicated on a symptomatic basis. The prognosis of this form is excellent.

Virus is shed in feces up to 2 weeks before the icteric phase, when close contacts may become infected with the virus. Overall improvements in habitation and sanitation reduce transmission. Passive and active immunization are both available in the United Kingdom; the former is offered to the occasional traveler to endemic areas or close personal contacts of sufferers, while seronegative individuals who frequently travel to endemic areas are candidates for active vaccination.

Hepatitis B

The carrier rate of HBsAg varies worldwide from 0.1–0.2% in United Kingdom and Scandinavia to 3% in Greece and southern Italy and up to 10–15% in Africa and the Far East. The numbers exposed to hepatitis B, as denoted by presence of anti-HBs, is much higher in any given community than the numbers with HBsAg. The incubation period of HBV is 60–120 days. Transmission of HBV may occur horizontally or vertically. Horizontal transmission follows parenteral exposure to HBV and is associated particularly with homosexuality and drug abuse.

The course may be anicteric; indeed, many who are seropositive for HBsAg give no history of an acute hepatitis. The non-icteric patient is more likely to become a carrier of the virus than the icteric patient. In those who have a clinical attack,

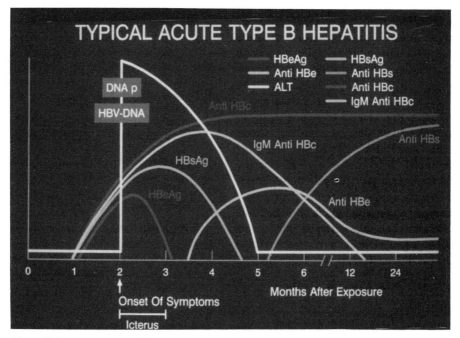

Figure 2-5. A schematic representation of the typical serological course of acute hepatitis B infection.

the disease course tends to be more severe than in acute hepatitis A or C. Features suggesting immune complex disease are often present, characterized by constitutional upset, fever, skin rash, and transitory nonmigratory arthropathy affecting the small joints.

Occasionally the disease runs a fulminant course, as the result of a brisk immune response to the virus, with more rapid clearing of HBV. Antibodies to surface antigen may be in low titer or absent and the only positive serology may be IgM anti-HB core.

Most frequently acute HBV disease is self-limiting (Figure 2-5) with clearance of the HBsAg; however, approximately 10% of adults and 90% of neonates who contract hepatitis B fail to clear HBsAg from serum within 6 months. By definition these patients are carriers, and in many patients this status will persist. There are estimated to be 300 million carriers worldwide.

Chronic infection carries the risk of transmitting the disease and also of developing chronic hepatitis, cirrhosis, or hepatocellular carcinoma. Patients who are apparently healthy carriers may have biopsy changes ranging from mild nonspecific changes to chronic active hepatitis or cirrhosis.

Interferon therapy is indicated in some patients with chronic HBV infection of greater than 6 months duration.[42,43] Therapy may "convert" pa-tients from "e" antigen (HBeAg) positive to negative. Trials assessing the benefit of interferon alpha therapy report around 40% success; however, multivariate analysis has shown that certain patients are more likely to respond.[44] These are patients with a history of recent acute hepatitis of short duration and transmitted nonvertically, with active histologic change and elevated serum transminases and a serum HBV DNA level of < 100 ng/l. In carefully selected cases, the response rate should exceed 50%.

The development of an acute exacerbation of chronic HBV disease and even apparent "fulmi-nant" hepatic failure may occur following super-added infection with delta virus (HDV).[45,46] This is a defective RNA virus that is dependent on the presence of HBV for its infectivity. Diagnosis can be confirmed serologically.

Prevention

Neonates born to HBV carriers should receive active immunization if the mother is surface antigen positive. The first dose of 10 μg is given by deep intramuscular injection within 48 hours of delivery, and this is repeated at 1 month, 2 months, and 12 months. Serology should be checked at 12 months. Neonates born to HBeAg-positive mothers should also receive passive immunization with hepatitis B immune globulin (HBIg) 200 IU into the contralateral thigh. This treatment regimen has an efficacy in excess of 90%.[47] Individuals at risk of occupational exposure to HBV should also receive active immunization. Antibody levels (HBsAb) maintained in excess of 1/100 are considered protective.

Hepatitis C

Identification of non-A, non-B (NANB) hepatitis as a distinct clinical entity was first made about 15 years ago.[48] Hepatitis C virus (HCV) accounts for much of the disease previously described as NANB hepatitis. Many infections were previously acquired by exposure to blood and blood products. Donors are now screened for HCV. High-risk groups include homosexuals and intravenous drug abusers, but a small proportion of the population has developed infection in the absence of defined risk factors.

Infection may run an acute self-limiting course, but a chronic carrier state probably develops in at least 50% of patients. Pathologic studies divide chronic HCV into chronic active hepatitis, chronic persistent hepatitis, and chronic lobular hepatitis. In these aspects HCV resembles chronic HBV or autoimmune hepatitis and, although there are histological patterns characteristic of HCV, none is diagnostic. In general, chronic HCV disease appears more benign than chronic HBV, although those who are chronically infected are at risk of developing cirrhosis and HCC.

A variety of diagnostic tests are available,[49] which have differing sensitivities and specificities, so it is important to know which test is being used. The earliest test developed, the ELISA using an HCV-related antigen, C-100, is limited by a lack of sensitivity and specificity.[50] False-positive results were noted in patients with autoimmune hepatitis. These were attributed to the associated hypergammaglobulinemia, since they reversed as disease activity was reduced by effective immunosuppression. A subsequent test, the recombinant immunoblot assay (RIBA), has increased both specificity and sensitivity. This detects antibodies to three recombinant antigens: C-100, also present in the ELISA assay; 5-1-1 polypeptide; and superoxide dismutase. A second-generation RIBA test (4-RIBA) has been validated and is also highly specific and sensitive. The presence of a positive antibody test for HCV is important, since it corresponds to ongoing infection and infectivity. The polymerase chain reaction (PCR) for HCV RNA is the most sensitive test and is becoming more available.

Controlled therapeutic trials of interferon therapy are in progress. Clearance of HCV occurs in approximately 25% of patients with chronic disease, although the long-term outcome of these patients is uncertain, since many of the apparent responders have relapsed following the cessation of therapy.

Hepatitis E

Hepatitis E is a recently recognized enterically transmitted virus infection endemic in much of the developing world. There is no chronic carrier state. Disease is most severe if HEV is contracted during the third trimester of pregnancy.

Other Viruses

Other viruses such as cytomegalovirus, herpes simplex virus, and adenovirus are not primarily hepatotropic but may cause an associated hepatitis. Effects on the liver are usually minor and transitory, except in neonates and immunocompromised individuals.

Infectious mononucleosis, due to the Epstein-Barr virus, frequently affects the liver. It causes hepatitis in 90%, but jaundice in only around 10%. Associated hemolysis may contribute to the hyperbilirubinemia. Liver tests are most abnormal between the second and fourth week. Disease is usually mild, short, and self-limiting, but a case of fatal fulminant hepatic failure has been reported, as has a case of chronic hepatitis.

Other Infections of the Liver

Pyogenic liver abscess may result from portal pyaemia, biliary sepsis, or trauma. Many abscesses, however, occur in the absence of apparent risk factors. *Streptococcus milleri* is a common pathogen; others include *Escherichia coli* and staphylococci. Patients present with malaise, fever, anorexia, and weight loss. Diagnosis is made by ultrasound examination. A sample of pus should be aspirated before starting antibiotic therapy and processed for culture and sensitivity. Percutaneous drainage followed by a prolonged course of appropriate antibiotics eradicates the organism in the majority of patients.

Entamoeba histolytica may cause a liver abscess, which can develop many years after the original infection. Diagnosis is made ultrasonographically. Aspiration may reveal *E. histolytica,* or the ameobic hemagglutination test may be positive. Treatment is with metronidazole.

Hydatid disease is caused by the larval stage of the tapeworm *Echinococcus granulosus,* which lives in dogs. Humans, sheep, and cattle are intermediate hosts and the dog is the definitive host. Humans are infected by contact with excreta from dogs, which contains ova. Dogs are infected by eating the viscera of sheep, which contain hydatid cysts.

Ova are surrounded by an envelope, which is dissolved in gastric juice. The liberated ovum burrows through the intestinal mucosa and is carried by the portal vein to the liver, where it develops into an adult cyst. The disease is common in many sheep-raising countries, but is rare in the United Kingdom, other than some areas of Wales.

Clinical features depend on the site of the cyst and stage of development. A cyst may be found incidentally at autopsy. The only symptoms may be a dull ache in the right upper quadrant. A cyst may rupture into the peritoneal cavity, resulting in multiple cysts which can cause intestinal obstruction. Rupture into the colon may result in secondary infection, and rupture through the diaphragm into the lungs may also occur. Cysts can occur in lung, kidney, brain, and spleen, but the liver is usually the only organ involved.

Diagnosis may be based on positive serology or radiological demonstration of a cyst by ultrasound or CT. Cysts may become calcified and identified on plain abdominal x-ray. Because of the risk of rupture, hydatid disease should be treated. A single cyst should be excised surgically. Multiple cysts may be treated with mebendazole; however, viable cysts may persist despite 12 months therapy.

Tuberculosis frequently involves the liver following hematogenous spread. As in other organs, mycobacteria precipitate a granulomatous reaction, but most heal spontaneously. Culture of a liver biopsy is occasionally positive. Serious liver damage is unusual and treatment consists of eradication of the disease from the primary site.

Leptospirosis (Weil's disease) is caused by *Leptospira icterohaemorrhagiae.* Rats form the main reservoir, in which the organism is harbored in the renal tubules. Agricultural and sewerage workers are at most risk of infection.

Incubation is 6–15 days. The disease has three characteristic stages. The septicemic stage is associated with dissemination of the organism in the bloodstream. High fever develops rapidly and is associated with systemic effects including prostration, abdominal pain, headache, and meningism. Pneumonitis may occur and severe attacks are characterized by a hemorrhagic tendency, with bleeding into the lungs, gastrointestinal tract, or skin. Jaundice may develop within the first week and is an adverse prognostic indicator. The liver is enlarged, but the size of the spleen is normal. In the second week the temperature returns to normal, but without other signs of clinical improvement. Jaundice deepens and renal and myocardial damage develops. Severe illness is associated with hypotension, renal failure, and arrhythmias.

The convalescent phase begins during the third week. There is a great range in disease severity. A number of individuals have serologic evidence of past exposure, but no history of disease. Others suffer severe disease that is unresponsive to intensive supportive therapy and follow an inexorable decline to death.

Investigations may reveal the organism in the blood during the first week and in the urine during the second week. Serology is positive from around the first week. Antibody titers peak in the fourth week, but may be negative in those who die rapidly. Mortality is around 15%, but is negligible in the nonjaundiced patient. Treatment should be instituted with benzyl penicillin, although there is no conclusive evidence of benefit, since many of the manifestations are thought to be immune mediated.

Schistosomiasis

Schistosomiasis affects over 200 million people worldwide. *Schistosoma mansoni* and *S.japonicum* affect the liver; the latter is more pathogenic. There are three stages of infection. Initially there is local pruritus. Infection is subsequently characterized by fever, urticaria, and eosinophilia. In the third stage ova are deposited in the intestine, urinary tract, and liver. In the liver, the ova penetrate and obstruct portal branches provoking a granulomatous reaction that is proportional to the adult worm load.

Table 2-6. Biochemical Alterations in Normal Pregnancy

Alkaline phosphatase	Increases up to 3–4-fold at term
Gamma glutamyl transferase	No increase, may decrease and may not fluctuate in disease
Aminotransferases	Usual values, standard serological marker of hepatocellular damage
Bilirubin	Unchanged
Total protein	Mild progressive decline
Alpha and beta globulin	Tend to increase
Gamma globulins	Tend to decrease
Triglyceride and cholesterol	Increase substantially
Ceruloplasmin	Increase as consequence of increased hepatic synthesis
Transferrin	
Alpha-1-antitrypsin	
Fibrinogen	

Hepatic fibrosis leads to presinusoidal portal hypertension and splenomegaly. A collateral circulation develops which may manifest with hemorrhage from esophageal or gastric varices. Active infection is diagnosed by examination of stool or rectal biopsy. Treatment is with praziquantel.

The Liver in Pregnancy

A broad spectrum of liver disease may be encountered during pregnancy. Disease may arise as a direct consequence of pregnancy, but the conventional liver diseases may also occur. Some have an entirely benign course, whereas others may be associated with significant maternal and fetal mortality.

In pregnancy, physiologic and biochemical changes occur which affect the quoted normal ranges in the healthy adult. Results therefore need to be judged against revised baselines (Table 2-6).

Liver Disease Complicating Pregnancy

Hyperemesis gravidarum may be considered normal during early pregnancy, but when severe it may be associated with hepatic dysfunction and jaundice. The abnormalities settle as vomiting subsides.

Preeclampsia complicates up to 10% of pregnancies, and deranged liver tests occur in 10% of these. In more severe cases, disseminated intravascular coagulation may be present. The term *HELLP syndrome* has been coined[51] to refer to the cluster of hemolysis, elevated liver enzymes, and low platelet count that may occur in association with preeclampsia.

Hepatic hemorrhage and rupture are rare complications of pregnancy, mostly associated with eclampsia, and represent the extreme end of the spectrum of ischemic hepatocyte necrosis and hemorrhage.

Thrombotic thrombocytopenic purpura may rarely occur as a complication of pregnancy and create difficulties with the differential diagnosis from preeclampsia/eclampsia syndromes, since there may be associated derangement of liver function.[52] Correct diagnosis is particularly important because management of the two conditions is different. Diagnosis is based on the pentad of fever, microangiopathic hemolytic anemia, thrombocytopenia, fluctuating neurological symptoms, and renal abnormalities and may be assisted by the presence of subendothelial fibrin deposition on tissue biopsy. The prothrombin time (PT), partial thromboplastin time (PTT), and fibrinogen are normal.

Therapy involves the infusion of plasma or its high molecular weight fraction and plasmaphoresis. The prognosis for mother and fetus improves considerably with early diagnosis and appropriate therapy, without which it is almost universally fatal to both.

Intrahepatic cholestasis of pregnancy is a rare disorder of unknown etiology.[53] A familial tendency and a higher prevalence of this disorder in Scandinavia, Chile, and Bolivia suggest a genetic predisposition. Presentation is usually with pruritus in the third trimester, although some will present as early as the first trimester. Jaundice is frequently absent; if present, it tends to occur several weeks after the onset of pruritus. Laboratory features may include elevation of 5'-nucleotidase. Aspartate transaminase (AST) and alanine transaminase (ALT) are often normal, but may increase three-to-fourfold. Bile acid concentrations are inevitably elevated. Liver biopsy is not indicated, but characteristic centrilobular cholestasis has been reported in those biopsied. Prognosis for the mother is excellent. The condition always resolves rapidly after delivery. The effects on the fetus are less certain. Several authors report an increased incidence of premature labor, fetal distress, and neonatal death.[53a-c] Individuals who develop cholestasis frequently have recurrent cholestasis during subsequent pregnancies, with a fairly consistent time of onset in each pregnancy for any individual, and are prone to develop cholestasis in association with the estrogen-containing oral contraceptive pill.

Acute fatty liver of pregnancy[54] is a rare, but extremely serious complication of pregnancy. It occurs most commonly in primigravida with a male fetus and in twin pregnancies. The etiology is unknown. Clinical features initially consist of anorexia, nausea, abdominal pain, vomiting, and weight loss occurring between the 32nd and 38th week, most often in the setting of preeclampsia. There are no specific findings on examination, but the patient is frequently tender in the epigastrium and right hypochondrium. Progression to fulminant hepatic failure is rapid, with the onset of encephalopathy, coagulopathy, and hypoglycemia. Laboratory investigations confirm hepatocellular damage with elevated transaminases and bilirubin. Hyperuricemia is also present and can be useful diagnostically. Coagulopathy will progress rapidly, both as a result of reduced hepatic synthetic function and consumption of clotting factors due to DIC. Hematological parameters are likely to include thrombocytopenia, leucocytosis, and the presence of fragmented red cells and normoblasts on a blood film. Progressive renal impairment is usual. A liver biopsy is frequently precluded by poor coagulation,

but if performed, histology is most reliable by examination of a frozen section, revealing a microvesicular deposition of fat. CT scanning has been shown to be a reliable method of diagnosis[55] because of the abnormally low density of the liver due to the elevated fat content. Serial CT scans invariably show a resolution in the 2–3 weeks following delivery.

The mainstay of management is to support coagulopathy with fresh frozen plasma and platelet concentrate, the avoidance of hypoglycemia with adequate glucose supplementation, and expeditious delivery of the fetus. Its prompt diagnosis and recognition of the need for immediate delivery have resulted in a dramatic reduction in maternal mortality from around 90% to 10%, although fetal survival remains lower. Recurrence in subsequent pregnancies is exceedingly rare.

The Effects of Pregnancy on Preexistent Liver Disease

Cirrhosis and Portal Hypertension

Women with established cirrhosis have a reduced chance of conception.[56] Liver function frequently deteriorates with an elevation of bilirubin and transaminases. The more serious complication is the increased incidence of variceal bleeds, caused by a combination of factors resulting in elevated portal pressures, especially in the second and third trimesters. A successful outcome is, however, frequently obtained.

Gallstones may manifest during pregnancy, which itself enhances the lithogenicity of bile. This may be precipitated by impaired gallbladder contractility and a high rate of biliary sludge.[57] Patients developing biliary disease during pregnancy should ideally be managed conservatively, although surgery can be safely carried out if required.

References

1. Wilkinson, G.R. and Shand, G.D. (1975) A physiological approach to hepatic drug clearance. *Clinical Pharmacology and Therapeutics,* 18:377–90.
2. Bass, N.M. and Williams, R.L. (1988) Guide to drug dosage in hepatic disease. *Clinical Pharmacokinetics* 15:396–420.

3. Brosen, K. (1990) Recent developments in hepatic drug oxidation. Implications for clinical pharmocokinetics. *Clinical Pharmacokinetics* 18:220–39.

4. Child, C.G. and Turcott, J.G. (1964) Surgery and portal hypertension. In *The Liver and Portal Hypertension* (Child, C.G., ed). Philadelphia: WB Saunders Co.

5. Pugh, R.N.H., Murray-Lyon, I.M., Dawson, J.L., Pietroni, M.C. and Williams, R. (1973) Transection of the oesophagus for bleeding oesophageal varices. *British Journal of Surgery* 60:646–49.

6. Parsons-Smith, B.G., Summerskill, W.H.J., Dawson, A.M. and Sherlock, S. (1957) The encephalograph in liver disease. *Lancet* ii:867–71.

7. Moreno-Otero R., Lisker-Melman, M. and Jones, E.A. (1989) Primary biliary cirrhosis. *Medical Clinics of North America* 73:911–29.

8. Kaplan, M.M. (1987) Primary biliary cirrhosis. *New England Journal of Medicine* 316:521–28.

9. Butler P., Valle, F. and Burroughs, A.K. (1991) Mitochondrial antigens and antibodies in primary biliary cirrhosis. *Postgraduate Medical Journal* 67:790–97.

10. Beukers, R. and Schalm, S.W. (1992) Immunosuppressive therapy for primary biliary cirrhosis. *Journal of Hepatology* 14:1–6.

11. Wiesner, R.H. and LaRusso, N.F. (1980) Clinicopathologic features of the syndrome of primary sclerosing cholangitis. *Gastroenterology* 79:200–06.

12. Chapman, R.W.G., Arborgh, B.A.M., Rhodes, J.M. *et al.* (1980) Primary sclerosing cholangitis: A review of its clinical features, cholangiography and hepatic histology. *Gut* 21:870–07.

13. Chapman, R.W. (1991) Aetiology and natural history of primary sclerosing cholangitis—A decade of progress? *Gut* 32:1433–35.

13a. Harrison, R.F., Davies, M.H., Neuberger, J.M., and Hubscher, S.G. (1994) Fibrous and obliterative cholangitis in hepatic allografts: Evidence of recurrent primary sclerosing cholangitis. *Hepatology* (in press).

14. Macfarlane, I.G. and Eddleston, A.L.W.F. (1989) Chronic active hepatitis. In *Immunology and Immunopathology of the Liver and Gastrointestinal Tract.* (Targau F and Shanahau S, eds.) New York: Igaku-Shoin.

15. Macfarlane, I.G. and Williams, R. (1985) Liver membrane antibodies. *Journal of Hepatology* 1:313–19.

16. Read, A.E., Sherlock, S. and Harrison, C.V. (1963) Active 'juvenile' cirrhosis considered as part of systemic disease and the effect of corticosteroid therapy. *Gut* 4:378–93.

17. Keating, J.J., O'Brien, C.J., Stellon, A.J. et al. (1987) Influence of aetiology, clinical, and histological features on survival in chronic active hepatitis: an analysis of 204 patients. *Quarterly Journal of Medicine* 62:59–66.

18. Wilson, S.A.K. (1912) Progressive lenticular degeneration: A familial nervous disease associated with cirrhosis of the liver. *Brain* 34:295.

19. Dobyns, W.B., Goldstein, N.P. and Gordon, H. (1979) Clinical spectrum of Wilson's disease. *Mayo Clinic Proceedings* 54:35–42.

20. Frydman, M., Bonne-Tamir, B., Farrer, L.A., *et al.* (1985) Assignment of the gene for Wilson disease to chromosome 13: Linkage to the esterase D locus. *Proceedings National Association of Science* 82:1819–21.

21. Fleming, C.R., Dickson, E.R., Hollenhorst, R.W. *et al.* (1975) Pigmented corneal rings in a patient with primary biliary cirrhosis. *Gastroenterology* 69:220–25.

22. Weintraub, L.R., Edwards, C.O. and Krikker, M. (eds.) (1988) Haemochromatosis. Proceedings of the first international conference. *Annals of the New York Academy of Sciences* 526.

23. Bassett, M.L., Halliday, J.W. and Powell, L.W. (1984) Genetic Hemochromatosis. *Seminars of Liver Disease* 4:217–27.

24. Simon, M., Bourel, M., Fauchet, R. and Genetet, B. (1976) Association of HLA-A3 and HLA-B14 antigens with idiopathic haemochromatosis. *Gut* 17:332–34.

25. Brissot, P. and Deugnier, Y. (1990) Les porphyries vues par l'hepatologue. *Gastroenterol Clin Biol* 14:74–79.

26. Lelbach, W.K. (1985) Epidemiology of alcoholic liver disease; Continental Europe. In *Alcoholic Liver Disease.* (Hall, P. ed). London: Edward Arnold Ltd.

27. Lau, H.H. (1975) Cost of alcoholic beverages as a determinant of alcohol consumption. In *Research Advances in Alcohol and Drug Problems.* (Gibbins, R.J., Israel, Y., Kalant, H., Popham, R.E., Schmidt, W. and Smart, R.G., eds) New York: John Wiley & Sons.

28. Doffoel, M., Tongio, M.M., Gut, J.-P., et al. (1986) Relationship between 34 HLA-A, HLA-B, and HLA-DR antigens and three serological markers of viral infections in alcoholic cirrhosis. *Hepatology* 6:457–63.

29. Tamburro, C.H., Fortwengler, M.P., Miller, B., Mendenhall, C.L. and Mendenhall, V.A. (1986) Cooperative study group on alcoholic hepatitis. Histocompatibility antigens (HLA) in alcoholic hepatitis. *Hepatology* 6:777.

30. Lieber, C.S. (1988) Biochemical and molecular basis of alcohol-induced injury to liver and other tissues. *New England Journal of Medicine* 319:1639–50.

31. Kawachi, I., Robinson, G.M., and Stace, N.H. (1990) A combination of raised AST:ALT ratio and erythrocyte mean cellular volume detects excessive alcohol consumption. *New Zealand Medical Journal* 103:145–48.

32. Munoz, N. and Bosch X. (1987) Epidemiology of hepatocellular carcinoma. In *Neoplasms of the Liver.* (Okuda, K. and Ishak, K.G., eds.) Tokyo: Springer Verlag. pp. 3–19.

33. Yamada, R., Sato, M., Kawabata, M. et al. (1983) Hepatic arterial embolisation in 120 patients with unresectable hepatoma. *Radiology* 148:397–401.

34. Konno, T., Maeda, H., Iwai, K. et al. (1983) Effect of administration of high-molecular-weight anticancer agent SMANCS with lipid lymphographic agent on hepatoma.

A preliminary report. *European Journal of Cancer and Clinical Oncology* 19:1053–65.

35. Ohto, M., Ebara, M., Yoshikawa, M. and Okuda, K. (1987) Radiation therapy and percutaneous ethanol injection for the treatment of hepatocellular carcinoma. In *Neoplasms of the Liver.* (Okuda, K. and Ishak, K.G., eds.) Tokyo: Springer Verlag. pp. 3–19.

36. Glenner, G.G. (1980) Amyloid deposits and amyloidosis. *New England Journal of Medicine* 302:1283–92.

37. Zemer, D., Pras, M., Sohar, E. et al. (1986) Colchicine in the prevention and treatment of amyloidosis of familial Mediterranean fever. *New England Journal of Medicine* 314:1001–07.

38. Simon, H.B. and Wolff, S.M. (1973) Granulomatous hepatitis and prolonged fever of unknown origin: A study of 13 patients. *Medicine* 52:1–22.

39. James, D.G. and Jones Williams, W. (1985) *Sarcoidosis and Other Granulomatous Disorders.* Philadelphia: WB Saunders.

40. McNeil, M., Hoy, J.F., Richards, M.J. et al. (1984) Aetiology of fatal viral hepatitis in Melbourne. A retrospective study. *Medical Journal of Australia* 2:637–40.

41. Gordon, S.C., Reddy, R., Schiff, L. and Schiff, E.R. (1984) Prolonged intrahepatic cholestasis secondary to acute hepatitis A. *Annals of Internal Medicine* 101:635–37.

42. Dusheiko, G., Dibisceglie, Bowyer, S. et al. (1985) Recombinant leukocyte interferon treatment of chronic hepatitis B. *Hepatology* 5:556–60.

43. Alexander, G.J.M., Brahm, J., Fagan, E.A. et al. (1987) Loss of HBsAg with interferon therapy in chronic hepatitis B virus infection. *Lancet* ii:66–68.

44. Brook, M.G., Karayiannis, P. and Thomas, H.C. (1989) Which patients with chronic hepatitis B infection will respond to alpha-interferon therapy? A statistical analysis of predictive factors. *Hepatology* 10:761–63.

45. Rizetto, M., Canese, M.G., Arico, S. et al. (1977) Immunofluorescence detection of a new antigen-antibody system (delta/anti delta) associated with hepatitis B virus in liver and in serum of HBsAg carriers. *Gut* 18:997–1003.

46. Rizetto, M., Verne, G., Gerin, J.L. and Purcell, R.H. (1986) Hepatitis delta virus disease. In *Progress in Liver Disease.* (Popper H, Schaffner E, eds.) New York: Grune Stratton.

47. Beasley, R.P., Hwang, L.-Y., Lee, G.C. et al. (1983) Prevention of perinatally transmitted hepatitis B virus infections with hepatitis B immune globulin and hepatitis B vaccine. *Lancet* ii:1099–102.

48. Gerber, M.A. (1992) Chronic hepatitis C: The beginning of the end of time-honored nomenclature. *Hepatology* 15:733–34.

49. Gumucio, J.J. (1992) Hepatitis C: Improving the diagnostic armamentarium. *Hepatology* 14:736–38.

50. Alter, H.J., Purcell, R.H., Shih, J.W. et al. (1989) Detection of antibody to hepatitis C virus in prospectively followed transfusion recipients with acute and chronic non-A non-B hepatitis. *New England Journal of Medicine* 321:1494–500.

51. Weinstein, L. (1982) Syndrome of hemolysis, elevated liver enzymes and low platelet count: A severe consequence of hypertension in pregnancy. *American Journal of Obstetrics and Gynecology* 142:159–67.

52. Ambrose, A., Welham, R.T., and Cefalo, R.C. (1985) Thrombotic thrombocytopenic purpura in early pregnancy. *Obstetrics and Gynecology* 66:267–72.

53. Reyes, H., Taboada, Ribalta, J. (1979) Prevalence of intrahepatic cholestasis of pregnancy in La Paz, Bolivia. *Journal of Chronic Diseases* 32:499–504.

53a. Reid, R., Ivey, K.J., Rencoret, R.H., and Storey, B. (1976) Fetal complications of obstetric cholestasis. *British Medical Journal* 1:870–2.

53b. Fish, N.M. and Storey, G.N.B. (1988) Fetal outcome in obstetric cholestasis. *British Journal of Obstetrics and Gynaecology* 95:1137–43.

53c. Johnston, W.G. and Baskett, T.F. (1979) Obstetric cholestasis. A 14 year review. *American Journal of Obstetrics and Gynecology* 133:299–301.

54. Sheehan, H.L. (1990) The pathology of acute yellow atrophy and delayed chloroform poisoning. *Journal of Obstetrics and Gynaecology of the British Empire* 47:49–61.

55. McKee, C.M., Weir, P.E., Foster, J.H. et al. (1986) Acute fatty liver of pregnancy and diagnosis by computed tomography. *British Medical Journal* 292:291–92.

56. Schreyer, P., Caspi, E., El-Hindu, J.M., and Eschar, J. (1982) Cirrhosis, pregnancy and delivery: A review. *Obstetrics and Gynecology Surveys* 37:304–12.

57. Angelico, M., De Santis, A., and Capocaccia L. (1990) Biliary sludge: A critical update. *Journal of Clinical Gastroenterology* 12:656–62.

Chapter 3
Liver Function Tests

Paul G. Roe and Dagmar Schaps

The liver has a wide range of functions that may be disturbed in different ways by the many diseases that affect it. Consequently, a large number of tests have been developed that are affected in different ways by different diseases. Specific diagnoses are made using a range of clinical, biochemical, histologic, and radiologic methods. In this chapter, we have divided tests of liver function into tests that show hepatic damage, cholestasis, and impaired synthetic function, respectively. In addition, a series of quantitative liver function tests are described that do not form part of routine testing (Table 3-1) Their role is described later. Measurement of the plasma concentration of alanine aminotransferase (ALT, SGPT), gamma-glutamyl transpeptidase (GGT), and albumin are particularly valuable as these substances are specifically affected by liver disease. Their elevation can reveal increases in the membrane permeability of hepatocytes (ALT), cholestasis and toxic damage (GGT), or an impairment of liver protein synthesis and secretion (albumin). If their activities remain within the normal range, the likelihood of significant liver disease is less than 2%.

Table 3-1. Classification of Liver Function Tests

Markers of hepatic damage
Aspartate aminotransferase (AST)
Alanine aminotransferase (ALT)
Lactate dehydrogenase (LDH)
Glutamate dehydrogenase (GDH)
Markers of Cholestasis
Bilirubin
Alkaline phosphatase (AP)
Gamma-glutamyl transferase (GGT)
5-Nucleotidase (5-NT)
Lipoprotein-X (LPX)
Markers of reduced synthetic junction
Albumin
Cholinesterase (CHE)
Clotting factors
Quantitative liver function tests
Bromsulphthalein clearance
Indocyanine green clearance
Galactose elimination capacity
Antipyrine/aminopyrine clearance
Caffeine clearance
Serum bile acids
Lignocaine metabolites (MEGX)
Hexobarbital clearance
Tryptophan tolerance[15]
[15]NH_3 clearance

Indicators of Hepatic Damage

After cell damage, intracellular enzymes from organs with low capillary protein permeability reach the blood after passing through the lymphatic system. The slow lymphatic flow will result in a delayed increase in plasma concentrations of enzymes. In organs with average capillary permeability, for example the heart, the molecular weight of each enzyme determines whether it will be drained directly into the blood or indirectly through the lymphatic system. Consequently, patients with an acute myocardial infarct show an early increase in creatine phosphokinase (CK, molecular weight 80,000) as opposed to a late increase in lactate dehydrogenase (LDH, molecular weight 130,000). In the liver the capillaries and sinusiods do not have a basement membrane, the endothelial cells are fenestrated, and the surface of hepatic cells consists of deep intercellular columns. Almost all (90%) of the surface of a hepatocyte has direct contact with plasma, and as a result, the intracellular parenchymal enzymes reach the blood almost as quickly as enzymes liberated from circulating blood cells. This unique anatomical characteristic of the liver is responsible for the high serum concentration of enzymes that occurs after comparatively moderate cell damage.

The amount of intracellular substances released into the extracellular space depends on the number of cells injured and the extent of cellular injury. Only severely injured cells release *insoluble* mitochondrial enzymes.

The degree of injury depends on whether the damage occurs acutely or chronically. Cell structures can adapt to a slowly changing situation. Following an acute hypoxic insult, the injury predominantly occurs in the center of the hepatic lobules. Depending on the degree of cellular damage, large amounts of enzymes may be released which persist only for a short period, as the dead cells do not continue to liberate enzymes. In contrast, the parenchymal cells of patients with chronic, slowly progressing hepatic venous stasis will adapt their metabolism to this state, and the degree of membrane damage and enzyme release will be low.

Patterns and ratios of the various enzymes indicative of liver damage have, in the past, been investigated as possible diagnostic indicators. In practice, however, most patients have a mixed and varying picture not easily resolved into theoretical components. In most patients measurement of serum concentrations of ALT, aspartate aminotransferase, and LDH give little further information than measurement of ALT alone.

Aspartate aminotransferase (AST) occurs in many different tissues and is therefore not liver specific. It is, however, a sensitive indicator of liver damage and becomes elevated after 8 hours with a peak at 24–36 hours. Its plasma concentrations are proportional to the degree of hepatocellular damage and may increase 50-fold when the damage is severe, for example in acute hepatitis. In extrahepatic obstruction and inactive cirrhosis, when there is little new parenchymal damage, plasma concentrations are low.

Alanine aminotransferase (ALT) is more liver specific than AST, but is less sensitive. It has a longer plasma half-life than AST.

Lactate dehydrogenase (LDH) is an insensitive and nonspecific indicator of liver damage. Isoenzyme electrophoresis will distinguish cardiac, renal, and erythrocyte injury (LDH 1 and 2) from liver and skeletal muscle injury (LDH 4 and 5).

Glutamate dehydrogenase (GDH) has high activity in the center of the hepatic lobule, whereas LDH and ALT have a higher concentration in the periphery of the lobule. Therefore, in hypoxic liver damage, with predominant injury of the centrilobular regions, high plasma concentrations of GDH occur with only a moderate increase of ALT. This enzyme pattern does not occur in patients with an acute viral hepatitis or other inflammatory diseases which affect the entire liver cell in a diffuse way.

With severe cellular damage, insoluble mitochondrial substances such as GDH and the mitochondrial isoenzyme of aspartate aminotransferase (AST, SGOT) are released. The ratio of poorly soluble to highly soluble enzymes shows the degree of cell damage.

After release, enzymes are eliminated from the plasma at different rates. The relatively short half-life of AST and GDH, in comparison to that of ALT, is of diagnostic importance. This is illustrated in patients with an acute illness such as acute viral hepatitis, where the increased elimination of AST in comparison to ALT becomes evident as a decrease in the AST/ALT ratio. A low AST/ALT ratio can, however, occur with mild acute viral hepatitis. LDH activity is useful to differentiate between hepatitis in regression and hepatitis of low severity. Liver LDH (LDH-4 and 5 fractions) has an extremely short serum half-life and its serum concentration becomes normal early in the course of an acute hepatitis.

Liver cells react to acute and chronic damage with a change of their metabolism and a subsequent change in the intracellular distribution of enzymes. Liver-specific functions are down-regulated in favor of general metabolic needs. In an acute illness these changes are rapidly reversible, whereas in a chronic illness they persist for its duration. During the transition of chronic hepatitis to cirrhosis, the activity of the relatively hepatospecific enzymes ALT and GDH in liver tissue decreases while the activity of the nonspecific enzymes AST and LDH show no change. In patients with advanced liver disease, the activity of AST is characteristically higher than that of ALT, and GDH activity is often completely normal. The peak serum concentration of enzymes is related to the absolute hepatic cell mass.

Indicators of Cholestasis

Bilirubin

Hemoglobin released during the breakdown of erythrocytes is converted to bilirubin by the reticuloendothelial system. It is then taken up by hepatocytes and conjugated with glucuronide molecules for excretion in the bile. Two pigment fractions of bilirubin are measured: a water-soluble conjugated fraction (direct reaction) and a lipid-soluble unconjugated fraction (total minus direct). Bilirubin concentrations may be elevated with haemolysis, biliary obstruction, and liver cell damage. Jaundice occurs when the total bilirubin exceeds 3 mg/dL.

Elevations of conjugated bilirubin indicate impaired secretion into the bile. They occur in the majority of hepatobiliary disorders regardless of whether the cholestasis is caused by bile duct or hepatic parenchymal disturbance.

Acute biliary obstruction is characterized by an increase in conjugated bilirubin. Hepatocyte damage secondary to cholestasis results in an increase in unconjugated bilirubin. Hepatocellular damage as a result of hepatitis, cirrhosis, or infiltration results in increases in both conjugated and unconjugated bilirubin. The conjugated fraction is a result of intrahepatic cholestasis caused by bile duct plugging by damaged cell debris. The unconjugated fraction is the result of a reduction in the population of hepatocytes available for conjugation. As cholestasis may lead to hepatocellular damage, and vice versa, measurement of conjugated and unconjugated bilirubin fractions is of limited diagnostic value. Total bilirubin is therefore now generally used in standard liver function test profiles.

Elevations of unconjugated bilirubin occur in hemolytic anemia and in hepatic defects of conjugation. Gilbert's disease is characterized by chronic, unconjugated hyperbilirubinemia, which may be the result of a defect in hepatic uptake or, more commonly, a defect in conjugation. In physiologic, neonatal jaundice there are several causes, including decreased erythrocyte lifespan, disturbed hepatic uptake, conjugation and excretion, and a rapid enterohepatic biliary recirculation. In type I and II Crigler-Najjar syndrome there is an absolute and partial deficiency of glucoronyl transferase, respectively. This is responsible for the high levels of unconjugated bilirubin seen in this condition. In Dubin-Johnson and Rotor syndrome an impaired excretion of bilirubin is the cause of increased serum concentrations of unconjugated and conjugated bilirubin.

Alkaline Phosphatase

Alkaline phosphatase (AP) is a membrane-bound enzyme found in bone, liver, intestine, and placenta. It has a half-life of 1 to 10 days. In the absence of pregnancy and bone disease, a raised AP usually indicates biliary tract dysfunction. Plasma concentrations of AP are increased in the presence of an obstruction of a single hepatic duct branch, although the plasma concentration will return to normal as atrophy of the obstructed part of the liver occurs.[1] Hyperbilirubinemia would not occur in this situation. Alkaline phosphatase is only slightly elevated in infiltrative disease. In patients with portal hypertension an increased plasma activity of intestinal phosphatase, an additional isoenzyme of AP, can be found.

Gamma-Glutamyl Transferase

Gamma-glutamyl transferase (GTT) is also a membrane-bound cellular enzyme. It is not actively released into the plasma and its half-life is 4 days. An increase in GGT in the liver can be seen in a multitude of diseases. Synthesis of this enzyme is induced by obstructive cholestasis, alcohol, various drugs, and active and chronic inflammation of viral and toxic origin. Only slight damage to the membrane may be sufficient to result in a release of GGT, which is probably bound to the exterior of the membrane. Therefore GGT is one of the most sensitive markers of hepatobiliary disease. The type and degree of changes in GGT enzyme activity are distinct from those of alkaline phosphatase, although the two correlate well in biliary tract disease.

Lipoprotein-X

Lipoprotein-X (LPX) is a specific indicator for cholestasis but is not indicative of the underlying cause. LPX is a lipoprotein of the class of low-density lipoproteins (LDL). It consists of equal amounts of unesterified cholesterol and lecithin and appears in the plasma following regurgitation from the obstructed biliary tract.

Impairment of Synthesizing Capacity

Proteins

The liver regulates the concentrations and patterns of plasma proteins and amino acids, and their plasma concentrations vary within narrow limits in hepatic venous blood. This regulation can be impaired by disturbances of oxidative deamination, transamination, the urea cycle, and protein synthesis. The analysis of methionine concentration is a sensitive variable for recognition of changes in amino acid pattern. Ammonia concentration is a less sensitive marker, as its concentration is affected by hepatic breakdown, the degree of protein metabolism in other organs, the failure to excrete it in patients with alkalosis and hypokalemia, and varying intestinal absorption. The measurement of urea excretion in a 24-hour urine sample is not now used as a liver function test, but it may be used to estimate protein breakdown as a guide for nutritional replacement.

Albumin is made in the liver and released into the plasma. Its synthesis is regulated through negative feedback mechanisms. During shortage of amino acids, albumin synthesis is reduced to a lesser extent than the synthesis of other proteins. Additional compensatory mechanisms that maintain the plasma concentration include a reduction of albumin metabolism and mobilization of albumin from extravascular to intravascular space. In addition, the plasma concentrations are influenced by the volume of distribution, which changes in severe liver disease and after surgery. A net dislocation of intravascular water into the tissues occurs, compromising both cerebral and pulmonary function.[2] The contracted plasma volume stimulates the renin–aldosterone system with renal retention of sodium and water.

Albumin concentrations decrease during acute illness largely as a result of protein catabolism. This is a more important cause of reduced albumin than impaired hepatic synthesis in this situation.[3] Albumin is decreased in moderately severe and severe hepatocellular disease and is associated with a poor prognosis. Alpha and beta globulins are also increased in both cirrhosis and biliary obstruction.

The synthesis and release of cholinesterase (CHE) is decreased in patients with severe liver damage, and this is responsible for the reduced fraction in the serum. This reduction has been used as a prognostic indicator. The assay of cholinesterase activity has been used as an indicator of decreased protein synthesis and secretion in the liver, especially after liver transplantation. However, an increase in synthesis may occur in alcoholic fatty liver, primary or secondary hyperlipemia, and occasionally in patients with a protein-losing enteropathy. The activity of CHE may be a sensitive and valuable indicator of the severity of liver disease in some circumstances.

A variety of specialized plasma proteins may also have reduced plasma concentrations in patients with severe hepatocellular dysfunction, including transferrin, ceruloplasmin, thyroid-binding globulin, alpha-2 antitrypsin, and pseudocholinesterase. Acute phase reactants, including haptoglobulin, alpha-1 antitrypsin, C-reactive protein, C3, and fibrinogen, may be increased with acute hepatocellular injury. Acute phase reactants are also increased following surgical trauma when the liver is stimulated to switch from synthesis of albumin to production of acute phase proteins. Their use has been investigated to monitor the synthetic function of the liver after transplantation, where their value was found to be limited.[4]

The coagulation factors, which are all made by the liver except factors VIII, are better indicators of decreased protein synthesis than CHE because of their short-plasma half-lives. However, the coagulation system, with its many feedback mechanisms, can minimize any decrease in coagulation factor activity, and loss of one-third of functional hepatic mass is required before any abnormality is seen. Coagulation may therefore be completely normal despite severe liver cirrhosis. With these limitations a prolonged prothrombin time (deficiency of factors II, VII, and X) or partial thromboplastin time (deficiency of factors II, IX, and X) shows a reduced synthetic capacity of the liver. Coagulopathy is a relatively late sign of slowly evolving hepatic dysfunction but is useful in following the course of acute hepatic failure.[5] With a half-life of less than 4 hours, factor VII is a sensitive indicator of reduced hepatic synthetic capacity because its concentration declines earlier, more rapidly, and more regularly than any of the other coagulation enzymes.

The activity of factor VIII is normally increased in liver disease, regardless of severity and duration. This is also true of factor-VIII–related antigen, which is synthesized in the vascular endothelium. A discrepancy in the activity of factor-VIII–related antigen and factor VIII as seen in patients with liver cirrhosis may be due to intravascular coagulation. A reduction of factor XIII has been described in patients with acute hepatitis and acute liver failure. Decreased, normal, or even increased activity of this factor can be seen with chronic liver disease.

The synthesis of fibrinogen is rarely influenced by liver disease. The concentration of this protein may be increased in cirrhosis. Decreased fibrinogen activity is found only in patients with severe liver damage.

Carbohydrates

The large reserve of hepatic glycogen ensures glucose homeostasis even with only 20% liver tissue remaining. This equilibrium may be disrupted in severe liver disease. An absolute increase of the serum glucose after a bolus of glucagon is a good predictor of the quantity of glycogen reserves in the liver. This reserve is decreased in patients with advanced liver disease. Hypoglycemia is rare and is seen only with severe liver damage and primary liver carcinoma. However, glucose tolerance is often reduced in patients with liver disease. Impaired glucose tolerance can be a reversible feature of acute hepatitis or cirrhosis. Lactate and pyruvate are often increased in patients with liver disease. This is caused by a reduced hepatic clearance and increased synthesis.

Fats

Although liver function is essential for fat metabolism, specific changes resulting from liver disease are not of specific diagnostic importance.

Connective Tissue Formation

During the change to the chronic phase of an illness, there is an increase in the synthesis of substances that form fibrous tissue, such as collagens and proteoglycans. Collagen, a structural protein, is the most frequently found protein in the human. However, normal human liver contains only small amounts of collagen (approximately 7–9 mg/g wet weight). It contains collagen types I, II, and IV in almost equivalent amounts. During fibrosis there is an increase mostly in types I and III. The concentration of proteoglycans and glycosaminoglycans also increase.

While normal concentrations of enzymes are found in acute and chronically persistent hepatitis, a significant increase in enzyme activity of monoamine oxidase and collagen-peptidase can be shown in 60% of patients with chronic progressive hepatitis and 80% of patients with liver cirrhosis. Among the various metabolites of collagen metabolism the concentration of the *N*-terminal propeptide of procollagen III shows the best correlation to fibrosis activity. Determination of N-acetyl-β-D-glucosaminidase activity allows the best evaluation of fibrosis formation from glycosaminoglycan and proteoglycan metabolism.[6]

Reticuloendothelial System Function

Kupffer cells have a key position in the reticuloendothelial system because of both their cell mass and strategic position between portal blood and systemic circulation. Their specific task is the elimination of bacteria, viruses, tumor cells, fatty acids, and toxic and antigenic material by means of phagocytosis and pinocytosis, followed by degradation, transformation, and excretion. They are involved in the regulation of microcirculation and can prolong the survival of isolated hepatic cells.

The functional capacity of Kupffer cells depends on hepatic blood flow. The phagocytic capacity of the reticuloendothelial system can be impeded by saturation with colloids; administration of cyclophosphamide, halothane, morphine, and pentobarbital; and after higher doses of corticosteroids and alcohol. Small doses of corticosteroids and alcohol, however, stimulate the Kupffer cells. Phagocytic capacity is decreased by endotoxins. Stimulation of phagocytosis occurs in bacterial infections but is reduced in viral infections.

The rate of elimination of different radioactively labeled colloids is used to determine the immediate phagocytic capacity. Approximately 90% of colloids are eliminated by Kupffer cells, the remainder by phagocytes situated in the spleen.

Normal phagocytic function is often seen in patients with hepatitis A and chronic hepatitis. The same is true for patients with primary biliary cirrhosis, although in these patients hepatic blood flow is reduced. The ability of the liver to clear toxins in toxic alcoholic disease is decreased, even before severe morphologic changes occur. This is possibly because of the direct effect of alcohol on the Kupffer cell. In alcoholic cirrhosis there is a negative correlation of phagocytic activity with the markers of parenchymal cell damage, while a positive correlation exists with the extent of portal hypertension. In patients with extrahepatic obstructive jaundice, the clearance of toxins is also reduced.

Quantitative Tests of Liver Function

A large number of tests have been developed that quantitatively evaluate the capacity of hepatic function by testing a single metabolic pathway or function within the liver. It was hoped that these tests would give information about the degree of impairment and progress of liver function. The disadvantage of such an approach is that because only one aspect of liver function is measured there is an inconsistent relationship between the degree of impairment and subsequent progress. Studies evaluating various quantitative tests in patients with cirrhosis using regression analysis have recently been carried out. Merkel and colleagues[7] found that, although all the quantitative tests studied were prognostic indicators, only galactose elimination capacity added any further prognostic information to that obtained from the Child-Pugh classification.[8,9] Albers and coworkers[10] found that no new diagnostic information was found using quantitative tests.

The Child-Pugh classification uses a series of measurements that are graded from one to three according to severity (see Table 2-2). It was first proposed to assess risk before surgery for portal hypertension. It has subsequently been shown to be a good prognostic indicator in cirrhosis.[11–13] The indicators used in the Child-Pugh classification are part of the clinical picture of decompensation, and

their high prognostic value can be attributed to their indication that the specific complications of advanced disease are already occurring.

In contrast, quantitative liver function tests reflect functioning liver cell mass and parenchymal blood flow. It is not known, however, at what critical level decompensation occurs and recent studies[14] have failed to show a close correlation between galactose elimination capacity (GEC), indocyanine green (ICG) elimination, and complications of cirrhosis.

Quantitative tests of liver function have some use in a variety of other situations, for example predicting survival after partial hepatic resection (ICG) and detection of metastases (carcinoembryonic antigen).[15] Recent work using lignocaine metabolite formation has shown promise in the assessment of liver function in children awaiting transplantation,[16] and in predicting organ survival after transplantation.[17]

The following quantitative liver function tests remain under evaluation and have been the subject of recent publications.

Bromsulphthalein and Indocyanine Green Clearance

Two substances, bromsulphthalein (BSP) and indocyanine green (ICG), may be injected intravenously and their elimination measured. As their uptake and excretion are rapid, liver blood flow is an important rate-limiting factor. During a single liver passage 15–50% of the BSP is eliminated. After absorption into the hepatic parenchymal cell by active transport mechanisms, it is conjugated with glutathione and to a smaller extent with cysteine. ICG has fewer adverse effects than BSP. In the liver ICG is excreted in the bile without conjugation or transformation. There is practically no enterohepatic circulation or urinary excretion of this substance. ICG has been shown to be a good predictor of survival after hepatic resection in cirrhotic patients.[18]

In view of the high hepatic extraction ratio of ICG, clearance is blood flow dependent and is used as a measure of this. The use of higher doses of ICG saturates the enzymes involved and results in zero-order kinetics, in which elimination is independent of blood flow. This is commonly used as a test of functional hepatic mass.[19] This distinction is important in the critically ill patient where hepatic blood flow is commonly reduced.

Galactose Elimination Capacity

Galactose is mainly metabolized in the liver and a small percentage is excreted in the urine. In healthy humans the liver will metabolize approximately 2.5 mmol/min of this substance. After oral or intravenous administration of galactose, its blood and urine concentrations can be measured (galactose tolerance test). This has been developed into a test that uses expired air. [14]C and ^{13}C galactose are given and the [14/13]CO_2 ratio in expired air is measured. In patients with cirrhosis it has been shown to add prognostic information to that already obtained from the Child-Pugh classification.[7] It has also been used as a prognostic indicator in patients with fulminant hepatic failure.[20]

Antipyrine/Aminopyrine Clearance

The capacity of the mixed-function oxygenase system, the main biotransformation system of the liver, can be estimated by the assessment of the metabolism rate of the two drugs aminopyrine and antipyrine. The hepatic extraction of aminopyrine and antipyrine is low and only a small percentage is bound to plasma proteins. Therefore their clearance rates are not influenced by liver perfusion, but represent the metabolic capacity of the liver. Aminopyrine clearance can also be measured in expired air. Patients with cirrhosis show approximately a 50% reduction in clearance.[21–24]

Caffeine Clearance

When caffeine is given orally, plasma concentrations can be monitored noninvasively using saliva samples. Its clearance has been shown to be reduced in all subjects with liver disease and particularly in those with alcoholic liver disease where its sensitivity was found to be 100%.[25]

Bile Acids

The uptake of bile acids by the normal hepatocyte is highly efficient, and the determination of serum concentrations of bile acids has been proposed as a test of early changes of liver function not associated with cytotoxicity. They have been of use in detecting subclinical hepatic damage in subjects with occupational exposure to toxins.[26] Serum bile acid measurements are also reliable indicators of enterohepatic circulation.

Lignocaine Metabolism

The local anesthetic lignocaine is de-ethylated in the liver by cytochromes P_{450} to form monoethylglycinexylidide (MEGX). The plasma concentration of this metabolite has been found to be inversely proportional to the severity of liver disease in children measured using a standard clinical scoring system,[16] and may therefore be used as a quantitative assessment of liver function in children awaiting transplantation.[27] Of particular interest is the finding that the MEGX test carried out in donors before hepatectomy predicts 120-day posttransplant graft survival. Standard liver function tests, ICG clearance, and GEC were all inefficient in this regard.[17]

Hexobarbital clearance,[28] tryptophan tolerance,[29] 15N-ammonia clearance,[30] and a redox tolerance test[31] are also being evaluated as quantitative tests of hepatic function.

Hepatic Function in the Critically Ill Patient

There are several ways in which hepatic transformation of lipophilic substances into polar, readily excreted, metabolites may be disrupted in critically ill patients. The liver is supplied with 20% of the cardiac output. This is usually reduced in the critically ill patient either because of a reduction in cardiac output (cardiogenic or hypovolemic shock) or because of diversion of blood away from the liver (septic shock). The use of vasoactive drugs, for example vasopressin,[32–34] may reduce hepatic blood flow. Reduced hepatic blood flow reduces oxygen supply. Ischemic hepatitis is well recognized in the critically ill patient.[35] "ICU jaundice" is also common in the critically ill patient in association with intra-abdominal sepsis, trauma, and major surgery.[36] It is characterized by intrahepatic cholestasis and an inability of the hepatocyte to excrete bilirubin into bile canaliculi. Biliary sludge has been shown by ultrasonography to be present in 47% of patients who have been in intensive care for longer than two days.[37] The anatomical position of the liver ensures that early in the development of multiple organ failure, hepatic macrophages are in contact with endotoxin released into the portal system secondary to increases in gut permeability. Albumin decreases and acute phase proteins increase in severe illness.[38] This affects the presentation of protein-bound substances and drugs to the liver.

Phase I (oxidation and hydroxylation) and phase II (glucuronidation, sulphation, and acylation) enzymes may be interfered with during hepatic dysfunction. Phase I reactions involve the cytochromes P450, which are present in small amounts and are therefore affected more by disease processes than phase II reactions. For example, the metabolism of lignocaine forms the basis of a recent test of hepatic function (see above), but involves mostly cytochrome P450 3A4. Thirty other P450 cytochromes have so far been described in man and many more may exist.

The levels of hepatic metabolizing enzymes may also be affected by a series of factors present in critical illness that are not related primarily to hepatic function. Interleukin 1 may reduce levels of cytochrome P450[39,40] as may interferon.[41-44] Serum from critically ill patients has been shown to reduce the conjugation of ^{14}C-progesterone in isolated human hepatocytes.[45] It has been shown in animals[46] that stress results in both reduced liver blood flow (indocyanine green) and drug elimination (antipyrine clearance).

The liver derives its oxygen supply from both hepatic arterial and portal venous blood. Hence, there are wide variations in the oxygen partial pressure to which hepatocytes are exposed. The distribution of different types of metabolizing enzymes is determined by these variations, and changes in oxygen gradients affect the capacity of different enzymes differently.[49] Exposure of isolated hepatocytes to hypoxia for four days has been shown to produce a five- to tenfold decrease in cytochrome P450 3A but not in cytochrome P450 2E1.[45] The resistance of cytochrome P450 2E1 to hypoxia is explained by its concentration in the pericentral region of the hepatic lobule, which is the most hypoxic area.[50] Studies of drug metabolism using an isolated perfused liver model have confirmed that an acute reduction in oxygen supply results in inhibition of hepatic drug elimination.[51] This effect has been shown to be exacerbated by many drugs used in the critically ill.[52]

Drug interactions are common in the critically ill patient. The activity of hepatic metabolizing enzymes may be induced by many drugs, for example phenobarbitone. Substrate competition for enzymes may also occur, particularly with phase I enzymes. Erythromycin, nifedipine, cortisol, cyclosporin, and midazolam are all metabolized by cytochrome P450 3A, and some are also inducers or inhibitors of this enzyme.

In conclusion, the most useful tests for inclusion in an all-purpose liver function test profile are ALT, AP, total bilirubin, and albumin (possibly also GGT). These all complement each other functionally and are based on robust, easily automated methods. Quantitative liver function tests must be shown to give significantly better information to the routine profile before their use can be justified. It is likely, in view of their specificity, that they will be restricted to specific situations where their benefits are of value, for example, MEGX testing in liver transplantation.

References

1. Hadjis, N.S., Blenkharn, J.I., Hatzis, G., Adam, A., Beacham, J. and Blumgart, L.H. (1990) Patterns of serum alkaline phosphatase activity in unilateral hepatic duct obstruction: A clinical and experimental study. *Surgery* 107:193–200.
2. Elwyn, D.H, Bryan-Brown, C.W. and Shomaker, W.C. (1975) Nutritional aspects of body water dislocations in postoperative and depleted patients. *Annals of Surgery* 182:76–85.
3. Starker, P.M., Gump, F.E. and Askanazi, J. (1982) Serum albumin levels as an index of nutritional support. *Surgery* 91:194–99.
4. Burns, A.M., Shelly, M.P., Walker, S. and Park, G.R. (1990) Serum acute phase proteins after orthotopic liver transplantation. *British Journal of Anaesthesia* 65:418–20.
5. Strunin, L. (1978) Preoperative assessment of the patient with liver dysfunction. *British Journal of Anaesthesia* 50:25–31.
6. Severini, G., Aliberti, L.M., Capurso, L. and Tarquini, M. (1990) Clinical evaluation of serum N-acetyl-beta-D-glucosaminidase as a liver function test. *Biochemical Medicine and Metabolic Biology* 44:247–51.
7. Merkel, C., Gatta, A., Zoli, M. et al. (1991) Prognostic value of galactose elimination capacity, aminopyrine breath test, and ICG clearance in patients with cirrhosis. Comparison with the Pugh Score. *Digestive Diseases and Sciences* 36:1197–203.
8. Child, C.G. and Turcotte, J.G. (1964) Surgery and portal hypertension. In *The Liver and Portal Hypertension*, Child, C.G. ed. W.B. Saunders Co., Philadelphia.

9. Pugh, R.N.H., Murray-Lyon, I.M., Dawson, J.L., Pietroni, M.C. and Williams, R. (1973) Transection of the oesophagus for bleeding oesophageal varices. *British Journal of Surgery* 60:646–49.

10. Albers, I., Hartmann, H., Bircher, J. and Creutzfeldt, W. (1989) Superiority of the Child-Pugh classification to quantitative liver function tests for assessing prognosis of liver cirrhosis. *Scandinavian Journal of Gastroenterology* 24:269–76.

11. Sauerbruch, T., Weinzierl, M., Kopcke, W. and Paumgartner, G. (1985) Long term sclerotherapy of bleeding oesophageal varices in patients with liver cirrhosis. *Scandinavian Journal of Gastroenterology* 20:51–58.

12. Infante-Rivard, C., Esnaola, S. and Villeneuve, J.P. (1987) Clinical and statistical validity of conventional prognostic factors in predicting short term survival among cirrhotics. *Hepatology* 7:660–64.

13. Pascal, J.P., Cales, P. and a multicenter study group. (1987) Propranolol in the prevention of first upper gastrointestinal tract hemorrhage in patients with cirrhosis of the liver and esophageal varices. *New England Journal of Medicine* 317:856–61.

14. Albers, I., Hartmann, H. and Creutzfeldt, W. (1988) Vergleich quantitativer Leberfunktionsprufungen Zu Klinischen, laborchemischen und bioptischen Befunden bei Patienten mit Lebererkrankungen. *Zeitschrift Für Gastroenterologie* 26:130–36.

15. Rocklin, M.S., Senagore. A.J. and Talbott, T.M. (1991) Role of carcinoembryonic antigen and liver function tests in the detection of recurrent colorectal carcinoma. *Diseases of the Colon and Rectum* 34:794–97.

16. Gremse, D.A., A-Kader, H.H., Schroeder, T.J. and Balistreri, W.F. (1990) Assessment of lidocaine metabolite formation as a quantitative liver function test in children. *Hepatology* 12:565–69.

17. Oellerich, M., Burdelski, M., Ringe, B. et al. (1989) Lignocaine metabolite formation as a measure of pretransplant liver function. *Lancet* i:640–42.

18. Hemming, A.W., Scudamore, C.H., Shackleton, C.R., Pudek, M. and Erb, S.R. (1992) Indocyanine green clearance as a predictor of successful hepatic resection in cirrhotic patients. *American Journal of Surgery* 163:515–18.

19. Gottlieb, M., Stratton, H., Newell, J. and Shah, D. (1984) Indocyanine green. Its use as an early indicator of hepatic dysfunction following injury in man. *Archives of Surgery* 119:264–8.

20. Ranek, L., Andreasen, P.B. and Tygstrup, N. (1976) Galactose elimination capacity as a prognostic index in patients with fulminant liver failure. *Gut* 17:959–63.

21. Saunders, J.B., Wright, N. and Lewis, K.O. (1980) Predicting outcome of paracetamol poisoning by using [14] C-aminopyrine breath test. *British Medical Journal* 280:279–80.

22. Schneider, J.F., Baker, A.L., Haines, N.W., Hatfield, G. and Boyer, J.L. (1980) Aminopyrine N-demethylation. A prognostic test of liver function in patients with alcoholic liver disease. *Gastroenterology* 79:1145–50.

23. Villeneuve, J.P., Infante-Rivard, C., Ampelas, M., Pomier-Layrargues, G., Huet, P.M. and Marleau, D. (1986) Prognostic value of the aminopyrine breath test in cirrhotic patients. *Hepatology* 6:928–31.

24. St. Peter, J. V. and Awni, W. M. (1991) Quantifying hepatic function in the presence of liver disease with phenazone (antipyrine) and its metabolites. *Clinical Pharmacokinetics* 20:50–65.

25. McDonagh, J.E., Nathan, V.V., Bonavia, I.C., Moyle, G.R. and Tanner, A.R. (1991) Caffeine clearance by enzyme multiplied immunoassay technique: A simple, inexpensive, and useful indicator of liver function. *Gut* 32:681–84.

26. Franco, G. (1991) New perspectives in biomonitoring liver function by means of serum bile acids: Experimental and hypothetical biochemical basis. *British Journal of Industrial Medicine* 48:557–61.

27. Balistreri, W.F., A-Kader, H.H., Setchell, R.D., Gremse, D., Ryckman, F.C. and Schroeder, T.J. (1992) New methods for assessing liver function in infants and children. *Annals of Clinical and Laboratory Science* 22:162–74.

28. Zilly, W. and Richter, E. (1992) Drug clearance as a decision aid for further invasive liver diagnosis-studies with hexobarbital as a model substrate [German]. *Zeitschrift Für Gastroenterologie* 30:325–28.

29. Zhu, S.S., Hu, F., Li, D.G. et al. (1990) Intravenous tryptophan tolerance test for liver function. *Chinese Medical Journal-Peking* 103:146–51.

30. Jung, K., Faust, H. and Matkowitz, R. (1989) [15N] ammonium test for liver function diagnosis. *Zeitschrift Für Medizinische Laboratoriumsdiagnostik* 30:169–74.

31. Mori, K., Ozawa, K., Yamamoto, Y. et al. (1990) Response of hepatic mitochondrial redox state to oral glucose load. Redox tolerance test as a new predictor of surgical risk in hepatectomy. *Annals of Surgery* 211:438–46.

32. Edmunds, R. and West, JP. (1962) A study of the effect of vasopressin on portal and systemic blood pressure. *Surgery Gynecology and Obstetrics* 114:459–62.

33. Hanson, K.M. (1970) Vascular response of intestine and liver to intravenous infusion of vasopressin. *American Journal of Physiology* 219:779–84.

34. Silva, Y.J., Moffat, R.C. and Walt, A.J. (1969) Vasopressin effect on portal and systemic hemodynamics. *Journal of the American Medical Association* 210:1065–8.

35. Gibson, P.R. and Dudley, F.J. (1984) Ischemic hepatitis: Clinical features, diagnosis and prognosis. *Australian and New Zealand Journal of Medicine* 14:822–5.

36. Te Boeckhorst, T., Urlus, M., Doesburg, W., Yap, S. and Goris, R. (1984) Etiologic factors of jaundice in severely ill patients. *Journal of Hepatology* 7:111–7.

37. Murray, P.E., Stinchcombe, S.J., and Hawkey, C.J. (1993) Development of biliary sludge in patients on intensive care unit: Results of a prospective ultrasonographic study. *Gut* 33:1123–5.

38. Burns, A.M., Shelly, M.P., Walker, S., and Park, G.R. (1990) Serum acute phase proteins after orthotopic

liver transplantation. *British Journal of Anaesthesia* 65:418–20.

39. Sujita, K., Okuno, F., Hirano, Y., Inamoto, Y., Eto, S. and Arai, M. (1990) Effect of interleukin 1 (IL-1) on the levels of cytochrome P450 involving IL-1 receptor on the isolated hepatocytes of rat. *Biochemical and Biophysical Research Communications* 168:1217–22.

40. Shedlofsky, S.I., Swim, A.T., Robinson, J.M., Gallicchio, V.S., Cohen, D.A. and McClain, C.J. (1987) Interleukin-1 (IL1) depresses cytochrome P450 levels and activity in mice. *Life Sciences* 40:2331–6.

41. Bailey, P.L., Pace, N.L., Ashburn, M.A., Moll, J.W.B., East, K.A. and Stanley, T.H. (1990) Frequent hypoxemia and apnoea after sedation with midazolam and fentanyl. *Anesthesiology* 73:826–30.

42. Moochhala, S.M. and Renton, K.W. (1989) Effects of the interferon inducing agent, PolyrI.rC on the synthesis of hepatic cytochrome P450. *Asia and Pacific Journal of Pharmacology* 4:83–8.

43. El Azhary, R., Renton, K.W. and Mannering, G.J. (1980) Effect of interferon inducing agents (polyriboinosinic acid, polyribocytidylic acid and tilorone) on the heme turnover of hepatic cytochrome P450. *Molecular Pharmacology* 17:395–9.

44. Morgan, E.T. and Norman, C.A. (1990) Pretranslational suppression of cytochrome P-450h (IIC11) gene expression in rat liver after administration of interferon inducers. *Drug Metabolism and Disposition* 18:649–53.

45. Park, G.R., Pichard, L., Tinel, M., et al. (1994) What changes drug metabolism in critically ill patients? Two preliminary studies in isolated hepatocytes. *Anaesthesia* 49:188–91.

48. Pollack, G.M., Browne, J.L., Marton, J. and Haberer, L.J. (1991) Chronic stress impairs oxidative metabolism and hepatic excretion of model xenobiotic substrates in the rat. *Drug Metabolism and Disposition* 19:130–4.

49. Jones, D.P. and Mason, H.S. (1978) Gradients of O_2 concentration in hepatocytes. *Journal of Biological Chemistry* 253:4874–80.

50. Tsutsumi, M., Lasker, J.M., Shimizu, M., Rosman, A.S. and Lieber, C.S. (1989) The intralobular distribution of ethanol-inducible P450 IIEI in rat and human liver. *Hepatology* 10:437–46.

51. Wu, Y.R., Kauffman, F.C., Qu, W., Ganey, P.E. and Thurman, R.G. (1990) Unique role of oxygen in regulation of hepatic monooxygenation and glucuronidation. *Molecular Pharmacology* 38:128–33.

52. Becker, G.L. (1988) Effects of nonvolatile agents on oxygen demand and energy status in isolated hepatocytes. *Anesthesia and Analgesia* 67:923–8.

TWO

Pharmacology

Chapter 4
Volatile Anesthetics and the Liver

Steven R. Rettke

Introduction

The pharmacology of volatile anesthetic agents in patients with liver disease is difficult to evaluate because of the paucity of information in the medical literature. Data obtained from animal studies may not be transferable to humans because of qualitative and quantitative differences in anesthetic metabolism or the sensitivity of the liver to the products of metabolism.[1] Difference in species may result in different findings: livers of rats obtained from Zivic-Miller were injured; specific pathogen-free rats from Charles River were not injured or were less injured by enflurane, thiopental, or fentanyl. Furthermore, minor changes in experimental conditions can substantially affect results.[2]

Human studies are mostly anecdotal or retrospective in nature and they are complicated by several issues. First, the degree of hepatic dysfunction may vary widely among patients even with similar liver disease, and statistical analysis is difficult unless large and often unobtainable group sizes are used. Second, clinical and laboratory criteria to evaluate the severity of liver dysfunction are relatively inaccurate and assessing small to moderate changes in liver function is difficult. Third, patients frequently have complications of coexisting disease such as shock, pulmonary edema, renal failure, hypoxia, or sepsis. Fourth, patients with chronic liver disease often receive drugs, raising the possibility of confounding drug-to-drug interactions. Finally, separating the effects of anesthesia on postoperative liver function from those of surgery is extremely difficult.[3] For example, the incidence of postoperative liver failure that occurs after patients receive halothane (one per 10,000 administration) is considerably lower than that of unexpected liver disease found in routine laboratory testing of patients scheduled for elective surgical procedures.[4]

But the topic, the pharmacology of volatile anesthetics in patients with liver disease, is pertinent because acute and chronic liver disease are among the most prevalent underlying disorders found in surgical patients,[5] and the incidence of chronic liver disease and the mortality rate from this condition have progressively increased over the past three decades in the United States.[6] A greater increase in the number of patients with hepatic dysfunction has been seen in Canada where cirrhosis is now one of the leading causes of death for men aged 25–64 years.[6] Viral hepatitis, by chance, can be incubating in about 1 of 4,000 patients, and residual damage by a previous infection may still be present.[7] The per capita ingestion of potentially cirrhogenic quantities of alcohol continues to escalate, and two-thirds of all chronic liver disease in the United States is alcohol induced.[8–10] In addition, industrial chemicals are widely discussed as hepatotoxins (Chapter 18).

Therefore, more cirrhotic patients are presenting for anesthesia and surgery and a greater number can be expected in the future.[11]

The question of the safety of these agents in this patient population is also pertinent, since patients with preexisting liver disease develop postoperative hepatic complications more commonly than do those with normal livers:[12,13] between 4% and 16% of all cirrhotic patients[14,15] and 9.5% of those with viral hepatitis[16] die from postoperative complications. However, modern anesthetic drugs and techniques have not been investigated adequately.[3] The estimation of operative risk in patients with liver disease is hampered by a lack of large prospective studies, and most data are derived from relatively small retrospective studies of cirrhotic and hepatitis patients undergoing abdominal surgery.[17]

In this chapter, the following are reviewed: effects of volatile anesthetics on systemic and hepatic arterial circulation; metabolism of anesthetics; effects of inhalation anesthetics on hepatic metabolism; interaction between inhalation anesthetics and other agents; and clinical relevance of inhalation anesthetics.

Effects of Inhalation Anesthetics and Hepatic Blood Flow and Oxygen Consumption

All anesthetic agents, including those administered by the spinal or epidural routes, reduce hepatic blood flow (HBF) and result in decreased oxygen uptake by the liver and splanchnic organs.[5,18] This is true with volatile anesthetics,[19] and altered systemic hemodynamics (perfusion pressure, cardiac output, systemic vascular resistance), neural/hormonal balance ("stress" hormones), and a direct effect on hepatic circulation are responsible for the changes (Table 4-1). In most instances, the decrements in HBF produced by anesthetics are in proportion to the reduction in systemic blood pressure. It appears that all inhalation anesthetics dilate the intestinal vasculature by direct or centrally mediated effects. In the isolated liver, perfusion of halothane, chloroform, and ether through the hepatic artery and the portal vein at constant rates does not change perfusion pressure significantly, thereby suggesting that vascular resistances within the liver are not affected by these inhalation agents.[20] However, in the intact animal, portal blood flow is frequently reduced. This reduction is apparently associated with a de-

Table 4-1. Factors Altering Hepatic Blood Flow in Surgical Patients

1. Extent of surgical trauma to splanchnic nerves
2. Position
3. P_aCO_2
4. pH
5. Blood volume deficits
6. Anesthesia technique and drugs
7. Positive-pressure ventilation
8. P_aO_2
9. Preexisting pathology (i.e., hepatitis, intra-abdominal tumors, cirrhosis)
10. Presence of vascular acting drugs (e.g., beta-adrenergic blockers; sympathomimetics; vasodilators)
11. Surgical packs, retractors

From Brown, B. R., Jr (1988a) Effects of anesthetics on hepatic blood flow. In: *Anesthesia in Hepatic and Biliary Tract Disease.* Philadelphia: F. A. Davis, pp. 49–60. By permission of F. A. Davis Company.

crease in cardiac output and partially with a reduction in intestinal oxygen requirement.

Generally, the decrease in HBF is relatively greater than the reduction in oxygen uptake. Therefore, anesthetics possibly produce splanchnic hypoxia, although the oxygen extraction by the liver is increased at low HBF.[21] The inequality of HBF and oxygen consumption varies with the anesthetic agent employed, and the oxygen supply to the liver depends to a large extent on the hepatic arterial blood flow,[19] so the ratio of hepatic arterial to portal blood flow becomes important (Table 4-2).

Nitrous oxide and thiopental anesthesia produces little decrease in hepatic blood flow when decrease in blood pressure is minimal.[22] Nitrous oxide with hypocarbia decreases HBF and a greater reduction in oxygen consumption has been reported.[23] During the surgical plane of cyclopropane anesthesia, HBF decreases 33%[24] secondary to an increase in regional vascular resistance. Excess lactate is produced by the splanchnic viscera during cyclopropane anesthesia, and this affect can be abolished by a beta-adrenergic blocking drug.[25] Therefore, excess lactate apparently resulted not from splanchnic ischemia but from metabolic action associated with increased visceral sympathetic nervous activity.

Halothane markedly reduces HBF in a dose-dependent fashion by reducing systemic arterial pressure[25] and myocardial depression: a slight increase in HBF is seen during 1 minimum alveolar concentration (MAC) of halothane anesthesia and a significant decrease during 2 MAC of halothane anesthesia in dogs. In a study of healthy volunteers,

Table 4-2. Changes (%) in Liver Circulation during Inhalation Anesthesia

Anesthetic	Dose (%)	Species	Baseline anesthetic	Method	MAP	CO	PBF	HABF	Reference
Halothane		Dog	Barb	el-m		−20		−32	Galindo 1965
Halothane	1.5	Dog	Barb	el-m	−40	−27	−40	−46	Thulin 1975
Halothane	1.5	Dog	Barb	el-m	−43		−40	−47	Andreen et al. 1975
Halothane	1	Dog	Barb	el-m	−42	−36	−50	−59	Andreen et al. 1977
Halothane	1	Dog	Barb	el-m	−38	−21	−30	−37	Hughes et al. 1980
Halothane	1.5	Dog	Barb	el-m	−50	−46	−45	−60	Hughes et al. 1980
Halothane	2	Dog	Barb	el-m	−72	−57	−55	−65	Hughes et al. 1980
Halothane	0.9	Dog	Barb	el-m	−42		−44	−59	Andreen 1982
Halothane	1	Dog	Barb	el-m	−10	−10	−10	−15	Thomson et al. 1983
Halothane	2	Dog		el-m	−20		−49	−37	Matsumoto et al. 1982
Halothane	0.5	Dog		el-m	0		−45	+49	Matsumoto et al. 1982
Halothane	0.6	Monkey	Local	m-Sph	−22	−20	−7	+24	Lees et al. 1971
Halothane	1.8	Monkey	Local	m-Sph	−65	−59	−31	−27	Less et al. 1971
Halothane	0.8	Monkey	None	m-Sph	−45	−25	−25	−15	Amory et al. 1971
Halothane	0.8	Rabbit	Hal	m-Sph	−25	−37	−37	−28	Wyler 1974
Halothane	1.5	Cat	Barb	Cineangiography			−57	+30	Gelman 1975
Halothane	0.8	Monkey	None	m-Sph	−45	−18	−25	−15	Amory et al. 1971
Halothane (30 min)	1.5	Dog	Barb	m-Sph	−25	−43	−21	−67	Ahlgren et al. 1978a
Halothane (120 min)	1.5	Dog	Barb	m-Sph	−27	−17	−37	−58	Ahlgren et al. 1978a
Halothane	0.6	Rat	None	m-Sph		−27	−8	−20	Ross and Daggy 1981
Halothane	1.2	Rat	None	m-Sph	−27	−36	−32	0	Seyde and Longnecker 1984b
Halothane	2.3	Pig	None	m-Sph	−47	−52	−60	+32	Tranquilli et al. 1982
Halothane	0.9	Dog	None	m-Sph	−9	−15	−30	+13	Gelman et al. 1984a
Halothane	1.8	Dog	None	m-Sph	−31	−44	−54	−46	Gelman et al. 1984a
Halothane	1.5	Sheep	Barb	[125I] iodo-hippurate	−11	−32	−28	−73	Runciman et al. 1984
Halothane + nitrous oxide	1.3	Pig	None	m-Sph	−23	−24	−45	+54	Tranquilli et al. 1982
Enflurane	2.2	Dog	Barb	el-m	−46	−35	−36	−35	Irestedt and Andreen 1979a
Enflurane	2	Dog	Barb	el-m	−58	−33	−35	−25	Hughes et al. 1980
Enflurane	2.2	Dog	Barb	el-m	−46		−36	−36	Andreen 1982
Enflurane	4	Pig	None	m-Sph	−43	−41	−50	+45	Tranquilli et al. 1982
Enflurane	2.2	Rat	None	m-Sph	−34	−17	−9	−43	Seyde and Longnecker 1984b
Isoflurane	1.5	Pig	None	m-Sph	−25	−19	−25	+82	Lundeen et al. 1983
Isoflurane	2.2	Pig	None	m-Sph	−41	−29	−25	+47	Lundeen et al. 1983
Isoflurane	1.4	Dog	None	m-Sph	−10	0	−26	+97	Gelman et al. 1984a
Isoflurane	2.8	Dog	None	m-Sph	−42	−35	−42	+81	Gelman et al. 1984a
Isoflurane	1.4	Rat	None	m-Sph	−22	+2	+2	+3	Seyde and Longnecker 1984b
Nitrous oxide	30	Dog	Barb	el-m	0	0	−11	−12	Thomson et al. 1982
Nitrous oxide	50	Dog	Barb	el-m	+8	−8	−9	−16	Thomson et al. 1982
Nitrous oxide	70	Dog	Barb	el-m	+9	−8	−15	−24	Thomson et al. 1982
Nitrous oxide	50	Pig	None	m-Sph	0	0	−25	+43	Lundeen et al. 1983
Nitrous oxide	70	Rat	Hal, 1.5%	m-Sph	+1	−14	−21	−4	Seyde et al. 1986

Note: MAP, mean arterial pressure; CO, cardiac output; PBF and HABF, portal blood flow and hepatic arterial blood flow, respectively; − and +, decrease and increase, respectively; Hal, halothane; Barb, barbiturates; el-m, electromagnetic flowmeters; m-Sph, microspheres. From Gelman, S. (1987) General anesthesia and hepatic circulation. *Canadian Journal of Physiology and Pharmacology* 65:1762–1779. By permission of the National Research Council of Canada.

the use of 1.5% halothane diminishes splanchnic blood flow, but the lactate-to-pyruvate ratio does not change, indicating no anoxic metabolism in this patient population.[25] Therefore, oxygen debt does not appear to occur in the splanchnic viscera during halothane anesthesia. Methoxyflurane decreases HBF by a reduction in mean arterial pressure and perhaps by a direct effect on the hepatic arterial tone.

Enflurane and isoflurane decrease HBF in a dose-dependent manner by a combination of peripheral vasodilation and myocardial depression.[18,26] Enflurane, in intact animals, reduces portal blood flow,[27] apparently by a decrease in cardiac output resulting from a decrease in oxygen requirement in the preportal area. Isoflurane anesthesia increases HBF substantially at 1 MAC and 2 MAC levels of anesthesia in a dog model. In another animal study, relatively severe arterial hypotension produced by isoflurane and piritramid anesthesia was associated with a constant hepatic arterial inflow, a decrease in portal blood flow, and an increase in hepatic oxygen extraction.[28] These effects were more pronounced at higher isoflurane concentrations. In other studies, the total HBF was unchanged[29] or even slightly increased[30] during isoflurane anesthesia. Therefore, isoflurane appears to facilitate oxygen supply to the liver better than halothane because isoflurane dilates the hepatic arterial vascular bed and/or better preserves the hepatic autoregulatory ability to increase hepatic arterial blood flow in response to decreased portal blood flow.[31] This may be a possible explanation why halothane is more destructive to the liver than isoflurane in anesthesia-induced hepatotoxicity rat models.[32,33]

However, other important factors affect HBF adversely. Preexisting liver disease reduces HBF on a mechanical basis[34] and surgery itself decreases HBF. There is evidence that hypocapnia significantly decreases HBF, and that hypercapnia has the opposite effect.[22] Portal, pulmonary, and intrapulmonary shunting are presumed to contribute to these changes.[35] Positive pressure ventilation, hypotension, hemorrhage, systemic hypoxemia, and vasoactive drugs also reduce blood flow. In addition, traction on abdominal viscera during surgery reduces HBF by producing reflex-mediated dilatation of splanchnic capacitance vessels and systemic hypotension.

Metabolism of Volatile Anesthetics

Drug metabolism occurs in many organs and tissues such as the kidneys, lungs, and intestinal wall. How-

ever, the liver plays a central role in drug metabolism by containing the highest concentration of drug metabolizing enzymes.[36,37] In general, the liver converts drugs and other compounds into products that are more easily excreted and that usually have a lower pharmacologic activity and toxicity than the parent compound,[37] although metabolites may have a higher activity and/or greater toxicity than the original drug. Similarly, lipid soluble inhalation anesthetic agents are transformed to water-soluble (polar) compounds in the liver to excrete in the bile.[17,18] Hepatic metabolism of inhalation agents hinges on the oxidation reactions that are catalyzed by a group of mixed oxidases, the cytochromes P450, contained within the endoplasmic reticulum.[36,37] The general scheme of this enzyme system is shown in Figure 4-1. The relative amounts of biotransformation of the several halogenated drugs are listed in Table 4-3.

Halothane (CF_3CC BrH) receives most attention for its biotransformation since man is one of the species most capable of converting halothane to its potentially hepatotoxic metabolites (Figure 4-2).[36] Halothane undergoes oxidative and reductive metabolism. Oxidative metabolites, bromide and trifluoroacetic acid, are not hepatotoxic. This metabolic pathway is enhanced by enzyme inducers such as phenobarbital. During reductive metabolism of halothane, however, reactive intermediate compounds probably form and they bind to liver protein and phospholipids to alter the cellular constituents. This reductive pathway is enhanced by low oxygen tension in the liver and by certain drugs such as polychlorobiphenyl. It may also be enhanced in certain genetically susceptible individuals, and they may develop hepatitis after exposure to halothane.

Fifty percent of the inhaled dose of methoxyflurane (CH_3-O-CF_2H) undergoes metabolism. Its biotransformation is more complex than that of

Table 4-3. Approximate Amount of Biotransformation of Halogenated Inhalation Anesthetics in Humans

Anesthetics	Biotransformation (%)
Halothane	46
Methoxyflurane	75
Enflurane	8.5
Isoflurane	<1%

From Brown, B. R., Jr (1988c) Hepatotoxicity of inhalation anesthetics. In: *Anesthesia in Hepatic and Biliary Tract Disease*. Philadelphia: F. A. Davis, pp. 93–111. By permission of F. A. Davis Company.

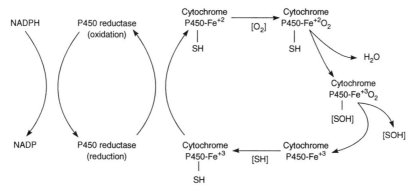

Figure 4-1. Scheme of events that are believed to occur in oxidation of drugs. Adapted from Van Dyke, R. A. (1973) Biotransformation of volatile anaesthetics with special emphasis on the role of metabolism in the toxicity of anaesthetics. *Canadian Anaesthesia Society Journal* 20:21–33.

halothane, because the molecule can be metabolized by different enzyme systems at either the dichloromethyl group or at the ether linkage.[38] Metabolites of methoxyflurane found in human urine are inorganic fluoride, dichloroacetic acid, methoxydifluoroacetic acid, and oxalic acid. Based on these products, the route of breakdown of methoxyflurane is as follows:[36]

$$CH_3\text{-}O\text{-}CF_2\text{-}CCl_2H \quad CH_3\text{-}O\text{-}CF_2\text{-}COOH + 2Cl^-$$
$$[O]$$
$$HCHO + 2F^- + HCCl_2\text{-}COOH$$
$$HCHO + 2F^- + HOOC\text{-}COOH$$
$$[O]$$
$$2Cl^- + HOOC\text{-}COOH$$

An elevated inorganic fluoride level above 50 μmol/L has been shown to be associated with renal damage,[18] and metabolites of methoxyflurane have been associated with hepatotoxicity.[39]

Biotransformation pathway of enflurane ($CHF_2OCF_2CHC F$) is shown in Figure 4-3. Its metabolism is much slower than that of halothane and a small amount of inorganic fluoride is found in the urine. Enflurane is only a weak enzyme inducer in rats.[40]

Isoflurane ($CHF_2OCHC CF_3$) is the least metabolized volatile anesthetic agent. Although the exact metabolic pathway for isoflurane has not been discovered, inorganic fluoride and trifluoroacetic acid are the main metabolic products. Stevens and colleagues did not detect increases in serum fluoride level in volunteers anesthetized with isoflurane for several hours.[41] Isoflurane anesthesia does not result in glutathione depletion in mice, suggesting that significant amounts of reactive metabolites are not produced.[42] A potential oxidative pathway is shown in Figure 4-4.

Effects of Inhalation Anesthetics on Hepatic Function and Hepatotoxicity

Effects of inhalation anesthetics on hepatic function, particularly on hepatotoxity, is controversial. The degree of liver injury varies from agent to agent and from species to species, and experimental study results range from no effects on hepatic function to structural changes in the hepatocytes.

Effects of Inhalation Anesthetics on Normal Liver

The type of anesthetic may result in aberrations of liver function.[43,44] In contrast to halothane, isoflurane does not alter bromsulphalein (BSP) retention in volunteers.[41] In this respect, isoflurane is similar to enflurane. On the other hand, isoflurane or halothane anesthesia does not increase lactate dehydrogenase (LDH) and serum glutamic oxaloacetic transaminase (SGOT), while both indices increase with enflurane anesthesia. Thus, halothane and enflurane appear to produce subtle changes in liver function or integrity. These relationships are not consonant with the degree of biodegradation of the three anesthetic agents.[41]

Effects of Subanesthetic Concentration on Normal Liver

Effects of subanesthetic concentration of inhalation anesthetics on hepatic function is controversial. Rats and guinea pigs that were given up to 0.1 MAC of isoflurane, enflurane, ether, or nitrous oxide

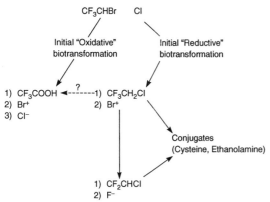

Figure 4-2. Biotransformation of halothane. Adapted from B. R. Brown, Jr. (1988) Hepatotoxicity of inhalation anesthetics. In *Anesthesia in Hepatic and Biliary Tract Disease.* Philadelphia: F. A. Davis.

fared reasonably well and tended to gain as much weight as the control group. In contrast, rats given 0.1 MAC halothane or 0.003 MAC fluroxine failed to thrive. The failure to thrive was associated with the development of degenerative hepatic lesions.[45]

Hepatotoxicity

Several mechanisms have been proposed for the development of inhalation anesthetic induced hepatitis, particularly with halothane. Suggestions that anesthetics such as halothane are true hepatotoxins have never been substantiated.[46] An allergic basis for the hepatitis was supported by certain clinical features, such as the increased risk after repeated exposures, eosinophilia, and case reports of two anesthesiologists who developed abnormal liver function after reexposure to halothane. However, the lack of pediatric patients with the disease, the occurrence of hepatitis after a single exposure to halothane, and the pathologic features that are unusual for an allergic response have limited the enthusiasm for the allergic concept.[47]

There are indications that abnormal reductive metabolites produced by an alternate pathway with enzyme induction are capable of causing liver damage,[37] evidenced by the liver damage caused in rats by the combination of halothane, enzyme induction, and hypoxia.[48] In addition, rats fed ethanol that received halothane at 10% oxygen concentration showed patchy necrosis in the centrilobular regions with parenchymal lipid accumulation in the liver. A milder degree of necrosis was seen at am-

bient oxygen concentrations. These data suggest that halothane is hepatotoxic to rats chronically pretreated with ethanol, especially under hypoxic conditions.[49] It is possible that alcohol enhances hepatic hypoxia, thereby promoting the reductive pathway of halothane.

It is hypothesized that the metabolites of the reductive pathway are potentially more hepatotoxic than the oxidative metabolites, based upon the increased covalent binding of halothane metabolites under hypoxic conditions;[50] or reductive metabolites produced in this abnormal condition could act as haptens and might be responsible for an immune response leading to subsequent liver damage on further exposure to the drug.[18] The binding capacity of reactive intermediate compounds may be cumulative and multiple exposures result in hepatitis in susceptible individuals. This reductive biotransformation of halothane to free radicals is known to occur in patients with obesity, with decreased HBF, and with specific genetic amplification of the reductive pathway which interplays with various inducing drugs and environmental chemistry.[51] In addition, it can be enhanced by enzyme-inducing agents, halothane itself,[52] and by stress of surgery that releases steroids, enzyme inducers.[53] Also defluorination of halothane occurs during hypoxic conditions.

This hepatotoxity of halothane does not appear to occur with other anesthetic agents. Liver injury that occurred in rats pretreated with phenobarbital and anesthetized with halothane and low oxygen tension (8%) was not seen with enflurane or isoflurane anesthesia.[54] The lesser hepatotoxicity of enflurane and isoflurane may be related to the lesser degree of biotransformation[55] and far less formation of free radicals or reactive intermediates.[51]

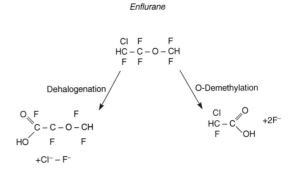

Figure 4-3. Biotransformation of enflurane. Adapted from B. R. Brown, Jr. (1988) Hepatotoxicity of inhalation anesthetics. In *Anesthesia in Hepatic and Biliary Tract Disease.* Philadelphia: F. A. Davis.

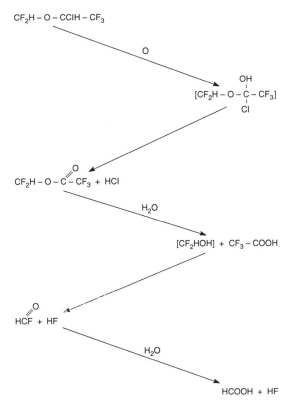

Figure 4-4. A potential oxidative pathway of isoflurane. Adapted from Edger, E. I. II. (1981) Metabolism of isoflurane. In Isoflurane (Forane), edited by Eger E. I. II. Madison WI. : Airco Inc.

Factors Affecting Hepatotoxicity of Anesthetics

The hyperthyroid state has been shown to potentiate centrilobular injury in rodents caused by chloroform, carbon tetrachloride, 1-1-dichloroethylene, and acetaminophen.[56] However, this hepatotoxicity seen in T3-treated rats may be caused by hypoxic damage resulting from hypermetabolic centrilobular cells in combination with isoflurane- and enflurane-induced depression of splanchnic blood flow. This concept is supported by the observations that T3 decreases liver cytochrome P450, that isoflurane and enflurane are relatively inert, and that the central area of the liver is exquisitely sensitive to low oxygen tensions.[57]

Periods of hypoxia, shorter than those previously described,[58] can produce hepatic injury in starved enzyme-induced rats. The threshold for injury in these animals is as little as 5 minutes. If these results apply to humans, patients who are deprived of food preoperatively and who are taking drugs that induce hepatic enzymes may be at risk for even brief periods of hypoxia during anesthesia. However, caution

must be exercised when relating animal data to humans. The slower human metabolic rate may make them less vulnerable to hepatic injury. In addition, the 24-hour period of starvation in animals usually is longer than that seen in humans.[59]

Effects of Inhalation Anesthetics on Other Drugs

Two issues are of clinical relevance concerning interactions of potent volatile anesthetics on biotransformation: the acute effects of an inhalation anesthetic may inhibit clearance of intravenously administered drugs by binding with and reversibly inhibiting the function of microsomal cytochrome P450;[36,60] and chronic effects of an inhalation anesthetic on hepatic microsomal enzyme activity.[60]

Effects of Inhalation Agents on Intravenous Drugs

Effects of inhalation agents on intravenous drugs vary. Twenty-four hours after a 7-hour exposure to 0.3% isoflurane, rats given hexobarbital had a shortened sleeping time.[61] A similar finding was observed with halothane, enflurane, and ether, but not with cyclopropane or nitrous oxide, suggesting that halothane, enflurane, and isoflurane may induce liver enzymes. The increased metabolic capacity of liver microsomes following ether or halothane anesthesia adds support to this suggestion.[61]

On the other hand, a study by Wood and Wood using carbon-labeled aminopyrine breath test as an index of drug biotransformation in rats found that isoflurane and enflurane did not cause any decrement of aminopyrine metabolism 24 hours after anesthesia.[62] However, halothane produced significant depressions of this biotransformation index.

In a human study, Loft and associates studied the aminopyrine breath test in fit subjects following knee arthrotomies during which patients were given two different types of anesthesia: halothane-oxygen or spinal.[53] Both groups of patients displayed identical increases in the rate of biotransformation of aminopyrine. Therefore, hepatic microsomal enzyme induction may occur after minor surgery in humans, but factors other than the anesthetic agents seem to be responsible.

Effects of Intravenous Agents on Inhalation Agents

It is a clinical impression that the dose requirement of inhalation anesthetic is increased in patients with chronic ethanol abuse. In fact, MAC of halothane in chronic alcoholic patients is 1% compared with 0.75% in the controls.[63] A decrease in the dose requirement of inhalation anesthetics appears to be associated with a proliferation of hepatic smooth endoplasmic reticulum that enhances a variety of microsomal drug metabolizing enzymes in man[64] and rat.[65]

Effects on Volatile Anesthetics

Volatile anesthetics can inhibit the metabolism of other volatile anesthetics.[66] Isoflurane is shown to inhibit acutely the oxidative pathway of halothane metabolism. This inhibition appears to be caused by suppression of hepatic microsomal and somatic function rather than a reduction in HBF.

Effects of Inhalation Anesthetics on Patients with Hepatic Dysfunction

Hepatic blood flow is reduced in patients with hepatic dysfunction,[67] and portal blood flow is remarkably reduced in patients with portal hypertension[17] and portacaval shunt.[18] Further reductions in HBF and hepatic hypoxia secondary to stress of surgery and anesthetics may precipitate hepatic decompensation and result in increased morbidity and mortality,[17] including overt liver dysfunction or even hepatic failure. Most clinicians believe that liver function in cirrhotic patients is made worse by anesthesia and surgery, whether performed under general (cyclopropane or ether) or regional anesthesia, although little work has been done to determine the causes.[3]

In general, anesthetics themselves may have only minor hepatotoxic and hemodynamic effects, but marginal changes in HBF and oxygenation may become clinically significant when other intraoperative factors further compromise hepatic function.[5] A patient with preexisting liver disease and already reduced HBF is much more likely to have an elevation in liver enzymes after anesthesia and surgery, and animals show markedly increased hepatic oxygen consumption after liver injury.[68]

A study by Maze, Smith, and Baden showed that halothane did not exacerbate hepatic dysfunction in cirrhotic rats.[11] Furthermore, Baden and coworkers compared effects of anesthetics on their potential to exacerbate liver dysfunction in rats with preexisting cirrhosis.[3] The study results showed that halothane, enflurane, isoflurane, and fentanyl were associated with the same minimal degree of postanesthetic hepatic dysfunction and that the dysfunction was similar in both cirrhotic and noncirrhotic rats. Therefore, these anesthetics do not appear to have acute effects on hepatic function in the presence of preexisting cirrhosis, although the authors noted that the relatively large variance in the liver function test, the small group sizes, and the comparison of multiple groups might have caused a beta-type error in analysis.

The administration of halothane to a patient with known liver disease poses a dilemma, although there are no data that show halothane accentuates underlying liver disease. Specifically, there is no evidence that patients with preexisting compensated (Child's class A) liver disease are at any greater risk of developing halothane hepatitis, although factors that favor reductive metabolism of halothane may be more likely to be present in the patient with liver disease (especially ethanol produced) than in a normal patient. For example, chronic ethanol abuse may induce hepatic microsomal enzymes, whereas fibrotic parenchymal changes characteristic of cirrhosis predictably decrease hepatic blood flow and jeopardize hepatocyte oxygenation.[63] On the contrary, it has been suggested that an immunoregulatory defect in a patient with chronic liver disease may make the individual more susceptible to the hepatotoxic effect of halothane.[69] In general, there is a very strong case for avoiding anesthesia with or without halothane and surgery in patients with active hepatitis from any cause unless absolutely essential: these patients may develop a serious hepatic dysfunction postoperatively, resulting in fulminant hepatic failure.[70]

Single or repeated administration of isoflurane in the presence of preexisting hepatic disease does not necessarily aggravate hepatic injury as illustrated in a patient with ascending cholangitis.[71] This negligible effect of isoflurane and enflurane on hepatic function compared with halothane appears to be associated with their better oxygen delivery to the liver, mainly by a more effective preservation of hepatic arterial blood flow.[19,25]

In conclusion, volatile agents have distinct advantages over intravenous anesthetic agents in patients with liver disease. First, they can be used with a high inspired oxygen concentration, which may be important in some cirrhotic patients with severe intrapulmonary shunting.[72] Second, alterations in pharmacokinetics of intravenous anesthetics may occur in patients with liver disease secondary to changes in HBF, drug binding, volume of distribution, and biotransformation.[73] Third, hepatic dysfunction after exposure to inhalation anesthestics is mild and inconsequential, if it occurs. Finally, isoflurane may be the preferred agent in patients with liver disease[1,18] because it undergoes the least metabolism and has no or little hepatotoxicity.

References

1. Eger, E.I., II (ed) (1981) Effects on the liver. In *Isoflurane (Forane)*. Madison: Airco Inc., pp. 78–82.
2. Shingu, K., Eger, E.I. II, Johnson, B.H., Van Dyke, R. A., Lurz, F. W. and Cheng, A. (1983) Effect of oxygen concentration, hyperthermia, and choice of vendor on anesthetic-induced hepatic injury in rats. *Anesthesia and Analgesia* 62:146–50.
3. Baden, J.M., Kundomal, Y.R., Luttropp, M.E., Maze, M. and Kosek, J.C. (1985) Effects of volatile anesthetics or fentanyl on hepatic function in cirrhotic rats. *Anesthesia and Analgesia* 64:1183–88.
4. Schemel, W.H. (1976) Unexplained hepatic dysfunction found by multiple laboratory screening. *Anesthesia and Analgesia* 55:810–12.
5. Brown, F.H., Shiau, Y-F. and Richter, G.C. (1982) Anesthesia and surgery in the patient with liver disease. In *Medical Care of the Surgical Patient. A Problem-Oriented Approach to Management*. (Goldmann, D.R., Brown, F.H., Levy, W.K., Slap, G.B. and Sussman, E.J., eds). Philadelphia: J.B. Lippincott, pp. 326–42.
6. Schmidt, W. (1977) The epidemiology of cirrhosis of the liver: A statistical analysis of mortality data with specific reference to Canada. In *Alcohol and the Liver*, (Fisher, M.N. and Rankin, J.G., eds). New York: Plenum Press, pp. 1–260.
7. Parker, E.O., III. (1985) Anesthetic management of the patient with hepatic dysfunction. *Anesthetic Reviews* 12:9–16.
8. Martin, G.A. and Bode, C.H. (1970) The epidemiology of cirrhosis of the liver. In *Alcoholic Cirrhosis and Other Toxic Hepatopathies*. Stockholm: Nordiska Bkhandelis Forag, p. 315.
9. Zakin, D., Boyer, T.D., Montgomery, C. and Kanas, N. (1982) Alcoholic disease. In *Hepatology*, (Zakin, D. and Boyer, T.D. eds). Philadelphia: W.B. Saunders, pp. 739–40.
10. Saunders, J.B. (1983) Alcoholic liver disease in the 1980's. *British Medical Journal* 187:1819–21.
11. Maze, M., Smith, C.M. and Baden, J.M. (1985) Halothane anesthesia does not exacerbate hepatic dysfunction in cirrhotic rats. *Anesthesiology* 62:1–5.
12. Keeri-Szanto, M. and Lefleur, F. (1963) Postanesthetic liver complications in a general hospital: A statistical study. *Canadian Anaesthetists Society Journal* 10:531–38.
13. Herber, R. and Specht, N. (1965) Liver necrosis following anesthesia. *Archives of Internal Medicine* 115:266–72.
14. Ratnoff, O.D. and Patek, A.J. (1942) Natural history of Laennec's cirrhosis. *Medicine* 21:259.
15. Jackson, F.J., Christopher, E.G., Peternel, W.W. and Kirimli, B. (1968) Preoperative management of patients with liver disease. *Surgical Clinics of North America* 48:907–30.
16. Harville, D.D. and Summerskill, W.H.J. (1963) Surgery in acute hepatitis. Causes and effects. *Journal of the American Medical Association* 184:257–61.
17. Friedman, L.S. and Maddrey, W.C. (1987) Surgery in the patient with liver disease. *Medical Clinic of North America* 71:453–76.
18. Strunin, L. (1985) Anaesthetic management of patients with liver disease. In *Liver and Biliary Disease*. (Wright, R., Millward-Sadler, G.H., Alberti, K.G.M.M. and Karran, S. eds). London: W.B. Saunders, pp. 1379–1394.
19. Gelman, S. (1987) General anesthesia and hepatic circulation. *Canadian Journal of Physiology and Pharmacology* 65:1762–99.
20. Bombeck, C.T., Aoki, T., Smuckler, E.A. and Nyhus, L. M. (1969) Effects of halothane, ether, and chloroform on the isolated, perfused, bovine liver. *American Journal of Surgery* 117:91–107.
21. Lutz, J., Henrich, H. and Bauereisen, E. (1975) Oxygen supply and uptake in the liver and the intestine. *Pflugers Archiv. Euro. J. Physiol.* 360:7–15.
22. Brown, B.R., Jr (1988a) Effects of anesthetics on hepatic blood flow. In *Anesthesia in Hepatic and Biliary Tract Disease*. Philadelphia: F.A. Davis, pp. 49–60.
23. Price, H.L. and Pauca, A.L. (1971) Effects of anesthesia on the peripheral circulation. In *A Decade of Clinical Progress*. (Fabian, L. ed). Philadelphia: F.A. Davis pp. 73–90.
24. Price, H.L., Deutch, S., Cooperman, L.H., Clement, A.J. and Epstein, R.M. (1965) Splanchnic circulation during cyclopropane anesthesia in normal man. *Anesthesiology* 26:312–19.
25. Price, H.L., Deutsch, S., Davidson, I.A., Clement, A.J., Behar, M.G. and Epstein, R.M. (1966) Can general anesthetics produce splanchnic visceral hypoxia by reducing regional blood flow? *Anesthesiology* 27:24–32.
26. Epstein, R.M., Deutsch, S., Cooperman, L.H., Clement, A.J. and Price, H.L. (1966) Splanchnic circulation during halothane anesthesia and hypercapnia in normal man. *Anesthesiology* 27:654–61.
27. Irestedt, I. and Andreen, M. (1979) Effects of enflurane on haemodynamics and oxygen consumption in the dog with special reference to the liver and preportal tissues. *Acta Anaesthesia Scandinavica* 23:13–26.

28. Conzen. P.F., Hobhahn, J., Goetz, A.E. et al. (1988) Splanchnic oxygen consumption and hepatic surface oxygen tensions during isoflurane anesthesia. *Anesthesiology* 69:643–51.

29. Gelman, S., Fowler, K.C. and Smith, L.R. (1984a) Liver circulation and function during isoflurane and halothane anesthesia. *Anesthesiology* 61:726–30.

30. Lundeen, G., Manohar, M. and Parks, C. (1983) Systemic distribution of blood flow in swine while awake and during 1.0 and 1.5 MAC isoflurane anesthesia with and without 50% nitrous oxide. *Anesthesia and Analgesia* 62:499–512.

31. Gelman, S., Fowler, K.C. and Smith, L.R. (1984b) Regional blood flow during isoflurane and halothane anesthesia. *Anesthesia and Analgesia* 63:557–65.

32. Eger, E.I., II, Shingu, K. and Johnson, B.H. (1983) Hypoxia and halothane hepatotoxicity (letter). *Anesthesia and Analgesia* 62:861.

33. Shingu, K., Eger, E.I., II and Johnson, B.H. (1983) Hepatic injury induced by anesthetic agents in rats. *Anesthesia and Analgesia* 62:140–65.

34. Crosti, P.F., Giovannelli, C.A., Bardi, U. and Vigo, P.L. (1971) Hepatic blood flow in cirrhosis. *Lancet* ii:322.

35. Stoelting, R.K. (1976) Estimation of hepatic function—Effects of the anesthetic experience. In *American Society of Anesthesiologists Refresher Courses in Anesthesiology*, 149–50.

36. Van Dyke, R.A. (1973) Biotransformation of volatile anaesthetics with special emphasis on the role of metabolism in the toxicity of anaesthetics. *Canadian Anaesthesicts Society Journal* 20:21–33.

37. Poppers, P.J. (1980) Hepatic drug metabolism and anesthesia. *Anaesthetist* 29:55–58.

38. Van Dyke, R.A. and Wood, C.L. (1973) Binding of radioactivity from ^{14}C-labeled halothane in isolated perfused rat livers. *Anesthesiology* 38:328–32.

39. Brown, B.R. Jr, Sipes, I.G., Jee, R.C. and Gandolfi, A.J. (1979) Characterization of hypoxic model for halothane hepatotoxicity. *Anesthesiology* 51:S239.

40. Dale, O., Nielsen, K., Westgaard, G. and Nilsen, O.G. (1983) Drug metabolizing enzymes in the rat after inhalation of halothane and enflurane. *British Journal of Anaesthesia* 55:1217–23.

41. Stevens, W.C., Eger, E.I., II, Joas, T.A., Chomwell, T.H., White, M.A. and Dolan, W.M. (1973) Comparative toxicity of isoflurane, halothane, fluroxene and diethyl ether in human volunteers. *Canadian Anaesthetists Society Journal* 20:357–68.

42. Zumbiel, M.A., Fiserova-Bergerova, V., Malinin, T.I. and Holaday, D.A. (1978) Glutathione depletion following inhalation anesthesia. *Anesthesiology* 49:102–08.

43. Gelman, S.I. (1976) Disturbances in hepatic blood flow during anesthesia and surgery. *Archives of Surgery* 111:881–83.

44. Kalow, B., Rogoman, E. and Sims, F.H. (1976) A comparison of the effects of halothane and other anesthetic agents on hepato-cellular junction in patients submitted to elective operations. *Canadian Anaesthetists Society Journal* 23:71–79.

45. Stevens, W.C., Eger, E.I., II, White, A., et al. (1975) Comparative toxicity of halothane, isoflurane, and diethyl ether at subanesthetic concentrations in laboratory animals. *Anesthesiology* 42:408–19.

46. Simpson, B.R., Strunin, L. and Walton, B. (1974) Evidence for halothane hepatotoxicity is equivocal. In *Controversy in Internal Medicine II*. (Ingelfinger, F.J., Ebert, R.V., Finland, M., and Relman, A.S. eds). Philadelphia: W. B. Saunders, pp. 580–94.

47. Cooperman, L.H., Wollman, H. and Marsh, M.L. (1977) Anesthesia and the liver. *Surgical Clinics of North America* 57:421–28.

48. McLain, G.E., Sipes, I.G. and Brown, B.R. (1979) An animal model of halothane hepatotoxicity: Role of enzyme induction and hypoxia. *Anesthesiology* 51:321–26.

49. Takagi, T., Ishii, H., Takahashi, H. (1983) Potentiation of halothane hepatotoxicity by chronic ethanol administration in rat: An animal model of halothane hepatitis. *Pharmacology and Biochemical Behavior* 18:461–65.

50. Widger, L.A., Gadolfi, A.J. and Van Dyke, R.A. (1976) Hypoxia and halothane metabolism in vivo: Release of inorganic fluoride and halothane metabolite binding to cellular constituents. *Anesthesiology* 44:197–201.

51. Brown, B.R., Jr (1988c) Hepatotoxicity of inhalation anesthetics. In *Anesthesia in Hepatic and Biliary Tract Disease*. Philadelphia: F.A. Davis, pp. 93–111.

52. Cascorbi, H.F., Vesell, E.S., Blake, D.A. and Helrich, M. (1971) Halothane biotransformation in man. *Annals of the New York Academy of Science* 179:244–48.

53. Loft, S., Boel, J., Kyst, A., Rasmussen, B., Hansen, S.H. and Dossing, M. (1985) Increased hepatic microsomal enzyme activity after surgery under halothane or spinal anesthesia. *Anesthesiology* 62:11–16.

54. Harper, M.H., Johnson, B.H., Collins, P. and Eger, E.I. II. (1980) Hepatic injury following halothane, enflurane, and isoflurane anesthesia in rats (abstract). *Anesthesiology* 53:S242.

55. Carpenter, R.L., Eger, E.I., II, Johnson, B.H., Jashavant, A.B., Unadkat, D. and Sheiner, L.B. (1986) The extent of metabolism of inhaled anesthetics in humans. *Anesthesiology* 65:201–05.

56. Berman, M.L., Kuhnert, L., Phythyon, J.M. and Holaday, D.A. (1983) Isoflurane and enflurane-induced hepatic necrosis in triiodothyronine-pretreated rats. *Anesthesiology* 58:1–5.

57. Lemasters, J.J., Sungchul, J. and Thurman, R.G. (1981) Centrilobular injury following hypoxia in isolated, perfused rat liver. *Science* 213:661–63.

58. Shingu, K., Eger, E.I. II and Johnson, B.H. (1982) Hypoxia per se can produce hepatic damage without death in rats. *Anesthesia and Analgesia* 61:820–23.

59. Fassoulaki, A., Eger, E.I., II, Johnson, B.H. et al. (1984) Brief periods of hypoxia can produce hepatic injury in rats. *Anesthesia and Analgesia* 63:885–87.

60. Brown, B.R., Jr (1988b) Drug biotransformation by the liver. In *Anesthesia in Hepatic and Biliary Tract Disease*. Philadelphia: F.A. Davis, pp. 67–91.

61. Linde, H.W. and Berman, M.L. (1971) Nonspecific stimulation of drug-metabolizing enzymes by inhala-

tion anesthetic agents. *Anesthesia and Analgesia* 50:656–65.

62. Wood, M. and Wood, A.J.J. (1984) Contrasting effects of halothane, isoflurane, and enflurane on in vivo drug metabolism in the rat. *Anesthesia and Analgesia* 63:709–14.

63. Stoelting, R.K. (1980) Anesthetic considerations in the patient with liver disease. *Current Reviews in Clinical Anesthesia* 1:51–55.

64. Rubin, E. and Lieber, C.S. (1968) Hepatic microsomal enzyme in man and rat: Induction and inhibition by ethanol. *Science* 162:690–91.

65. Ishii, H., Joly, J.G. and Lieber, C.S. (1973) Effect of ethanol on the amount of enzyme activities of hepatic rough and smooth microsomal mechanisms. *Biochimica Biophysica Acta* 291:411–20.

66. Fiserova-Bergerova, V. (1984) Inhibitory effect of isoflurane upon oxidative metabolism of halothane. *Anesthesia and Analgesia* 63:399–404.

67. Bashour, F.A., McConnell, T. and Miller, W.F. (1967) Circulatory and respiratory changes in patients with Laennec's cirrhosis of the liver. *American Heart Journal* 74:569–77.

68. Brauer, R.W., Lesing, G.F. and Holloway, R.J. (1961) Oxygen uptake and hypoxia in the isolated rat liver preparation. *Federation Proceedings* 20:286.

69. Camilleri, M., Victorino, R.M.N. and Hodgson, H. J. F. (1984) Halothane aggravation of chronic liver disease. *Acta Medica Portuguesa* 5:194–96.

70. Powell-Jackson, P., Greenway, B. and Williams, R. (1982) Adverse effects of exploratory laparotomy in patients with suspected liver disease. *British Journal of Surgery* 68:449–51.

71. McLaughlin, D.R. and Eger, E.I., II. (1984) Repeated isoflurane anesthesia in a patient with hepatic dysfunction. *Anesthesia and Analgesia* 63:775–78.

72. Berthelot, P., Walker, J.G., Sherlock, S., and Reid, L. (1966) Arterial changes in the lungs in cirrhosis of the liver. *New England Journal of Medicine* 274:291–98.

73. Williams, R.L. (1983) Drug administration in hepatic disease. *New England Journal of Medicine* 309:1616–22.

Chapter 5
Sedative and Analgesic Drugs

Maire P. Shelly, Annie C. Elston, and Gilbert R. Park

Because the liver is a major site of drug metabolism, care should be taken when giving drugs to patients with liver disease. However, scientific evidence for altered drug metabolism is conflicting. Studies on patients with liver disease show that the pharmacokinetics of some drugs are severely deranged, while the pharmacokinetics of other drugs are unaffected by liver disease. In some of the earlier studies, poor analytical specificity may have contributed to these alterations, and the measurement of elimination half-life rather than clearance may have confused the issue. More recent studies using specific drug assays and measuring clearance have still produced inconsistent results. These inconsistencies arise because the liver is a complex organ that performs a wide range of functions. No generalizations can be made about the effects of impaired liver function on the pharmacokinetics and pharmacodynamics of drugs in patients with liver disease. The overall effect depends on the drug involved, the enzymes and cofactors necessary for the reactions, the type and severity of the liver disorder, and genetic variation.

Further difficulties arise because the sensitivity of receptors where the drugs act changes in liver disease.[1] There may also be changes in the amounts of neurotransmitters,[2] and other substances that may cause sedation.[3] Thus, patients with liver disease become more sensitive to the sedative effects of analgesic and sedative drugs.[4]

The response of a patient to a drug differs in acute and chronic liver disease. For example, lignocaine shows a decreased clearance in patients with cirrhosis, but its clearance is unchanged in patients with acute viral hepatitis.[5,5a] In chronic liver disease, clearance may be increased, decreased, or unchanged.[6]

Drug Metabolism

The purpose of drug metabolism is to turn an active, lipophilic substance into an inactive polar substance. A substance that changes from lipophilic to polar cannot cross membranes but can be excreted by the kidneys.

Two "phases" of drug metabolism have been described. Phase I metabolism usually adds molecular oxygen to the molecule. Phase II metabolism then adds a further group, such as glucuronic acid, to the phase I metabolite. Because some drugs (such as morphine) can go through phase II metabolism without first undergoing a phase I reaction (Figure 5-1), there is a trend toward doing away with the terms phase I and phase II and merely describing the reaction.

Phase I metabolite reactions are commonly performed by a super-family of enzymes, the cytochromes P450. So far 28 of these have been described, and they are thought to be responsible for the metabolism of 150–200,000 substances. Thus, one

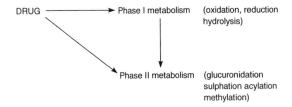

Figure 5-1. Drug metabolism.

enzyme metabolizes many compounds. For example, cytochrome P450 3A4 metabolizes erythromycin, midazolam, alfentanil, lignocaine, cyclosporin, and nifedipine among other compounds. The super-family of cytochromes P450 are described by an Arabic number (40% amino acid homology), a capital letter (55% amino acid homology), and the gene with a further Arabic number.[7]

In addition to their role in drug metabolism cytochromes P450 have other functions, including the manufacture of steroids and receptor regulation. They also convert procarcinogens into carcinogens. The cytochromes P450 are found in most cells in the body, commonly in the endoplasmic reticulum. There are high concentrations in the liver, adrenals, and nose. However, the greatest mass is found in the liver, explaining the importance of the liver in drug metabolism. Since they are a hemoprotein, they turn over in the same way as any other protein. Therefore, their expression may vary, depending on a variety of factors.[8]

Phase II metabolism is performed by enzymes located mostly in the cytoplasm. Less is known about their regulation compared to phase I enzymes. Their function appears to be less affected in liver disease than that of phase I enzymes. Drugs metabolized by their pathways are therefore less affected in liver disease.

The distribution of enzymes in the liver is not homogenous and varies according to many factors. For example, cytochrome P450 2E1, the enzyme that metabolizes volatile anesthetic agents, is concentrated in the most hypoxic area of the hepatic lobule, around the central vein, and so may be more resistant to hypoxia than others.[9]

Pharmacokinetic Alterations

Liver disease may affect the action of a drug by influencing a number of pharmacokinetic variables, such as hepatic clearance, protein binding, volume of dis-

tribution, biliary secretion, and absorption from the gastrointestinal tract. In patients with the hepatorenal syndrome, renal clearance will also be affected.

Hepatic Clearance

Hepatic clearance is defined as the volume of blood cleared of a drug by the liver, in unit time. Drugs are extracted from the blood by the liver and are then metabolized in the parenchyma to form hydrophilic substances that can be readily excreted in the urine or bile. Most drugs are rendered inactive by this process, but some have active metabolites.

The hepatic clearance of a drug depends on a number of factors:

- The intrinsic clearance; that is, the ability of the liver to remove a drug from the blood in the absence of any constraints such as protein binding or hepatic blood flow.
- The rate at which the drug is delivered to the liver; that is, the hepatic blood flow.
- Hepatic clearance also depends on the physicochemical properties of the drug, the fraction of unbound drug in the blood, the concentration of drug entering the liver, and the presence of any barriers to diffusion that may retard the accessibility of the drug into the liver.

Hepatic clearance may be defined by the equation:

$$Cl_H = Q_H \times ER$$

Where Cl_H = hepatic clearance, Q_H = hepatic blood flow, and ER = the extraction ratio. (see also chapter 1.)

The extraction ratio is the fraction of drug removed from the blood during its passage through the liver:

$$E = \frac{Ca - Cv}{Ca}$$

Where Ca = arterial concentration of drug and Cv = venous concentration of drug.

Drugs with a high extraction ratio are removed by the liver almost as rapidly as they are delivered, and hepatic clearance is equal to intrinsic clearance. For these drugs, hepatic clearance is sensitive to changes in hepatic blood flow. A decrease in hepatic blood flow results in a decreased clearance of drug by the liver.

Drugs with a low extraction ratio have a low intrinsic clearance. For these drugs, hepatic clearance is independent of hepatic blood flow but is dependent on the low intrinsic ability of the hepatic enzymes to metabolize the drug.[10] Plasma protein binding may also affect the hepatic clearance of drugs with a low extraction ratio, because only unbound drug crosses the plasma membrane and is available for drug metabolism. However, if the avidity of the hepatic enzymes for a particular drug is stronger than the drug's affinity for its protein binding sites, the drug can be effectively stripped from its binding sites during passage through the liver. This results in two types of extraction for drugs that are highly protein bound (>90%):

RESTRICTED EXTRACTION
Extraction is limited to unbound drug. The remainder is strongly bound to plasma protein (usually drugs with low intrinsic clearance).

UNRESTRICTED EXTRACTION
Both unbound and bound drugs are extracted. As unbound drug is cleared, bound drug dissociates from its low-affinity sites to replace it and is also cleared (usually drugs with a higher intrinsic clearance).

If the intrinsic clearance of free drug (intrinsic free clearance) is less than the hepatic blood flow, the extraction of the drug will be less than the free drug fraction. In this case, extraction will be restrictive regardless of the degree of protein binding. However, when the intrinsic free clearance exceeds liver blood flow, extraction of the drug will be greater than the free drug fraction and extraction will be nonrestrictive. As protein binding increases and the free drug fraction is decreased, extraction of some drugs changes from restrictive to nonrestrictive.

The greater the intrinsic free clearance, the larger is the free fraction at which the drug is nonrestrictively eliminated and the greater the range of binding over which this occurs.[10] It follows that the higher the intrinsic free clearance of a drug, the less sensitive its extraction is to changes in protein binding.

These clearance patterns apply in healthy subjects and in patients with mild liver disease. However, in patients with more severe liver disease, hepatic clearance may be changed by changes in either intrinsic clearance or hepatic blood flow, or both. Liver disease may also alter the extraction ratio of a drug.

In cirrhosis, the most widely studied chronic liver disease, the hepatic clearance of most drugs is decreased. This is mainly because of a reduction in hepatic enzyme capacity, which may reduce intrinsic clearance by as much as 83%.[11] To a lesser extent the decrease in hepatic clearance is caused by a reduction in hepatic blood flow. Hepatic perfusion is not consistently affected by cirrhosis, but on average there is 15% decrease[12] because of intra- and extrahepatic shunting. Three different types of shunt have been described:[12]

ANATOMIC SHUNTS
These occur between portal venules and hepatic veins.

PHYSIOLOGIC SHUNTS
These are caused by reducing perfusion of normal hepatocytes and continued perfusion of damaged hepatocytes.

EXTRAHEPATIC SHUNTS
These are portosystemic shunts that develop (or are surgically constructed) to relieve portal hypertension.

The reduction in hepatic clearance in cirrhosis is similar for drugs with both high and low extraction ratios. This has led to the development of a model of functional intrahepatic shunting to explain the phenomenon. The model suggests that the reduced drug clearance results from a reduced mass of perfused drug metabolizing hepatocytes.[11] Thus, drugs with a high extraction ratio have a decreased clearance caused by a reduction in perfusion, whereas those with a low extraction ratio have a decreased clearance owing to a reduced functional liver mass.

The effect of liver disease on hepatic clearance also depends on the distribution of disease within the hepatic lobule. Many of the drug metabolizing enzymes, including the cytochromes P450 system, are located on the smooth endoplasmic reticulum in zone 1. In conditions predominantly affecting this zone, such as acute viral hepatitis, impaired drug metabolism has been reported early in the disease process. However, in patients with primary biliary cirrhosis, which predominantly affects zone 3, drug metabolism is not impaired until the terminal stages of the disease.[13] Different metabolic pathways are affected by differing amounts. Phase I reactions such as oxidation, reduction, and hydrolysis are often severely impaired, while phase II conjugation reactions are relatively unaffected. Differential changes in the enzyme content of the liver have been described in liver disease,[14] but only very severe liver damage will completely destroy the capacity of the liver to metabolize drugs. The pharmacokinetics of drugs that undergo only phase II reactions will be less affected by liver disease than those of drugs that undergo phase I reactions.

This differentiation is particularly evident in benzodiazepines. The unsubstituted 3,1-4-benzodiazepines undergo phase I metabolism by the cytochrome P450 system, while the 3-hydroxy benzodiazepines undergo conjugation, with glucuronide, by a different set of enzymes. Liver disease therefore affects the pharmacokinetics of the unsubstituted benzodiazepines, such as diazepam, while the unsubstituted benzodiazepines, such as lorazepam, are relatively unaffected.[15]

Protein Binding

In liver disease, albumin synthesis decreases; thus, the number of binding sites available for acidic drugs is decreased and the free drug fraction is increased. They may also be qualitative changes in protein binding, caused by conformational changes in the albumin molecule, or alterations in its binding capacity caused by interference of endogenous substances such as bilirubin.[16]

Basic drugs are bound predominantly to the acute phase protein, α-1-acidglycoprotein. In liver disease, the plasma concentration of this protein may either decrease because of impaired synthesis, increase owing to coexisting inflammation, or remain unchanged. The binding capacity of α-1-acidglycoprotein may also be changed in patients with liver disease.[17] Decreased protein binding may result in changes in clearance and distribution, although the effects are unpredictable.[16] For this reason, it is important that clinical pharmacokinetic studies use analytical techniques that measure the concentration of free, rather than total, drug.

Volume of Distribution

In liver disease, the volume of distribution is increased because of changes in plasma and extracellular fluid volumes. For example, the development of ascites causes the volume of distribution of propanolol to double.[18] Changes in protein binding may also affect the volume of distribution, although the effect is unpredictable.

Bioavailability

The bioavailability of drugs given orally is increased in patients with liver disease. This is caused by the decrease in hepatic clearance, which decreases first-pass metabolism and increases the amount of drug reaching the systemic circulation. The contribution of the liver to the clearance of drugs given orally is difficult to measure, but in patients with liver disease it appears to depend more on intrinsic clearance than hepatic blood flow.

For these reasons, drugs given orally may produce a more profound and prolonged effect than normal. Therefore, the initial dose should be reduced in proportion to the severity of the liver disease, and subsequent doses titrated against the response. The effects of centrally acting agents may be particularly pronounced.

Absorption

Drug absorption from the gastrointestinal tract may alter in liver disease. This is an effect of portal hypertension that may cause edema and structural abnormalities of the small intestine.

Pharmacodynamic Alterations

The pathophysiological effects of liver disease may affect the pharmacodynamics of certain drugs. Thus, even if the pharmacokinetics are unchanged, alterations of the dose may still be necessary. For example, the reduced synthesis of clotting factors caused by liver dysfunction potentiates the action of anticoagulants. The dose of warfarin therefore needs careful evaluation in patients with impaired liver function.

Patients with liver disease show increased sensitivity to all central nervous system depressants. In addition, sedative drugs may precipitate hepatic encephalopathy and so must be used with extreme caution in patients with liver failure. Other groups of drugs may also precipitate hepatic decompensation and their doses may have to be reduced in the presence of liver disease. These include drugs that have the potential to reduce hepatic blood flow such as beta blockers and anesthetic agents, drugs that cause salt and water retention, and drugs such as the nonsteroidal anti-inflammatory agents that may precipitate gastrointestinal hemorrhage. However, renal disease is known to change the metabolism of drugs by the liver.[8]

The risk of hepatorenal syndrome should be kept in mind when prescribing potentially nephrotoxic drugs to patients with impaired liver function. Even if there is no evidence to suggest that renal function is impaired, nephrotoxicity from aminoglycosides is potentiated by liver disease. The mechanism for this is unclear because their elimination is almost entirely renal.

Liver disease may also cause pharmacodynamic changes by an effect on drug receptors. This may change the sensitivity of the patient to the drug.

Drug Interactions

Drug interactions are affected by liver disease. Induction and inhibition of cytochrome P450 may be reduced in the presence of impaired liver function. Acocella and colleagues have shown that after chronic dosing, serum concentrations of rifampicin decreased in normal patients because of induction, but increased in patients with cirrhosis.[19] This suggests that enzyme induction had not occurred in the cirrhotic patients.

Tolerance

Tolerance occurs whenever a central depressant is given repeatedly. It has been reported with thiopentone,[20] nitrous oxide,[21] midazolam,[22,23] and opioids.[24–28] However, tolerance to the different effects of a drug may occur at differing rates. For example, with opioids as tolerance to analgesia develops so does tolerance to respiratory depression, but not to the smooth muscle effects, such as constipation.

Tolerance to alcohol also occurs. A possible mechanism for this has been described involving a decrease in mRNA that is responsible for the synthesis of the $GABA_A$ receptor.[29]

The combination of tolerance and worsening encephalopathy in a patient with liver disease can make it difficult to judge the right dose of a sedative or analgesic drug. If the patient needs intensive care, and especially ventilatory support, the importance of using a sedation score routinely cannot be overemphasized.[30] Its use should help avoid unnecessary and dangerous oversedation.

Therapeutic Implications

Liver disease has a complex effect on the pharmacokinetics and pharmacodynamics of many drugs. Consequently, drugs should be prescribed with extreme caution to patients with liver disease. Monitoring of the plasma concentrations of some drugs is important in patients with liver dysfunction because the desired therapeutic effect may be achieved with a low concentration in the blood. This is particularly important with drugs with narrow therapeutic index. Unfortunately, it is of value only in drugs where the plasma concentration correlates with effect. In addition, changes in the bioavailability, protein binding, clearance, and volume of distribution of various drugs may not have a simple additive effect on drug pharmacokinetics. The pharmacodynamic result may be greater than the sum of the contributing factors, or one change may compensate for another.[16]

Attempts have been made to correlate pharmacokinetic changes with liver function tests. These have not met with any consistent success,[6] although a low serum albumin correlates with some changes in patients with chronic liver disease. More investigation into liver disease and drug metabolism is needed before generalizations can be made.

Benzodiazepines

These drugs are frequently used in patients with liver disease. The indications include sedation during minor procedures such as gastroscopy, premedication before operation, and sedation during postoperative intensive care.

As mentioned before, the effect of liver disease on the pharmacokinetics of an individual benzodiazepine will depend on the metabolic pathway it follows. Since phase I reactions are affected to a greater extent than phase II reactions, the pharmacokinetics of the substituted benzodiazepines will be less affected by liver disease than those of the unsubstituted benzodiazepines.[31]

Diazepam

Diazepam, although largely superseded by newer benzodiazepines, is still used to provide sedation in certain circumstances. It has a half-life of 24–57 hours in normal subjects and is metabolized primarily by phase I pathways. Two of its metabolites, des-methyldiazepam and oxazepam, are active. Oxazepam undergoes glucuronidation (phase II metabolism) and its pharmacokinetics are relatively unaffected by liver disease. However, because desmethyldiazepam is metabolized by a phase I reaction its metabolism is greatly altered in patients with liver disease.[31]

Several studies have shown changes in the pharmacokinetics of intravenous diazepam in patients with liver disease (Table 5-1). These studies show that hepatic clearance is decreased, elimination half-life is prolonged, and volume of distribution is increased in patients with cirrhosis, viral hepatitis, and chronic active hepatitis, but not in patients with extrahepatic cholestasis.[32] The results of these studies are summarized in the table. The protein binding of diazepam is also decreased in patients with cirrhosis.[33,34]

Klotz and colleagues[35] showed only small changes in the pharmacokinetics of diazepam after repeated oral dosing in patients with cirrhosis. However, accumulation of diazepam and desmethyldiazepam has been shown in patients with cirrhosis after repeated oral dosing over a long period. This resulted in increased sedation, although this was partly compensated for by the development of tolerance.[36,37]

Clinically, diazepam has been reported to produce more profound sedation and slower recovery in patients with severe liver disease.[38,39] The depth of sedation has been shown to correlate with the severity of liver dysfunction.[34,38] The response to diazepam has also been shown to correlate with the serum concentration of albumin.[40] This study also showed that for the same degree of sedation produced by diazepam, electroencephalographic changes were greater in patients with cirrhosis than in controls. The changes were greatest in patients with a history of encephalopathy.

The metabolism of diazepam may also be reduced by other drugs given to patients with liver failure. For example, cimetidine may be given to prevent gastrointestinal bleeding. This inhibits the cytochromes P450 responsible for the metabolism of diazepam. Rarely, diazepam causes a deterioration in liver function tests.[41]

Desmethyldiazepam

Desmethyldiazepam is the principal metabolite of diazepam. In patients with liver disease its production is decreased and is slower than in controls. Desmethyldiazepam is eliminated more slowly than diazepam; the clearance of diazepam is 32.3 mL/min and that of desmethyldiazepam is 11.3 mL/m. In patients with liver disease given a single intravenous dose of diazepam, the clearance of desmethyldiazepam decreased to 4.6 mL/min. The volume of distribution was unchanged and the elimination half-life was increased from 50.9 to 108.2 hours.[35]

Table 5-1. The Reported Pharmacokinetic Variables of Diazepam in Patients with Cirrhosis, Acute Viral Hepatitis and Chronic Active Hepatitis.

	$T_{1/2\beta}$ (h)	Cl (mL/min)	Vd Binding (L/kg)	Protein binding(%)	Study
Control	43.0 (3.2)	15.1 (3.1)	0.98 (0.18)	—	Branch and Shand, 1976[40]
	46.6 (14.2)	26.6 (4.1)	1.13 (0.28)	97.8 (1.0)	Klotz et al., 1975;[150] Klotz et al., 1973[151]
	32.1 (20.4)	35.0 (14.7)	—	—	Andreasen et al., 1976[152]
	46.6 (14.2)	32.3 (11.0)	1.04 (0.11)	—	Klotz et al., 1977[35]
Cirrhosis	48.7 (12.1)	10.6 (2.0)	0.69 (0.14)	—	Branch and Shand, 1976[40]
Cirrhosis + ascites	77.4 (4.3)	6.0 (1.47)	0.59 (0.10)	—	Branch and Shand, 1976[40]
Cirrhosis	105.6 (15.2)	13.8 (2.4)	1.74 (0.21)	95.3 (1.8)	
Cirrhosis	164.0 (152.0)	17.1 (6.5)**	—	—	Andreasen et al., 1976[152]
Cirrhosis	99.2 (23.2)	8.0	0.71	—	Klotz et al., 1977[35]
Acute viral hepatitis	74.5 (27.5)	—	—	—	Klotz et al., 1975;[150] Klotz et al., 1975[33]
Chronic active hepatitis	59.7 (23.0)	15.45	—	—	Klotz et al., 1977[35]

Values shown as mean (standard deviation). *p<0.05.
$T_{1/2\beta}$ = elimination half-life, Cl = clearance, vol = volume of distribution.

Oxazepam

The pharmacokinetics of oxazepam are unaltered in patients with cirrhosis and viral hepatitis.[42]

Midazolam

Midazolam is a water-soluble benzodiazepine with a short elimination half-life, a relatively large volume of distribution, and a high plasma clearance.[43] Its extraction ratio is in the intermediate range and its hepatic clearance depends on both hepatic blood flow and hepatic enzyme activity. In normal subjects, it has a rapid onset and short duration of action.[44] It undergoes phase I metabolism by the cytochrome P450 enzyme system, and its main metabolite is 1-hydroxy midazolam. This metabolite is pharmacologically active but has a shorter half-life than midazolam, so its activity is not clinically significant in normal subjects. 1-Hydroxy midazolam undergoes phase II conjugation to form a glucuronide that is eliminated in the urine.[43]

It has been suggested that about 6% of the population are poor metabolizers of midazolam, possibly because of a pharmacogenetic abnormality.[43a] However, we have shown in liver tissue from human organ donors that all have this cytochrome P450 and it is not, therefore, a pharmacogenetic abnormality. What does vary at least 100 times is the expression of this enzyme.[43b]

Since midazolam undergoes predominantly phase I metabolism, it would be expected that its pharmacokinetics would be significantly altered in patients with liver disease. However, the pharmacokinetic profile of oral midazolam in patients with compensated cirrhosis is similar to that of healthy volunteers.[45] Also, after liver transplantation, an acute hepatic injury, the pharmacokinetics of midazolam are unchanged, although the plasma concentration of 1-hydroxy midazolam is increased.[46] It is only in patients with severe cirrhosis that the pharmacokinetics of intravenous midazolam are altered. McGilchrist and colleagues[47] reported that in patients with severe cirrhosis, the clearance and elimination half-life of midazolam were significantly decreased, and the volume of distribution was slightly increased (Table 5-2).

A prolonged clinical effect of midazolam has been reported in patients with chronic liver disease.[38,45,47] The increase in sedation appears to correlate with the degree of liver impairment and a previous history of encephalopathy. This may be related to an increased sensitivity of these patients to the central effects of benzodiazepines.[47] The increased sedation does not correlate with the degree of protein binding, although a decrease in protein binding does increase the speed of onset of sedation.[48]

Investigation of patients during the anhepatic phase of liver transplantation has shown that metabolism of midazolam proceeds in the absence of a liver.[49] This suggests that extrahepatic sites are involved in the metabolism of midazolam, at least in patients with liver disease.

Acute liver injury occurs during septic shock. It is probably caused by the reduction in liver blood flow (causing hypoxia) and the release of inflammatory mediators. These may have direct effects on the drug-metabolizing enzymes.[8,9] These changes have been shown to change quickly as the patient's condition improves or worsens.[50]

Midazolam does not change liver function tests.[51] Although it does change both hepatic arterial and portal blood flow, the effects tend to cancel each other out, so no hepatic hypoxia occurs.[52]

Table 5-2. The Reported Pharmacokinetic Parameters of Midazolam in Patients with Cirrhosis and Following Liver Transplantation.

Intravenous	$T_{1/2\beta}$ (h)	Cl (mL/min/kg)	Vd (L)			Study
Controls	1.6 (0.3)	10.4 (1.3)	80.7 (10.3)			MacGilchrist et al., 1986[47]
Severe cirrhosis	3.9 (0.8)	5.4 (1.0)	106.2 (11.9)			MacGilchrist et al., 1986[47]
Post liver transplant	2.28 (0.43)	7.4 (2.7)	—			Shelly, Quinn, and Park, 1989[153]
Oral	$T_{1/2\beta}$ (h)	Tmax (h)	Cmax (ng/ml)	AUC (ng.h/ml)		Study
Cirrhosis	3.8 (1.0)	0.6 (0.14)	141 (41)	438 (244)		Rinetti et al., 1985[154]

Values shown as mean (standard deviation).
Tmax = Time to maximum concentration, Cmax = maximum concentration, AUC = area under the time/concentration curve

Lorazepam

Lorazepam is an effective sedative and a potent amnesic, but has a slow onset of action. Lorazepam has a terminal half-life of 2–3 hours in healthy individuals.[53] However, accumulation may occur after repeated doses. Lorazepam and its metabolites have been detected in significant plasma concentrations up to 24 hours after it has been given.[54] The metabolism of lorazepam is predominantly by phase II conjugation to lorazepam glucuronides.

In patients with cirrhosis, lorazepam has a prolonged elimination half-life owing to an increased volume of distribution. This in turn is attributable to a decrease in the protein binding of lorazepam. The total and unbound clearance of lorazepam is not changed in cirrhosis. However, in acute viral hepatitis the pharmacokinetics of lorazepam are unaltered (Table 5-3).[55] The metabolism of lorazepam remaining normal in liver disease supports the impression that phase II reactions are relatively spared in liver disease. Alternatively, lorazepam may undergo extrahepatic metabolism in the presence of liver disease.[56]

Temazepam

Temazepam is available only as an oral preparation and reports of its half-life range from 5 to 15 hours.[57] It is metabolized primarily to a glucuronide, although a small quantity of oxazepam and its glucuronide are found in the urine after temazepam has been given.

The pharmacokinetics of temazepam are unchanged in patients with cirrhosis.[57,58] However, one study reported a significant reduction in protein binding and a slight decrease in the free clearance of temazepam in patients with cirrhosis.[57] Another study demonstrated a decreased absorption half-life of temazepam in cirrhotic patients (Table 5-4), but no significant accumulation occurred during repeated dosing.[58]

Flumazenil

Flumazenil (Ro 15-1788) is a specific benzodiazepine antagonist. It has been shown to have an elimination half-life of about one hour in normal volunteers.[59] About 50% of flumazenil is bound to albumin at normal pH. Clinical trials have shown the efficacy of flumazenil in reversing the effects of benzodiazepine overdose,[60] single-dose therapeutic administration of benzodiazepines,[61] and after the longer term use of benzodiazepines for intensive care sedation.[62]

In liver disease the elimination of flumazenil is reduced. After similar doses plasma concentrations are increased in patients with cirrhosis and these increase further when humans are made anhepatic.[63,65]

Benzodiazepine-like substances have been shown in fulminant liver failure.[66] This has led to flumazenil being used to try to reverse hepatic encephalopathy. Unfortunately, most of the reports are anecdotal.[2,66–68] When all of the available evidence was reviewed a short-term improvement was seen in 72% of the patients given flumazenil.[68] Prospective, randomized trials are at the time of writing being done to see what place flumazenil has in routine treatment of hepatic encephalopathy.

Clinical Recommendations

During long-term oral therapy with diazepam in patients with liver disease, the dose should be reduced by 50%[37] or by 34%.[18] For oral use, lorazepam and temazepam are safe unless treatment is long-term or

Table 5-3. Pharmacokinetic Parameters of Lorazepam in Patients with Cirrhosis and Acute Viral Hepatitis

	$T_{1/2\beta}$ (h)	Cl (mL/min/kg)	Vd Binding (L/kg)	Protein (%)
Control	21.7 (7.6)	0.75 (0.23)	1.28 (0.34)	93.2 (1.8)
Cirrhosis	41.2 (24.5)*	0.81 (0.48)	2.01 (0.82)**	88.6 (2.5)**
Acute viral hepatitis	8.3 (8.9)	0.74 (0.34)	1.52 (0.61)	91.0 (1.9)

Values shown as mean (standard deviation). * = $p < 0.02$, ** = $p < 0.01$.
From Kraus et al.[55]

Table 5-4. The Pharmacokinetic Parameters of Temazepam in Patients with Cirrhosis.

	$T_{1/2}$abs (min)	$T_{1/2\beta}$ (h)	$T_{1/2\beta}$ (h)	Cl (mL/min/kg)	Vd (L/kg)	Study
Control	7.61 (5.42)	1.34 (0.63)	15.99 (5.76)	1.38 (5.87)	1.63 (1.26)	Ghabrail et al., 1986[57]
Cirrhosis	6.80 (3.40)	1.05 (0.83)	12.83 (5.73)	1.34 (1.02)	1.09 (0.39)	
	Tmax (h)	**Protein Binding (%)**	**$T_{1/2\beta}$ (h)**	**Cl (mL/min/kg)**	**Vd (1/kg)**	
Control	0.61 (0.1)	96.49 (0.5)	14.6 (1.5)	1.03 (0.15)	1.25 (0.17)	Ochs et al., 1986[58]
Cirrhosis	2.89 (0.9)**	96.11 (0.2)	10.6 (1.5)	1.03 (0.13)	0.96 (0.62)	

Values shown as mean (standard deviation) or mean (standard error). Cl = oral clearance, $T_{1/2}$abs = Absorption half-life, ** = $p < 0.05$.

the patient has hepatic encephalopathy. Intravenous benzodiazepines should be given cautiously and the effect monitored closely; midazolam is the agent of choice.

Chlormethiazole

Chlormethiazole is a sedative frequently used in patients with delirium tremens.[69] Initial recovery is by redistribution, and it is eliminated entirely by biotransformation. Prolonged infusion of chlormethiazole may lead to accumulation and delayed recovery.[70,71] This is because once the distribution space has been saturated, the drug can leave the plasma only as a result of hepatic metabolism.

In patients with cirrhosis the clearance of chlormethiazole is decreased.[72] This is thought to be caused by decreased hepatic blood flow. When chlormethiazole is given orally to patients with cirrhosis, the bioavailability is approximately ten times higher than that in healthy volunteers.[72] This results from a decrease in first-pass metabolism and correlates with serum concentrations of bilirubin and alkaline phosphatase. These results are summarised in Table 5-5.

Chlormethiazole has a protective effect against infection after burns.[73] Whether this also occurs with other injuries or illnesses is unknown. If it does then chlormethiazole could be an extremely useful agent.

Anesthetic Agents

Premedication is indicated only in patients with group A liver disease according to the Child-Turcotte classification. If centrally acting drugs are given to more seriously ill patients with liver disease, they may precipitate encephalopathy. A short-acting benzodiazepine such as temazepam is

appropriate. Intramuscular premedication is best avoided because of the coagulopathy associated with liver dysfunction.

The induction agents in common use are protein bound, and the free drug fraction is increased in liver disease when serum albumin is low, which leads to an enhanced effect. Thiopentone and etomidate are metabolized in the liver, but because their action is ended by redistribution, their duration of action is normal, unless large or repeated doses are given.

Fentanyl and alfentanil are suitable opioid analgesic agents for use during anesthesia in patients with liver failure because they have short half-lives and inactive metabolites.

Nitrous Oxide

Nitrous oxide, when used over several days to provide sedation and analgesia for patients suffering from tetanus, was shown to produce an aplastic anemia.[74] Amos and colleagues[75] prospectively studied 70 critically ill patients, 50 of whom had received nitrous oxide. Acute megaloblastic bone marrow changes were present in 22 of the 70 patients, 18 of whom had received nitrous oxide for 2 to 6 hours

Table 5-5. The Pharmacokinetic Parameters of Chlormethiazole in Patients with Cirrhosis.

	$T_{1/2\beta}$ (h)	Cl (mL/min/kg)	Oral Bioavailability (%)
Control	6.6 (1.0)	18.1 (1.2)	11.8 (2.9)
Cirrhosis	8.7 (1.4)	12.8 (1.7)*	136.0 (11.0)**

Values shown as mean (standard deviation). * = $p < 0.05$, ** = $p < 0.001$.
From Pentikainen, P.J., Neuvonen, P.J., Tarpila, S., and Sylvalahti, E. (1978) Effect of cirrhosis of the liver on the pharmacokinetics of chlormethiazole. *British Medical Journal* 2:861–63.

during anesthesia. Sixteen of the 18 patients who received nitrous oxide died. All the patients were also investigated with a deoxyuridine suppression test on the bone marrow aspirate, which indicated interference with the function of vitamin B_{12} and subsequently folate deficiency.

Skacel and colleagues[76] compared serial bone marrow changes in nine surgical patients who needed artificial ventilation and who received nitrous oxide for 4 to 36 hours with three patients who did not receive nitrous oxide. After 24 hours gross megaloblastic changes were seen that took one week to return to normal in the group that received nitrous oxide. No such changes were seen in the group that did not receive nitrous oxide. The rapidity of onset and similarity to animal work has been confirmed by Koblin and colleagues.[77]

The mechanism for these effects appears to be the irreversible interaction of nitrous oxide with vitamin B_{12}. This is an essential coenzyme for the enzymes methionine synthetase and methyl malonyl CoA mutase. These enzymes are essential for the synthesis of methionine and tetrahydrofolate,[78] and because they are inhibited after nitrous oxide anesthesia, plasma concentrations of methionine will decrease. Methionine is needed for methylation reactions and to produce 10-formyl tetrahydrofolate from folate, which is essential for the production of deoxythymidine and thus DNA. It is the inability to produce DNA that leads to the bone marrow changes.

The London group[79] has shown that the administration of 5-formyl tetra hydrofolinic acid can overcome the effects of nitrous oxide if given in sufficient doses.

Induction Agents

Thiopentone

Thiopentone is the most frequently used anesthetic induction agent. Its action is terminated by redistri-

bution to extravascular sites, and it is subsequently metabolized by several cytochromes P450. When infusions are used (such as in the management of raised intracranial pressure) metabolism becomes important as a way of ending its effects. After a subtotal hepatectomy (85–95%) in rats, recovery time from thiopentone was prolonged. This has been confirmed in man.[80,81] Patients with chronic or acute liver disease sleep longer than fit patients after thiopentone.

Although patients with mild to moderate cirrhosis have a normal total plasma clearance and volume of distribution, protein binding (normally 80%) is significantly decreased. The increased free fraction correlates with the decreased plasma concentration of albumin. After correction for the decrease in protein binding, the intrinsic clearance and volume of distribution of free drug are decreased, (Table 5-6), although the difference is not significant. This suggests that the metabolism of thiopentone may be reduced in patients with mild to moderate cirrhosis, and it may be impaired further in patients with more severe disease. This may have important consequences if repeated doses or an infusion are used in patients with liver failure.

Thiopentone does not change function tests, unless large doses (18 mg/kg) are given. Then there are changes in hepatocellular enzymes and plasma pseudocholinesterase. These return to normal over three or four days after the thiopentone is stopped. Giving thiopentone for a long time may induce cytochromes P450 and other enzymes.

Etomidate

Etomidate is a useful induction agent for patients with an unstable cardiovascular system. Thus, it may be useful in high-risk patients, such as those who are bleeding. However, continuous infusions of etomidate are no longer used to provide sedation for critically ill patients. This is because, when used in this way, it was associated with increased mor-

Table 5-6. The Pharmacokinetic Parameters of Thiopentone in Patients with Cirrhosis.

	$T_{1/2\beta}$ (h)	Cl (L/min)	Vd Binding (L/kg)	Protein (%)
Control	8.8 (1.6)	28.3 (9.0)	16.9 (4.6)	85.5 (3.4)
Cirrhosis	11.9 (4.2)	18.2 (10.5)	14.0 (6.9)	74.8 (3.9)*

Values shown as mean (standard deviation). * = p < 0.01.
From Pandele, G., Chaux, F., Salvadori, C., Farinotti, M., and Duvaldstein, P. (1983). Thiopental pharmacokinetics in patients with cirrhosis. *Anesthesiology* 59:123–26.

tality.[82] The increased mortality was subsequently shown to be caused by suppression of adrenal steroid synthesis.[83,84]

Propofol

Propofol is a substituted phenol solubilized in a fat emulsion. It has a short elimination half-life[85] and rapid termination of action. It is completely and rapidly metabolized to sulphate and glucuronide conjugates of propofol and of the corresponding quinol. The rapid clearance of propofol (1.3-2.1 L/min) exceeds hepatic blood flow (1.5 L/min) and extrahepatic sites of metabolism, particularly in the lung and gastrointestinal tract, have been suggested.[86–88] Extrahepatic metabolism of propofol has been shown to occur in man,[89] but the capacity of the extrahepatic sites appears to be small and does not include the lung.

Propofol is used not just for induction of anesthesia but also for sedation if a patient needs ventilatory support. Because it is metabolized almost exclusively by phase II enzymes it is little affected by liver disease. There are no significant changes in the pharmacokinetics of propofol in patients with cirrhosis after either a bolus dose[90] or an infusion [90,91] (Table 5-7). However, the recovery time has been shown to be prolonged in patients with cirrhosis, and the need for supplementary fentanyl was decreased.[90] Interestingly, patients with cirrhosis wake up with the same plasma concentration as normal controls.[91]

The hepatic circulation may be changed by propofol. Isolated strips of rat portal vein and hepatic artery exposed to propofol showed a dose-related relaxation.[92] Mather and colleagues[88] showed a 15% decrease in hepatic blood flow in sheep anesthetized with propofol.

Propofol in normal doses does not change liver function tests.[93,94] However, in large doses the solvent soya bean extract may interfere with these tests as part of the fat overload syndrome. This occurs only in critically ill patients given an intravenous infusion of propofol over several days. Some of the features of this are shown in Table 5-8.

To avoid the fat overload syndrome in patients needing long-term intravenous infusions, we recommend:

- Do not use both a fat emulsion as part of an intravenous feeding regimen and propofol for sedation.
- Measure the serum triglycerides before and after starting a propofol infusion. If the level is twice the upper limit of normal do not start, or stop, the infusion.
- Centrifuge a sample of serum each day. If it is lipemic stop or reduce the infusion.
- Do not give propofol to patients with metabolic abnormalities of fat metabolism, such as hyperlipidemia or hypothyroidism.

We also avoid propofol in patients who are hypoxemic ($F_1O_2 > 0.6$) since it may worsen shunting. In addition, we do not use it if the patient is thrombocytopenic ($< 20 \times 10^9$/L) because it may reduce platelet stickiness. These relative contraindications are controversial and need further investigation.[95]

Infection has been reported after the use of propofol in anesthesia.[96,97] These infections are thought to be related to the soya bean extract supporting microbiological growth. This might be important in the patient with liver disease, who is immunocompromised. However, we were unable to show any risk of infection when we studied this problem in a general intensive care unit.[98]

Table 5-7. The Pharmacokinetic Parameters of Propofol in Patients with Cirrhosis following Bolus and Infusion Administration

	$T_{1/2\beta}$ (h)	C1 (L/min)	Vd Binding (L/kg)	Protein Binding (%)	
Bolus control	0.62 (0.17)	2.2 (0.6)	6.3 (1.0)	97.8 (0.2)	
Cirrhosis	0.65 (0.3)	1.7 (0.6)	8.2 (5.2)	98.1 (0.2)	
	$T_{1/2\beta}$ (h)	C1 (L/min)	Vd (1)	Time to Waken (min)	Analgesic Supplement (e.g., fentanyl)
Infusion control	3.7 (1.1)	2.1 (0.42)	546 (169)	17 (5)	460 (240)
Cirrhosis	4.4 (1.5)	2.17 (0.64)	637 (349)	38 (34)*	270 (225)

Values shown as mean (standard deviation).
From Servin, F., Haberer, J.P., Cockshott, I.D., Farinotti, R., and Desmonts, J.M. (1986) Propofol pharmacokinetics in patients with cirrhosis. *Anesthesiology* 65:A554; Servin, F., Desmonts, J.M., Farinotti, R., Haberer, J.P., and Winckler, C. (1988) Pharmacokinetics of propofol administered by continuous infusion in patients with cirrhosis. *Anaesthesia* 43:23–24.

Table 5-8. The Fat Overload Syndrome

• Fever	• Tachycardia
• Jaundice	• Headache
↑ *transaminases*	
↑ *bilirubin*	
• Cerebral irritability	• Hepatosplenomegaly
• Hyperlipidemia	• Increased risk of hemorrhage
	↑ *prothrombin time*
	↑ *fibrin degradation products*
• Fatty infiltration	
of organs	
• Interference with labo-	
ratory measurements	

From Park, G. R. and Gempeler, F. (1993) Intravenous anaesthetic agents. In Sedation and Analgesia (pp. 209–53). London: Saunders.

Propofol is expensive and its use is justified only if the need for rapid and reliable assessment of conscious level is essential. Those patients who are encephalopathic or at risk of it are one such group. It is impossible to predict if they will accumulate alternative agents, such as benzodiazepines, that may then result in prolonged coma.

Ketamine

Ketamine has some properties that make it the induction agent of choice in certain circumstances: it maintains cardiovascular stability, it is a potent bronchodilator, in low doses it is a potent analgesic, and it is noncumulative. However, reports of hallucinations after its use as an induction agent limit its use in clinical practise. Ketamine undergoes oxidation metabolism in the liver, and drugs such as diazepam, secobarbital, and hydroxyzine are known to inhibit this metabolism.

No pharmacokinetic studies have yet been performed on ketamine in patients with liver disease. However, it has been shown that in patients with extrahepatic biliary obstruction, no significant changes take place in the metabolism or pharmacodynamics of ketamine.[99]

Opioids

Morphine

Morphine is commonly used to provide analgesia for critically ill patients, often by continuous intravenous infusion. Morphine undergoes extensive biotransformation, and less than 10% of a dose given parenterally is excreted unchanged in the urine. Only 30% is bound to albumin in the blood.

The principal metabolite is morphine-3-glucuronide (M3G), which is pharmacologically inactive. Morphine-6-glucuronide (M6G)[100] and normorphine[101,102] are both pharmacologically active metabolites of morphine. Morphine-6-glucuronide given parenterally to rats has an analgesic potency four times that of morphine and a duration of action twice that of morphine. Intracisternal administration of M6G reveals an analgesic potency 44 times that of morphine.[100]

It has been suggested that morphine may be at least in part a "prodrug," and some of its activity comes from the metabolites. The two metabolites are made by different pathways. Furthermore, although M6G is analgesic, M3G is antianalgesic.[103,104] The two pathways making these metabolites may be affected differently by disease, leading to a predominance of one metabolite and a change in effect. Indeed, one patient has been reported in whom there appeared to be a lack of the pathway for M6G. That patient did not get analgesia when given morphine.[105]

One of the purposes of drug metabolism is to make substances more polar and unable to cross membranes. It is therefore surprising that M6G and M3G are able to exert pharmacological effects. Carrupt and colleagues[106] have explained this apparent contradiction. They have shown that molecules of M6G and M3G are able to change the orientation of the polar groups. Thus, in a lipid environment they are fat soluble, while in aqueous surroundings they are water soluble.

The liver has long been thought to be the site of morphine metabolism.[107] However, studies performed in the anhepatic phase of liver transplantation have shown that a limited amount of extrahepatic metabolism of morphine occurs.[108] The kidney was postulated as a possible site of extrahepatic metabolism, based on studies on patients with renal failure.[109–111] However, the radioimmunoassay used for morphine in these studies was subsequently found to cross react with M3G and M6G.[112] More recent studies using high-performance liquid chromatography[113] and specific radioimmunoassay[114] to measure plasma concentrations of morphine have shown that the clearance of morphine is normal in patients with renal failure. This suggests that morphine is unlikely to undergo significant metabolism in the kidney. In contrast to these studies, the importance of the kidney in the elimination of morphine and its metabolites has been shown clinically.[115,116]

Recent investigations have shown both normal[117] and abnormal[118] morphine clearance in patients with cirrhosis. It has been suggested that these differences are related to differences in the severity of hepatic dysfunction in the two studies. Renal function is often compromised in patients with liver disease. Therefore, even if morphine is metabolized normally by these patients, either in the liver or at extrahepatic sites, the metabolites, which are all excreted by the kidneys, will accumulate. Accumulation of M6G, which is pharmacologically active, leads to clinical signs of opioid intoxication.[115,116]

Plasma concentrations of pancreatic enzymes may increase after morphine is given, because of spasm of the sphincter of Oddi.[119]

Pethidine

Pethidine is a synthetic opioid. It is metabolized principally to pethidinic acid and norpethidine by a cytochrome P450. Pethidinic acid is subsequently conjugated with glucuronic acid and is then excreted in the urine. Norpethidine is either excreted unchanged or further metabolized to norphethidinic acid. Norpethidine is thought to be the only pharmacologically active metabolite of pethidine, causing agitation and fits. It has a longer elimination half-life than pethidine and accumulates after repeated doses and in patients with renal failure.[120,121] About 64% of the total amount of pethidine in the blood is bound to plasma proteins.

The clearance of pethidine is decreased in patients with cirrhosis; the volume of distribution and degree of protein binding are unchanged (Table 5-9).[122–124] A similar pattern has been reported in patients with viral hepatitis.[122] The prolonged half-life of pethidine in these patients has therefore been attributed to impaired metabolism.[122] Norpethidine concentrations are lower than normal and its clearance is also decreased.[123,124]

Pethidine undergoes considerable presystemic elimination. In patients with liver disease this elimination is impaired, and oral bioavailability is increased by 81%.[123]

Pharmacodynamic studies of pethidine in patients with liver disease have not been performed, Prolonged activity has been reported,[125] but the influence of other contributing factors cannot be evaluated. The dose of pethidine should be reduced in patients with liver disease, and oral pethidine should be used with caution.

Phenoperidine

Phenoperidine is a synthetic opioid derived from pethidine. It has an elimination half-life of approximately 60 minutes and approximately half is metabolized to pethidine and norpethidine.

In patients with mild cirrhosis, phenoperidine has a prolonged elimination half-life and a reduced clearance (Table 5-10).[126] This appears to be caused by a decrease in hepatic metabolism since the proportion of the dose excreted as pethidine and norpethidine is decreased, whereas that excreted as phenoperidine is increased. Since these changes were observed in patients with mild cirrhosis, more severe pharmacokinetic and pharmacodynamic disturbances may be seen in patients with greater impairment of their liver function. Some cases of jaundice have been reported after its use.[127]

Table 5-9. The Reported Pharmacokinetic Parameters of Pethidine in Patients with Cirrhosis

Intravenous	$T_{1/2\beta}$ (h)	C1 (mL/min)	Vd (L/kg)		Study
Controls	3.21 (0.8)	1316 (383)	4.17 (1.33)		Klotz et al., 1974[122]
	5.20 (0.9)	900 (210)	4.70 (0.70)		Pond et al., 1981[124]
Cirrhosis	7.04 (0.9)**	664 (293)***	5.76 (2.55)		Klotz et al., 1974[122]
	11.4 (4.4)***	392 (105)***	5.20 (0.30)		Pond et al., 1981[124]
Oral	$T_{1/2\beta}$ (h)	C1 (mL/min)	Vd (1)	Bioavailability	Study
Control	3.55 (0.42)	900 (316)	232 (53)	0.48 (0.13)	Neal et al., 1979[123]
				0.53 (0.07)	Pond et al., 1981[124]
Cirrhosis	4.38 (1.28)*	573 (158)*	263 (28)	0.87 (0.27)*	Neal et al., 1979[123]
				0.85 (0.12)**	Pond et al., 1981[124]

Values shown as mean (standard deviation). $* = p < 0.05$, $** = p < 0.001$, $*** = p < 0.002$.

Table 5-10. The Pharmacokinetic Parameters of Phenoperidine in Patients with Cirrhosis.

	$T_{1/2}\beta$ (h)	Cl (mL/min/kg)	Vd (l/kg)
Control	1.01 (0.13)	26 (4)	2.4 (0.6)
Cirrhosis	1.53 (0.30)	17 (3)	2.1 (0.4)

Values shown as mean (standard error).

From Isherwood, C.N., Calvey, T.N., Williams, N.E., Chan, K., and Murray, G.R. (1984) Elimination of phenoperidine in liver disease. *British Journal of Anaesthesia* 56:843–46.

Fentanyl

Fentanyl is a synthetic opioid structurally related to pethidine. It is metabolized by hydrolysis and *N*-dealkylation to metabolites that are excreted in the urine. Only 4–7% is excreted unchanged in the urine. Its effects, however, are ended principally by rapid redistribution of the parent drug from the central compartment and its extensive tissue uptake. The slow reuptake of fentanyl from certain tissues is thought to be the rate-limiting step of its elimination from the body.[128] Fentanyl has a long elimination half-life of approximately 200 minutes, and its clearance is independent of protein binding (70% in the plasma).

The pharmacokinetics of a single bolus dose of fentanyl are not altered significantly in the presence of mild cirrhosis (Table 5-11).[129] The fact that the long terminal half-life of fentanyl probably reflects slow release from tissue depots rather than hepatic elimination[128] may explain the apparent lack of effect of cirrhosis on the pharmacokinetics of fentanyl.[129] It is possible that the pharmacokinetics of fentanyl may be altered in patients with more severely impaired liver function. Repeated doses of fentanyl lead to accumulation because of the prolonged elimination phase. In these circumstances, the biotransformation of fentanyl may became the rate-limiting step in its elimination, and impaired liver function may prolong clearance further.

Adequate liver function is needed for the metabolism of fentanyl, since the plasma clearance of fentanyl in anhepatic dogs is reduced from 45 to 4 mL/kg min. Extrahepatic sites of fentanyl metabolism have been suggested to explain the remaining clearance.[130]

Alfentanil

Alfentanil is a short-acting opiate structurally related to fentanyl. It has a small volume of distribution (0.4 L/kg) and a short elimination half-life of 98 minutes in healthy subjects.[131] Alfentanil is extensively redistributed, although not as extensively as fentanyl. It is rapidly metabolized to metabolites thought to be pharmacologically inactive.

Alfentanil is highly protein bound to α-1-acidglycoprotein, and the pattern of change in the concentration of this carrier protein in liver disease affects the pharmacokinetics of alfentanil.

A decreased clearance of alfentanil has been reported in patients with moderate cirrhosis (Table 5-12).[17,132] Similar changes have been seen after liver transplantation. In a study of seven patients given two doses of alfentanil 12 hours apart considerable variation in the pharmacokinetic variables was seen. Only one patient had normal pharmacokinetic variables. Four had an increased volume of distribution after the first dose that became normal after the second. Two patients showed a reduced plasma clearance of alfentanil.[133] These changes probably reflect recovery from anesthesia or surgery, as well as diminishing blood loss and fluid shifts.[134]

In patients with cirrhosis the degree of protein binding of alfentanil was decreased[132] while the concentration of α-1-acidglycoprotein itself was normal. This suggests a reduced binding capacity of alfentanil to α-1-acidglycoprotein in these patients.

A reduced clearance of alfentanil is also seen in the elderly.[135] Like midazolam it was suggested that

Table 5-11. The Pharmacokinetic Parameters of Fentanyl in Patients with Cirrhosis

	$T_{1/2}\beta$ (h)	Cl (mL/min/kg)	Vd (L/kg)	AUC (ng/mL/min)
Control	4.38 (0.82)	10.8 (1.2)	3.44 (64)	518 (53)
Cirrhosis	5.07 (1.23)	11.3 (1.6)	4.27 (65)	507 (63)

Values shown as mean (standard error). AUC = Area under the plasma concentration vs. time curve.

From Haberer, J.P., Schoeffler, P., Couderc, E., and Duvaldestin, P. (1982) Fentanyl pharmacokinetics in anaesthetised patients with cirrhosis. *British Journal of Anaesthesia* 54:1267–70.

Table 5-12. The Reported Pharmacokinetic Parameters of Alfentanil in Patients with Cirrhosis and following Liver Transplantation

	$T_{1/2\beta}$ (h)	C1 (mL/min/kg)	Vd (mL/kg)	Protein Binding (%)	Study
Controls	1.5 (0.3)	3.1 (1.6)	356 (167)	88.2 (4.1)	Ferrier et al., 1985[17]
	1.5 (0.3)	3.1 (1.6)	365 (165)	88.2 (4.4)	Hug and Chaffman, 1984[132]
Cirrhosis	3.65 (2.13)**	1.6 (1.0)**	404 (230)	80.5 (10.0)**	
	3.75 (1.72)**	1.3 (0.6)*	372 (131)	81.2 (9.5)	Hug and Chaffman, 1984[132]
Post Liver Transplant	4.7 (3.65)	4.34 (3.1)	1054 (486)	—	
	3.9 (2.15)	2.6 (1.6)	667 (339)	—	Shelly, Walker, and Park, 1989[133]

Values shown as mean (standard deviation). $* = p < 0.05$, $** = p < 0.01$

a subset of the normal population has a pharmacogenetic abnormality.[136] This is now known not to be so.[137]

No pharmacodynamic investigations of alfentanil in patients with liver disease have been performed. However, the pharmacokinetic alterations suggest that alfentanil would have a more profound initial effect and a more prolonged effect than normal in patients with liver disease. An increased severity of liver disease would be expected to cause more pronounced changes.

Codeine

This is a useful analgesic for less painful conditions than those needing powerful opioids. Codeine needs metabolism by cytochrome P450 2D6 to become morphine before it has significant analgesic potency. This particular cytochrome P450 is subject to a pharmacogenetic abnormality and is missing in about 10% of the population, who will not get good pain relief when codeine is given.

Codeine as a constituent of papaveretum and in the dihydrocodeine form has been associated with renal failure.[138,139] It has also been associated with life-threatening hypotension when given intravenously.[140,141]

Naloxone

This specific opiate antagonist has been investigated for a number of different conditions in the critically ill, including septic shock and acute spinal injury. To date its only proven indication is for the reversal of the effects of opiates.

Pharmacokinetic studies have been few because of difficulties in analyzing naloxone. In the normal subject naloxone has a high hepatic extraction giving a short elimination half-life of about one hour.[142]

No unchanged drug is seen in the urine. Studies in patients with septic shock have shown a profoundly decreased clearance, thought to be caused by decreased liver perfusion.[143] As functional liver perfusion is also decreased in liver disease, it is likely that the clearance of naloxone is also decreased in patients with liver failure.

Although useful in the diagnosis and treatment of opioid overdose, caution is needed when naloxone is given. Rapid reversal of sedation and analgesia is possible. The resulting pain and anxiety may cause a large outpouring of catecholamines. These are thought to be responsible for the life-threatening arrhythmias and pulmonary edema sometimes seen after it is given.[144,145]

Nonsteroidal Anti-Inflammatory Agents

Nonsteroidal anti-inflammatory drugs are used occasionally in the critically ill. Small intravenous doses of an anti-inflammatory agent may help to control pyrexia.[146] Also, there is current interest in their ability to modulate prostaglandin synthesis and the importance of this pathway in the cause of multiple organ failure. In patients with liver dysfunction, the limiting factors for their use are the dangers of gastrointestinal bleeding and renal dysfunction.[147] Because of this they are rarely used.

Regional Anesthesia

Pain relief may be provided by local anaesthetic agents injected around peripheral nerves. All major nerve trunks may be blocked, but common sites for injection are the intercostal nerves and the epidural space. However, if there is significant liver disease the accompanying coagulopathy usually prevents the use of regional analgesia.

Absorption of local anesthetic is rapid after injection. Altered pharmacokinetics in disease states are well studied for lignocaine when used as an antidysrhythmic agent. There is little information about the use of lignocaine in liver disease or for bupivacaine,[148] which has a longer duration of action and is more often used.

Accumulation of bupivacaine has been shown in patients after liver transplantation.[149] In this study, plasma concentrations of bupivacaine above the toxic level were found, although no signs of systemic toxicity were seen in any of the patients. Unfortunately, this study did not measure α-1-acidglycoprotein, the carrier protein for bupivacaine, and the free concentration is therefore unknown.

References

1. Ferenci, P., Pappas, S.C., Munson, P.J., Henson, K., and Jones, E. A. (1984) Changes in the status of neurotransmitter receptors in a rabbit model of hepatic encephalopathy. *Hepatology* 4:186–91.

2. Ferenci, P., Schafer, D.F., Kleinberger, G., Hoofnagle, J.H., and Jones, E.A. (1983) Serum levels of gamma-aminobutyric-acid-like activity in acute and chronic hepatocellular disease. *Lancet* 2(8354):811–14.

3. Bassett, M.L., Mullen, K.D., Skolnick, P., and Jones, E.A. (1987) Amelioration of hepatic encephalopathy by pharmacologic antagonism of the GABA$_A$-benzodiazepine receptor complex in a rabbit model of fulminant hepatic failure. *Gastroenterology* 93:1069–77.

4. Bakti, G., Fisch, H.U., Karlagnis, G., Minder, C., and Bircher, J. (1987) Mechanism of the excessive sedative response of cirrhotics to benzodiazepines: Model experiments with triazolam. *Hepatology* 7:629–38.

5. Thomson, P.D., Melmon, K.L., Richardson, J.A., Cohn, K., Steinbrunn, W., Cudihee, R., and Rowland, M. (1973) Lidocaine pharmacokinetics in advanced heart failure, liver disease and renal failure in humans. *Annals of Internal Medicine* 78:499–508.

5a. Williams, R.L., Blaschke, T.F., Meffin, P.J., Melmon, K.L., and Rowland, M. (1976) Influence of viral hepatitis on the disposition of two compounds with high hepatic clearance: Lidocaine and indocyanine green. *Clinical Pharmacology and Therapeutics* 20:290–99.

6. Rowland, M., Blasche, T.F., Meffin, P.J., and Williams, R.L. (1976) Pharmacokinetics in disease states modifying hepatic and metabolic function. In *The Effect of Disease States on Drug Pharmacokinetics* (L.Z. Benet, ed.). (pp. 53–75). Washington: American Pharmaceutical Association.

7. Nebert D.W., Nelson, D.R., Coon, M.J., Estabrook, R.W., Feyereisen, R., Fuji-Kuriyama, Y., Gonzalez,

F.J., Guengerich, F.P., Gunsalus, I.C., Johnson, E.F., Loper, J.C., Sato, R., Waterman, M.R., and Waxman, D.J. (1991) The P450 superfamily: Update on new sequences, gene mapping, and recommended nomenclature. *DNA and Cell Biology* 10:1–14.

8. Park, G.R. and Elston, A. (1991) What controls drug metabolism in the critically ill patient? *Care of the Critically Ill* 7:212.

9. Park, G.R., Pichard, L., Tinel, M., Larroque, C., Elston, A., Domerque, J., Dexionne, B., and Maurel, P. (1994) What changes drug metabolism in critically ill patients? Two preliminary studies in isolated hepatocytes. *Anaesthesia* 49:188–91.

10. Wilkinson, G.R. and Shand, D.G. (1975) A physiological approach to hepatic drug clearance. *Clinical Pharmacology and Therapeutics* 18:377–90.

11. Pessayre, D., Lebrec, D., Descatoire, V., Peignoux, M., and Benhamou, J-P. (1978) Mechanism for reduced drug clearance in patients with cirrhosis. *Gastroenterology* 74:566–71.

12. Shand, D. G. (1982) Presystemic hepatic drug metabolism in cirrhosis. In *Presystemic Drug Elimination* (C.F. George, D.G. Shand, and A.G. Renwick, eds.). (pp. 96–107). London: Butterworth Scientific.

13. Secor, J.W. and Schenker, S. (1987) Drug metabolism in patients with liver disease. *Advances in Internal Medicine* 32:379–406.

14. Schoene, B., Fleischmann, R.A., and Remmer, H. (1972) Determination of drug metabolizing enzymes in needle biopsies of human liver. *European Journal of Clinical Pharmacology* 4:65–73.

15. Reves, J. G. (1984) Benzodiazepines. In *Pharmacokinetics of Anaestheisa* (Prys-Roberts, C. and Hug, C.C., eds). Oxford: Blackwell, pp. 157–86.

16. Blascke, T.F. (1977) Protein binding and kinetics of drugs in liver disease. *Clinical Pharmacokinetics* 2:32–34.

17. Ferrier, C., Marty, J., Bouffard, Y., Haberer, J.P., Levron, J.C., and Duvaldestin, P. (1985) Alfentanil pharmacokinetics in patients with cirrhosis. *Anesthesiology* 62:480–84.

18. Branch, R.A. and Shand, D.G. (1976b) Hepatic drug clearance in chronic liver disease. In *The Effect of Disease States on Drug Pharmacokinetics* (L.Z. Benet, ed.), (pp. 77–86). Washington: American Pharmaceutical Association.

19. Acocella, G., Bonollo, L., Garimoldi, M., Mainardi, M., Tenconi, L.T., and Nicolis, F.B. (1972) Kinetics of rifampicin and isoniazid administered alone and in combination to normal subjects and patients with liver disease. *Gut* 13:47–53.

20. Dundee, J.W., Price, H.L., and Dripps, R.B. (1956) Acute tolerance to thiopentone in man. *British Journal of Anaesthesia* 28:344–52.

21. Whitwam, J.G., Morgan, M., Hall, G.M., and Petrie, A. (1976) Pain during continuous nitrous oxide administration. *British Journal of Anaesthesia* 48:425–28.

22. Lloyd-Thomas, A.R. and Booker, P.D. (1986) Infusion of midazolam in paediatric patients after cardiac surgery. *British Journal of Anaesthesia* 58:1109–15.

23. Shelly, M.P., Sultan, M.A., Bodenham, A., and Park, G.R. (1991) Midazolam infusions in critically ill patients. *European Journal of Anaesthesiology* 8:21–27.

24. McQuay, H.J., Bullingham, R.E.S., and Moore, R.A. (1981) Acute opiate tolerance in man. *Life Sciences* 28:2513–17.

25. Arnold, J.H., Truog, R.D., Scavone, J.M., and Fenton, T. (1991) Changes in the pharmacodynamic response to fentanyl in neonates during continuous infusion. *Journal of Pediatrics* 119:639–43.

26. Shafer, A.A., White, P.F., Schuttler, J., and Rosenthal, M.H. (1983) Use of fentanyl infusion in the intensive care unit: Tolerance to its anesthetic effects. *Anesthesiology* 59:245–48.

27. Marshall, H., Porteous, C., McMillan, I., McPherson, S.G., and Nimmo, W.S. (1985) Relief of pain by infusion of morphine after operation: Does tolerance develop. *British Medical Journal* 291:19–21.

28. Owen, H., Szekely, S.M., Plummer, J.L., Cushnie, J.M., and Mather, L.E. (1989) Variables of patient-controlled analgesia 2. Concurrent infusion. *Anaesthesia* 44:11–13.

29. Mhatre, M.C. and Ticku, M.K. (1992) Chronic ethanol administration alters GABA-$_A$ receptor gene expression. *Molecular Pharmacology* 42:415–22.

30. O'Sullivan, G. and Park, G.R. (1990) The assessment of sedation. *Journal of Clinical Intensive Care 1*.

31. Reves, J.G., Newfield, P., and Smith, L.R. (1981) Midazolam induction time: Association with serum albumin. *Anesthesiology* 55:A259.

32. Hoyumpa, A.M. (1978) Disposition and elimination of minor tranquilizers in the aged and in patients with liver disease. *Southern Medical Journal* 71:23–28.

33. Klotz, U., Avant, G.R., Hoyumpa, A., Schenker, S., and Wilkinson, G.R. (1975) The effects of age and liver disease on the disposition and elimination of diazepam in adult man. *Journal of Clinical Investigation* 55:347–59.

34. McConnell, J.B., Curry, S.H., Davis, M., and Williams, R. (1982) Clinical effects and metabolism of diazepam in patients with chronic liver disease. *Clinical Science* 63:75–80.

35. Klotz, U., Antoin, K.H., Brugel, H., and Bieck, P.R. (1977) Disposition of diazepam and its major metabolite desmethyl diazepam in patients with liver disease. *Clinical Pharmacology and Therapeutics* 21:430–36.

36. Greenblatt, D.J., Woo, E., Allen, M.D., Orsulak, P.J., and Shader, R.I. (1978) Rapid recovery from massive diazepam overdose. *Journal of the American Medical Association* 240:1872–74.

37. Ochs, H.R., Greenbalt, D.J., and Eckard, B. (1983) Repeated diazepam dosing in cirrhotic patients; cumulation and sedation. *Clinical Pharmacology and Therapeutics* 33:471–76.

38. Hamdy, N.A.T., Kennedy, H.J., Nicholl, J., and Triger, D.R. (1986) Sedation for gastroscopy: A comparative study of midazolam and Diazemuls in patients with and without cirrhosis. *British Journal of Clinical Pharmacology* 22:643–47.

39. Traeger, S.M. and Haug, M.T. (1986) Reduction of diazepam serum half life and reversal of coma by activated charcoal in a patient with severe liver disease. *Clinical Toxicology* 24:329–37.

40. Branch, R.A. and Shand, D.G. (1976a) Intravenous administration of diazepam in patients with chronic liver disease. *Gut* 17:975–83.

41. Tedesco, F. and Mills, L.R. (1982) Diazepam (Valium) hepatitis. *Digestive Diseases and Sciences* 27:470.

42. Shull, H.J., Wilkinson, G.R., and Johnson, R. (1976) Normal disposition of oxazepam in acute viral hepatitis and cirrhosis. *Annals of Internal Medicine* 84:420–25.

43. Allonen, H., Zeigler, G., and Klotz, U. (1981) Midazolam kinetics. *Clinical Pharmacology and Therapeutics* 30:653–61.

43a. Dundee, J.W., Collier, P.S., Carlisle, R.J.T., and Harper, K.W. (1986) Prolonged midazolam elimination half-life. *British Journal of Clinical Pharmacology* 21:425–29.

43b. Tarbett, M.M., Bayliss, M., Herriott, D., Mood, S.R., Mutson, J.L., Park, G.R., and Serabjit, C.J. (1993) Applications of molecular biology and in vitro technology to drug metabolism studies: An industrial perspective. *Biochemical Society* Transactions 21:1018–23.

44. Dundee, J.W., Halliday, N.J., Harper, K.W., and Brogden, R.N. (1984) Midazolam. A review of its pharmacological properties and therapeutic use. *Drugs* 28:519–43.

45. Binetti, M., Ascalone, V., Colombi, A., Zinelli, L., and Cisternino, M. (1985) A pharmacokinetic study on midazolam in compensated liver cirrhosis. *International Journal of Clinical Pharmaceutical Research* 6:405–11.

46. Shelly, M.P., Dixon, J.S., and Park, G.R. (1989) The pharmacokinetics of midazolam following orthotopic liver transplantation. *British Journal of Clinical Pharmacology* 27:629–33.

47. MacGilchrist, A.J., Birnie, G.G., Cook, A., Scobie, G., Murray, T., Watkinson, G., and Brodie, M.J. (1986) Pharmacokinetics and pharmacodynamics of intravenous midazolam in patients with severe alcoholic cirrhosis. *Gut* 27:190–95.

48. Halliday, N.J., Dundee, J.W., Collier, P.S., Loughran, P.G., and Harper, K.W. (1985) Influence of plasma proteins on the onset of hypnotic action of intravenous midazolam. *Anaesthesia* 40:763–66.

49. Park, G.R., Manara, A.R., and Dawling, S. (1989) Extrahepatic metabolism of midazolam. *British Journal of Clinical Pharmacology* 27:634–37.

50. Shelly, M.P., Park, G.R., and Mendel, L. (1987) Failure of critically ill patients to metabolise midazolam. *Anaesthesia* 42:619–26.

51. Cote, S. and Shalit, M.N. (1975) Effects of diazepam on cerebral blood flow and oxygen uptake after head injury. *Anesthesiology* 43:117–22.

52. Gelman, S., Reves, J.G., and Harris, D. (1983) Circulatory responses to midazolam anaesthesia: Emphasis on canine splanchnic circulation. *Anesthesia and Analgesia* 62:135–39.

53. Dundee, J.W., Liliburn, J.K., Toner, W., and Howard, P.J. (1978) Plasma lorazepam levels. *Anaesthesia* 33:15–19.

54. Elliott, H.W. (1976) Metabolism of lorazepam. *British Journal of Anaesthesia* 48:1017–23.

55. Kraus, J.W., Desmond, P.V., Marshall, J.P., Johnson, R.F., Schenker, S., and Wilkinson, G R. (1978) Effects of aging and liver disease on disposition of lorazepam. *Clinical Pharmacology and Therapeutics* 24:411–19.

56. Gerkens, J.F., Desmond, P.V., Schenker, S., and Branch, R.A. (1981) Hepatic and extrahepatic glucuronidation of lorazepam in the dog. *Hepatology* 1:329–35.

57. Ghabrail, H., Desmond, P.V., Watson, K.J.R., Gijsbers, A.J., Harman, P.J., Breen, K.J., and Mashford, M.L. (1986) The effects of age and chronic liver disease on the elimination of temazepam. *European Journal of Clinical Pharmacology* 30:93–97.

58. Ochs, H.R., Greenblatt, D.J., Verburg-Ochs, B., and Matlis, R. (1986) Temazepam clearance unaltered in cirrhosis. *American Journal of Gastroenterology* 81:80–84.

59. Roncari, G., Ziegler, W.H., and Guentert, T.W. (1986) Pharmacokinetics of the new benzodiazepine antagonist Ro 15-1788 in man following intravenous and oral administration. *British Journal of Clinical Pharmacology* 22:421–28.

60. Geller, E., Niv, D., Silbiger, A., Halpern, P., Leykin, Y., Rudick, V., and Sorkin, P. (1985) Ro 15-1788 in the treatment of 34 intoxicated patients. *Anesthesiology* 63:A157.

61. Darragh, A., Lambe, R., Brick, I., and Downie, W.W. (1981) Reversal of benzodiazepine-induced sedation by intravenous Ro 15-1788. *Lancet* 2:1042.

62. Kleinberger, G., Grimm, G., Laggner, A., Drume, W., Lenz, K., and Schneeweiss, B. (1985) Weaning patients from mechanical ventilation by benzodiazepine antagonist Ro 15-1788. *Lancet* 2(8449):268–69.

63. Janssen, U., Walker, S., Maier, K., von Gaisberg, U., and Klotz, U. (1989) Flumazenil disposition and elimination in cirrhosis. *Clinical Pharmacology and Therapeutics* 46:317–23.

64. van der Rijt, C.C.D., Drost, R.H., Schalm, S.W., and Schramel, M. (1991) Pharmacokinetics of flumazenil in fulminant hepatic failure. *European Journal of Clinical Pharmacology* 41:501.

65. Park, G.R. and Podkowik, A. (1992) Plasma concentrations of flumazenil during liver transplantation. *Anaesthesia* 47:887–89.

66. Mullen, K.D., Martin, J.V., Mendleson, W.B., Bassett, M.L., and Jones, E.A. (1988) Could an endogenous benzodiazepine ligand contribute to hepatic encephalopathy. *Lancet* 1:457–59.

67. Scollo-Lavizzari, G. (1983) First clinical investigation of the benzodiazepine antagonist Ro 15-1788 in comatose patients. *European Neurology* 22:7–11.

68. Gyr, K. and Meir, R. (1991) Flumazenil in the treatment of portal systemic encephalopathy—an overview. *Intensive Care Medicine* 17:S39–S42.

69. Glatt, M.M., George, H.R., and Frisch, E.P. (1965) Controlled trial of chlormethiazole in treatment of the alcoholic withdrawal phase. *British Medical Journal* 2:401–4.

70. Scott, D.B., Beamish, D., Hudson, I.N., and Jostell K-G, (1980) Prolonged infusion of chlormethiazole in intensive care. *British Journal of Anaesthesia* 52:541–45.

71. Robson, D.J., Blow, C., Gaines, P., Flanagan, R.J., and Henry, J.A. (1984) Accumulation of chlormethiazole during intravenous infusion. *Intensive Care Medicine* 10:315–16.

72. Pentikainen, P.J., Neuvonen, P.J., Tarpila, S., and Sylvalahti, E. (1978) Effect of cirrhosis of the liver on the pharmacokinetics of chlormethiazole. *British Medical Journal* 2:861–63.

73. Modig, J. (1988) Indications of chlormethiazole as a protective agent in experimental endotoxaemia. *European Surgical Research* 20:195–204.

74. Lassen, H.C.A., Henriksen, E., Neurkirch, F., Kristensen, H.S. (1956) Treatment of tetanus severe prolonged bone-marrow depression after prolonged nitrous oxide anaesthesia. *Lancet* 1:527–30.

75. Amos, R.J., Amess, J.A.L., Hinds, C.J., and Mollin, D.L. (1982) Incidence and pathogenesis of acute megaloblastic bone-marrow changes. *Lancet* 2:835–39.

76. Skacel, P.O., Hewlett, A. M., Lewis, J.D., Lumb, M., Nunn, J.F., and Chanarin, I. (1983) Studies on the haemopoietic toxicity of nitrous oxide in man. *British Journal of Haematology* 53:189–200.

77. Koblin, D.D., Waskell, L., Watson, J. E., Stokstad, E.L.R., and Eger, E.I. (1982) Nitrous oxide inactivates methionine synthetase in human liver. *Anesthesia and Analgesia* 61:75–78.

78. Nunn, V.F. (1987) Clinical aspects of the interaction between nitrous oxide and vitamin B_{12}. *British Journal of Anaesthesia* 59:3–13.

79. Amos, R.J., Amess, J.A.L., Nancekievill, D.G., and Rees, G.M. (1984) Prevention of nitrous oxide induced megaloblastic changes in bone-marrow using folinic acid. *British Journal of Anaesthesia* 56:103–7.

80. Shideman, F.E., Kelly, A.R., Lee, L.E., Lowell, V.F., and Adams, B.J. (1949) The role of the liver in the detoxication of thiopental (pentothal) by man. *Anesthesiology* 10:421–28.

81. Gibson, W.R., Swanson, E.E., and Doran, W.J. (1955) Pharmacology of a short-acting non-sulphur barbituric acid derivate (21788). *Proceedings of the Society for Experimental Biology and Medicine* 89:292–94.

82. Ledingham, I. McA. and Watt, I. (1983) Influence of sedation on mortality in critically ill multiple trauma patients. *Lancet* 1:1270.

83. Watt, I. and Ledingham, I. Mc.A. (1984) Mortality amongst multiple trauma patients admitted to an intensive therapy unit. *Anaesthesia* 39:973–81.

84. Lambert, A., Mitchell, R., Frost, J., Ratcliffe, J.G., and Robertson, W.R. (1983) Direct in vitro inhibition of adrenosteroidogenesis of etomidate. *Lancet* 2:1085–86.

85. Cockshott, I.D. (1985) Propofol ("Diprivan") pharmacokinetics and metabolism—an overview. *Postgraduate Medical Journal* 61(suppl. 3):45–50.

86. Cassidy, K.M. and Houston, J.B. (1984) In vivo capacity of hepatic and extrahepatic enzymes to conju-

gate phenol. *Drug Metabolism and Disposition* 12:619–24.

87. Dogra, S., Isaac, P.A., Cockshott, I.D., and Foy, J.M. (1989) Pulmonary extraction of propofol in post-cardiopulmonary bypass patients. *Journal of Drug Development* 2:133.

88. Mather, L.E., Selby, D.G., Runciman, W.B., and McLean, C.F. (1989) Propofol assay and regional mass balance in the sheep. *Xenobiotica* 19:1337–47.

89. Gray, P., Park, G.R., Cockshott, I.D., Douglas, E.D., Shuker, B., and Simons, P.J. (1992) Propofol metabolism in man during the anhepatic and reperfusion phases of liver transplantation. *Xenobiotica* 22:105–14.

90. Servin, F., Desmonts, J.M., Haberer, J.P., Cockshott, I.D., Plumer, G.F., and Farinotti, R. (1988) Pharmacokinetics and protein binding of propofol in patients with cirrhosis. *Anesthesiology* 69:887–91.

91. Servin, F., Cockshott, I.D., Farinotti, R., Haberer, J.P., Winckler, C., and Desmonts, J.M. (1990) Pharmacokinetics of propofol infusions in patients with cirrhosis. *British Journal of Anaesthesia* 65:177–83.

92. Bentley, G.N., Gent, J.P., and Goodchild, C.S. (1989) Vascular effects of propofol; smooth muscle relaxation in isolated veins and arteries. *Journal of Pharmacy and Pharmacology* 41:797–98.

93. Robinson, F.P. and Patterson, C.C. (1985) Changes in liver function tests after propofol (Diprivan). *Postgraduate Medical Journal* 61(Suppl 3):160–61.

94. Kawar, P., Briggs, L.P., Bahar, M., McIlroy, P.D.A., Dundee, J.W., Merrett, J.D., and Nesbitt, G.S. (1982) Liver enzyme studies with disopropofol (ICI 35,868) and midazolam. *Anaesthesia* 37:305–8.

95. Park, G.R. and Gempeler, F. (1993) Intravenous anaesthetic agents. In *Sedation and Analgesia* (pp. 209–53). London: Saunders.

96. Centers for Disease Control. (1990) Postsurgical infections associated with an extrinsically contaminated intravenous agent—California, Illinois, Maine and Michigan, 1990. *Morbidity and Mortality Weekly Report* 39:426–27, 433.

97. Daily, M.J., Dickey, J.B., and Paccko, K.H. (1991) Endogenous candida endophthalmitis after intravenous anesthesia with propofol. *Archives of Ophthalmology* 109:1081–84.

98. Farrington, M., McGuiness, J., and Park, G.R. (1994) Do infusions of propofol and midazolam pose a microbiological threat to critically ill patients? *British Journal of Anaesthesia* 72:415–8.

99. Idvall, J., Ahlgren, I., Aronsen, K.F., and Stenberg, P. (1979) Ketamine infusions: Pharmacokinetics and clinical effects. *British Journal of Anaesthesia* 51:1167–73.

100. Shimomura, K., Kamata, O., Ueki, S., Ida, S., Oguri, K., Yoshimura, H., and Tsukamoto, H. (1971) Analgesic effect of morphine glucuronides. *Tohoku Journal of Experimental Medicine* 105:45–52.

101. Lasagna, L. and De Kornfield, T.J. (1958) Analgesic potency of normorphine in patients with postoperative pain. *Journal of Pharmacology* 124:260–63.

102. Johannesson, T. and Milthers, K. (1962) Morphine and normorphine in the brain of rats. A comparison of subcutaneous, intraperitoneal and intravenous administration. *Acta Pharmacologica et Toxicologica* 19:241–46.

103. Smith, M.T., Watt, J.A., and Cramond, T. (1990) Morphine-3-glucuronide a potent antagonist of morphine analgesia. *Life Science* 47:579–85.

104. Gong, Q.L., Hedner, J., Bjorkman, R., and Hedner, T. (1992) Morphine-3-glucuronide may functionally antagonize morphine-6-glucuronide induced antinociception and ventilatory depression in the rat. *Pain* 48:249–55.

105. Morley, J.S., Miles, J.B., Wells, J.C., and Bowsher, D. (1992) Paradoxical pain. *Lancet* 340:1045.

106. Carrupt, P.A., Testa, B., Bechalany, A., El Tayar, N., Descas, P., and Perrissoud, D. (1991) Morphine 6-glucuronide and morphine 3-glucuronide as molecular chameleons with unexpected lipophilicity. *Journal of Medicinal Chemistry* 34:1272–75.

107. Stanski, D.R., Greenblatt, D.J., and Lowenstein, E. (1978) Kinetics of intravenous and intramuscular morphine. *Clinical Pharmacology and Therapeutics* 24:52–59.

108. Quinn, K.G., Manara, A.R., and Park, G.R. (1988) Failure to demonstrate in vitro metabolism of morphine in whole blood and plasma. *British Journal of Anaesthesia* 60:348.

109. McQuay, H. and Moore, A. (1984) Be aware of renal function when prescribing morphine. *Lancet* 2:284–85.

110. Moore, A., Sear, J., Baldwin, D., Allen, M., Hunniset, A., Bullingham, R., and McQuay, H. (1984) Morphine kinetics during and after renal transplantation. *Clinical Pharmacology and Therapeutics* 5:641–45.

111. Ball, M., McQuay, H.J., Moore, R.A., Allen, M.C., Fisher, A., and Sear, J. (1985) Renal failure and the use of morphine in intensive care. *Lancet* 1:784–86.

112. Moore, R.A., Baldwin, D., Allen, M.C., Watson, P.J.Q., Bullingham, R.E.S., and McQuay, J.H. (1984) Sensitive and specific morphine radioimmunoassay with iodine label: Pharmacokinetics of morphine in man after intravenous administration. *Annals of Clinical Biochemistry* 21:318–25.

113. Aitkenhead, A.R., Vater, M., Achola, K., Cooper, C.M.S., and Smith, G. (1984) Pharmacokinetics of single-dose I.V. morphine in normal volunteers and patients with end-stage renal failure. *British Journal of Anaesthesia* 56:813–17.

114. Chauvin, M., Sandouk, P., Scherrmann, J.M., Farinotti, R., Strumza, P., and Duvaldestin, P. (1987) Morphine pharmacokinetics in renal failure. *Anesthesiology* 66:327–31.

115. Shelly, M.P., Cory, E.P., and Park, G.R. (1986) Pharmacokinetics of morphine in two children before and after liver transplantation. *British Journal of Anaesthesia* 58:1218–23.

116. Osbourne, R.J., Joel, S.P., and Slevin, M.L. (1986) Morphine intoxication in renal failure: The role of Morphine 6 Glucuronide. *British Medical Journal* 292:1548–49.

117. Patwardhan, R.V., Johnson, R.F., Hoyumpa, A., Sheehan, J.J., Desmond, P.V., Wilkinson, G.R., Branch, R.A., and Schenker, S. (1981) Normal metabolism of morphine in cirrhosis. *Gastroenterology* 81:1006–11.

118. Mazoit, J.X., Sandouk, P., Zetalaoui, P., and Scherrmann, J.M. (1987) Pharmacokinetics of unchanged morphine in normal and cirrhotic subjects. *Anesthesia and Analgesia* 66:293–98.

119. Jaffe, J.H. and Martin, W.R. Opioid analgesics and antagonists. In *The Pharmacological Basis of Therapeutics* (Goodman Gilman, A., Rall, T.W., Nies, A.S., and Taylor, P., eds). New York: McGraw-Hill: pp. 485–521.

120. Szeto, H.H., Inturrisi, C.E., Houde, R., Saal, S., Cheigh, J., and Reidenberg, M.M. (1977) Accumulation of normeperidine, an active metabolite of meperidine, in patients with renal failure or cancer. *Annals of Internal Medicine* 86:738–41.

121. Inturrisi, C.E. and Umans, J.G. (1983) Clinics in Anesthesiology. In R.E.S. Bullingham (Ed.), (pp. 123–138). London: Saunders.

122. Klotz, U., McHorse, T.S., Wilkinson, G.R., and Schenker, S. (1974) The effect of cirrhosis on the disposition and elimination of meperidine in man. *Clinical Pharmacology and Therapeutics* 16:677–75.

123. Neal, E.A., Meffin, P.J., Gregory, P.B., and Blasche, T.F. (1979) Enhanced bioavailability and decreased clearance of analgesics in patients with cirrhosis. *Gastroenterology* 77:96–102.

124. Pond, S.M., Tong, T., Benowitz, N.L., Jacob, P., and Rigod, J. (1981) Presystemic metabolism of meperidine to normeperidine in normal and cirrhotic subjects. *Clinical Pharmacology and Therapeutics* 30:183–88.

125. Dundee, J. W. and Tinckler, L. F. (1952) Pethidine and liver damage. *British Medical Journal* 2:703–4.

126. Isherwood, C.N., Calvey, T.N., Williams, N.E., Chan, K., and Murray, G.R. (1984) Elimination of phenoperidine in liver disease. *British Journal of Anaesthesia* 56:843–46.

127. Davies, D.M. (1991) *Textbook of Adverse Drug Reactions.* Oxford: Oxford University Press.

128. McClain, D.A. and Hug, C.C. (1980) Intravenous fentanyl kinetics. *Clinical Pharmacology and Therapeutics* 28:106–14.

129. Haberer, J.P., Schoeffler, P., Couderc, E., and Duvaldestin, P. (1982) Fentanyl pharmacokinetics in anaesthetised patients with cirrhosis. *British Journal of Anaesthesia* 54:1267–70.

130. Hug, C.C., Murphy, M.R., Sampson, J.F., Terblanche, J., and Aldrete, J.A. (1981) Biotransformation of morphine and fentanyl in anhepatic dogs. *Anesthesiology* 55(Suppl):A 261.

131. Bower, S. and Hull, C.J. (1982) Comparative pharmacokinetics of fentanyl and alfentanil. *British Journal of Anaesthesia* 54:871–77.

132. Hug, C.C. and Chaffman, M. (1984) *Alfentanil: Pharmacology and Uses in Anaesthesia.* Auckland, New-Zealand: Adis Press.

133. Shelly, M.P., Walker, S., and Park, G.R. (1989) The pharmacokinetics of alfentanil in patients following liver transplantation. *Advances in the Biosciences* 75:643–46.

134. Burns, A. M., Hue, D.P., Wraight, E.P., and Park, G.R. (1993) Creatinine and ^{51}Cr-EDTA after liver transplantation. *Anaesthesia* 48:763–65.

135. Helmers, H., Van Peer, A., Woestenborghs, R., Noorduin, H., and Heykants, J. (1984) Alfentanil pharmacokinetics in elderly patients. *Clinical Pharmacology and Therapeutics* 36:239–43.

136. McDonnel, T.E., Bartkowski, R.R., and Kahn, C. (1982) Evidence for polymorphic oxidation of alfentanil in man. *Anesthesiology* 61:A284.

137. Meuldermans, W., Van Peer, A., Hendricks, J., Woestenborghs, R., Lauwers, W., Heykants, J., Vanden Bussche, G., Craeyvelt, H.V., and Van Der Aa, P. (1988) Alfentanil pharmacokinetics and metabolism in humans. *Anesthesiology* 69:527–34.

138. Hill, S.A., Quinn, K., Shelly, M.P., and Park, G.R. (1991) Reversible renal failure following opioid administration. *Anaesthesia* 46:938–39.

139. Park, G.R., Shelly, M.P., Quinn, K., and Roberts P. (1989) Dihydrocodeine: A reversible cause of renal failure? *European Journal of Anaesthesiology* 6:303–14.

140. Shanahan, E.C., Marshall, A.G., and Garrett, C.P.O. (1983) Adverse reactions to intravenous codeine phosphate in children. *Anaesthesia* 38:40–43.

141. Parke, T.J., Nandi, P.R., Bird, K.J., and Jewkes, D.A. (1992) Profound hypotension following intravenous codeine phosphate. *Anaesthesia* 47:852–54.

142. Stanski, D.R. (1982) *Narcotics and Naloxone.* New York: Grune and Stratton.

143. Groeger, J.S. and Inturrisi, C.E. (1987) High dose naloxone: Pharmacokinetics in patients in septic shock. *Critical Care Medicine* 15:751–56.

144. Andree, R.A. (1980) Sudden death following naloxone administration. *Anesthesia and Analgesia* 59:782–84.

145. Michaelis, L.L., Hickey, P.R., Clark, T.A., and Dixon, W.M. (1974) Ventricular irritability associated with the use of naloxone hydrochloride. *Annals of Thoracic Surgery* 18:608–14.

146. Pesenti, A., Riboni, A., Basilico, E., and Grossi, E. (1986) Antipyretic therapy in ICU patients: Evaluation of low dose diclofenac sodium. *Intensive Care Medicine* 12:370–73.

147. Zandstra, D.F., Stoutenbeek, C.P., and Alexander, J.P. (1983) Antipyretic therapy with diclofenac sodium. *Intensive Care Medicine* 9:21–22.

148. Tucker, G.T. and Mather, L.E. (1979) Clinical pharmacokinetics of local anaesthetics. *Clinical Pharmacokinetics* 4:241–78.

149. Bodenham, A. and Park, G.R. (1990) Plasma concentrations of bupivacaine after intercostal nerve block in patients after orthotopic liver transplantation. *British Journal of Anaesthesia* 64:436–41.

150. Klotz, U., Avant, G.R., Hoyumpa, A., Schenker, S., and Wilkinson, G.R. (1975) The effects of age and liver disease on the disposition and elimination of diazepam in adult man. *Journal of Clinical Investigation* 55:347–59.

151. Klotz, U., Avant, G.R., Wilkinson, G.R., Hoyumpa, A., and Schenkers, S. (1974) Altered disposition and elimination of diazepam in patients with liver disease. *Gastroenterology* 65:552.

152. Andreasen, P.B., Hendel, J., Greisen, G., and Hvidberg, E.F. (1976) Pharmacokinetics of diazepam in disordered liver function. *European Journal of Clinical Pharmacology* 19:115–20.

153. Shelly, M.P., Quinn, K., and Park, G.R. (1989) Pharmacokinetics of morphine in patients following liver transplantation. *British Journal of Anaesthesia* 63:375–79.

154. Rinetti, M., Ascalone, V., Colombi Zinelli, L., and Cisternino, M. (1985) A pharmacokinetic study on midazolam in compensated liver cirrhosis. *International Journal of Clinical Pharmacology Research* 6:405–11.

Chapter 6

Pharmacokinetics and Pharmacodynamics of Nondepolarizing Muscle Relaxants

D. Ryan Cook

Nondepolarizing muscle relaxants are large (molecular weight 600–1000), bulky molecules that contain one, two, or three quaternary nitrogen groups. Because the molecules are positively charged, highly ionized, and water soluble, they are largely distributed throughout the extracellular space but cross lipid membranes minimally. Conceptually there are five routes of elimination of nondepolarizing relaxants: metabolism, hepatobiliary uptake and excretion, renal excretion, redistribution, and a combination of these. The influence of a given degree of liver disease on the duration of effect (pharmadynamics) and the pharmacokinetics for a given muscle relaxant can generally be predicted if one is aware of its normal route(s) of elimination. These influences have been documented for most relaxants (Table 6-1). However, the type of liver disease (hepatocellular versus cholestatic), the severity of the liver disease, the associated surgical problem(s) and its pathophysiological perturbations, and the degree of corrective therapy can produce considerable variability in the response to relaxants. Because nondepolarizing muscle relaxants have low plasma protein binding capacity (i.e., <70%), disease-induced changes in plasma protein concentration have minimal effect on their pharmacologic effect. Tissue binding to cartilage and connective tissue, however, may play an important role in the distribution of some relaxants (i.e., *d*-tubocurarine and metocurarine).

Table 6-1. Elimination Routes of Muscle Relaxants

Agent	Metabolism in Plasma	Hepatobiliary Uptake and Metabolism	Renal Excretion
Mivacurium	XX		
Atracurium	XX		
Vecuronium		XX	X
Rocuronium		XX	X
d-Tubocurarine		X	XX
Pancuronium		XX	X
Pipecuronium		XX	X
Gallamine			XX
Metocurine			XX
Doxacurium			XX

XX (Major route); X (Alternative route).

Patients with severe liver disease often have seeming resistance to nondepolarizing relaxants that may be because of an increased volume of distribution, increased binding to stress proteins (such as alpha-1-glycoproteins, AAG), inhibitors, or increases in neuromuscular receptors. AAG levels are often normal in pediatric patients with cholestatic end stage liver failure, although serum albumin concentrations are decreased.[1] In addition, once one achieves adequate neuromuscular blockade, a prolonged but highly variable duration of effect may occur. For some long surgical procedures in which postoperative ventilation is usually required, this prolongation of effect can be of therapeutic benefit.

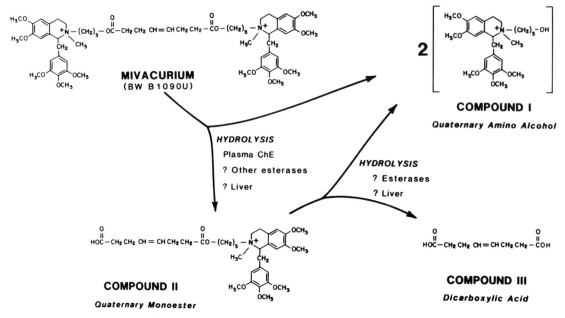

Figure 6-1. Major metabolic pathways for mivacurium. The quaternary amino alcohol and quaternary monoester have no pharmacological activity.

Severe liver disease may be associated with diminished hepatic uptake, storage, metabolism, and secretion of relaxants; impaired renal function; and significant physiologic changes. In addition, patients with severe liver disease may be taking a wide variety of drugs (steroids, H_2 blockers, immunosuppressive drugs, and antibiotics) that can effect neuromuscular transmission. The purpose of this chapter is to summarize the effects of liver disease on the pharmacodynamics and pharmacokinetics of short-acting, intermediate-acting, and long-acting nondepolarizing relaxants. The role of various elimination mechanisms for relaxants in normal patients and those with end stage liver disease (and renal disease) has recently been well reviewed by others.[2–4]

Characteristics of Specific Drugs

Relaxants of Short Duration

Mivacurium

Mivacurium, a potent short-acting nondepolarizing relaxant, consists of three stereoisomers: *trans-trans* (57.4% w/w), *cis-trans* (36.2% w/w), and *cis-cis* (6.4% w/w). The *cis-cis* isomer can be considered to be pharmacologically inactive. Some-

what like succinylcholine, the short duration of action of mivacurium is related to the hydrolysis of the active isomers by butyrylcholinesterase (plasma cholinesterase). Hydrolysis of mivacurium produces a quaternary monoester, a quaternary aminoalcohol, and a dicarboxylic acid. These breakdown products are also pharmacologically inactive (Figure 6-1).

Butyrylcholinesterases of human plasma are nonspecific and are capable of hydrolyzing a variety of substrates at different rates. For example, the Michaelis-Menten constants (Km) and the maximum velocities (Vmax) for succinylcholine differ significantly (Figure 6-2). These data represent only the active isomers of mivacurium. At equal multiples of the Km concentration (0.1–2), the rate of metabolism of mivacurium is about 70% that of succinylcholine. We demonstrated in vitro that the rate of metabolism of mivacurium is directly related to butyrylcholinesterase activity and that the estimated half-life of mivacurium increases as butyrylcholinesterase activity decreases (Figures 6-3 and 6-4).

Diminished activity of butyrylcholinesterase, a glycoprotein produced in the liver, may be caused by physiologic variation (e.g., age or pregnancy), disease, iatrogenic or environmental change, and genetic alteration. In patients heterozygous for the atypical butyrylcholinesterase gene, the clinically

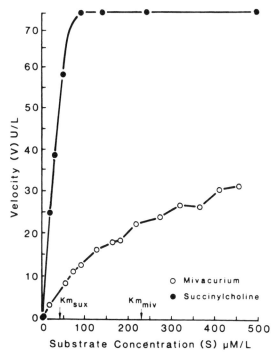

Figure 6-2. Relation between active isomers of mivac-urium (c) or succinylcholine (0) concentration in plasma and rate of in vitro metabolism in human plasma with normal butyrylcholinesterase activity.

effective duration of action from an intubating dose of mivacurium is 8–11 minutes longer than in geno-typically normal patients. Patients homozygous for the atypical butyrylcholinesterase gene (1 in 2500 patients) are extremely sensitive to mivacurium;

neuromuscular blockade may last 4–8 hours. In about half of patients with profound liver disease there is a marked reduction of butyrylcholinesterase activity; serum albumin and many clotting factors may be reduced as well. It is well known that the clinical duration of succinylcholine is prolonged to a variable degree from these conditions. Thus, one would expect comparable changes in the duration of effect from mivacurium and changes in its pharma-cokinetics. It is common, however, to administer large volumes of fresh frozen plasma to partially correct the bleeding problem which may increase butyrylcholinesterase activity.

We have recently noted that patients with liver failure exhibit markedly longer durations of neuro-muscular blockade with mivacurium and have slower drug clearance than those with normal liver function. The clinical duration (T_{25}), the time for neuromuscular transmissions to recover to 25% of control, and the recovery index (T_{25}–T_{75}) were prolonged and butyrylcholinesterase activity re-duced in the patients with liver failure. Patients with renal failure had intermediate values. There was a significant inverse relationship between butyryl-cholinesterase activity and the clinical duration of effect (Figure 6-5). Similar findings were noted by Phillips and Hunter.[5]

The analysis of the pharmacokinetic data was initially complicated by the presence of the three stereoisomers of mivacurium in the drug formula-tion and the lack of stereospecific assays for these

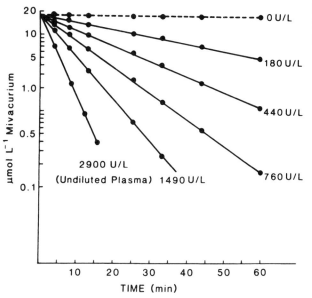

Figure 6-3. In vitro plasma decay curves of active isomers of mivacurium over time in normal human plasma with various butyrylcholinesterase activity.

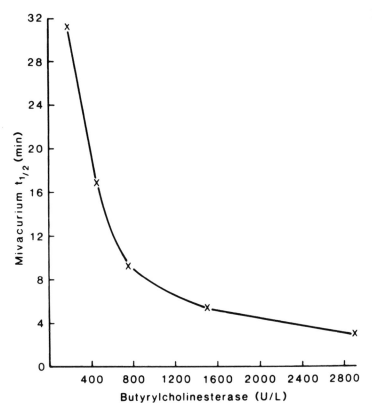

Figure 6-4. Mivacurium in vitro half-life at 0.1 km concentrations in normal plasma with various butyrylcholinesterase activity.

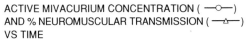

ACTIVE MIVACURIUM CONCENTRATION (—○—)
AND % NEUROMUSCULAR TRANSMISSION (—△—)
VS TIME

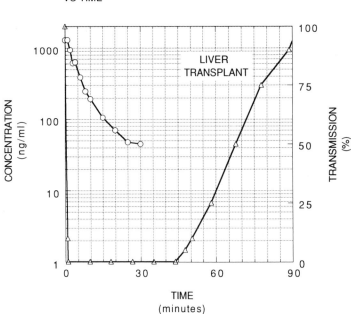

Figure 6-5. Correlation of estimated mivacurium plasma concentration and neuromuscular transmission over time.

Table 6-2. Pharmacokinetic Parameters of Pharmacologically Active Mivacurium Isomers

Parameter	Control Patients (n = 8)	Patients with Hepatic Failure (n = 9)	Patients with Renal Failure (n =9)
AUC (ng/min/ml)	2273 (864)	4868 (1847)*	2390 (1225)
Cl (ml/kg/min)	70.4 (28.1)	33.3 (13.8)*	76.6 (43.6)+
Vd$_{ss}$ (ml/kg)	112 (72)	124 (52)	150 (122)
MRT (min)	1.5 (0.8)	4.2 (2.6)*	1.9 (0.5)

Mean (SD). *Different from value in control patients (ANOVA). +Different from value in hepatic failure patients. AUC: area under concentration-time curve; Cl: clearance; Vd$_{ss}$: volume of distribution at steady-state; MRT: mean residence time. Irrespective of the distribution characteristics of a drug, MRT represents the time for 63.2% of a intravenous bolus dose to be eliminated.

isomers. Preliminary plots of mivacurium plasma concentration versus time revealed a long, relatively slow terminal elimination phase that was not consistent with the short clinical duration of the drug, clinical predictions of the half-life, or in vitro predictions of the half-life (see Figure 6-5). It is now clear that butyrylcholinesterase has a reduced affinity for the cis-cis mivacurium isomer. Estimates of mivacurium clearance, volume of distribution, and mean residence time were made after subtracting the presumed contribution of the cis-cis isomer. The estimated volume of distribution of mivacurium was not increased by liver failure but clearance was markedly reduced and mean residence time increased (Table 6-2). Reduced butyrylcholinesterase activity rather than organ failure per se is probably responsible for these changes. Further studies in end stage liver disease are needed to better define these kinetic issues.

Relaxants of Intermediate Duration

Atracurium

Atracurium, a potent intermediate-acting relaxant was designed to primarily undergo Hofmann degradation and to a lesser extent hydrolysis by nonspecific esterases (Figure 6-6). Acrylates and laudanosine are the potential end products of this degradation. Under physiologic conditions atracurium is continually inactivated by these dual pathways, although the relative role of each pathway is contentious.[6] The degradation of atracurium is enhanced by alkalosis and retarded by hypothermia. We noted that in vitro atracurium is degraded three times more rapidly in plasma than in buffer (at the same pH and temperature) and that laudanosine is formed more rapidly in plasma.[7] Probably two-thirds of atracurium is degraded enzymatically; a monoquaternary alcohol

and acid are intermediate breakdown products. This rapid degradation can be inhibited by esterase inhibitors. Most likely, nonspecific aliesterases but not butyrylcholinesterases facilitate the degradation of atracurium.

In patients, the degradation of atracurium is associated with the formation of two significant metabolites: a monoquaternary alcohol with an elimination half-life of about 40 minutes and laudanosine with an elimination half-life of about 4 hours. Laudanosine, a highly protein bound and highly lipid-soluble tertiary amine, is a glycine antagonist with convulsive effects or arousal effects in some experimental animals at high plasma concentrations (>17,000 ng/mL).[8-10] Laudanosine is metabolized by the liver and excreted by the kidney.[11] Whether laudanosine can cause convulsions in man, and if so under what conditions, has been the subject of great debate. Some have assumed that convulsions do occur at plasma concentrations greater than 17,000 ng/mL. To achieve such peak concentrations of laudanosine would require an initial bolus of atracurium of about 15 mg/kg; such a dose would probably be associated with severe hypotension from histamine release. It is more likely that high concentrations of laudanosine would occur during prolonged infusion in patients and particularly in patients with both renal and liver failure.

During a prolonged continuous infusion of atracurium (i.e., 16–20 hours) in the operating room or intensive care unit, laudanosine will be continuously formed and increase to a plateau concentration as atracurium is degraded. This plateau concentration has been estimated to be about 1000 µg/mL in normal patients and about 1600 µg/mL in patients with renal failure.[12] Few data are available for patients with liver failure, although we have seen two patients with laudanosine concentrations of 35,000–56,000 µg/mL after days of atracurium infusion (unpublished observations).

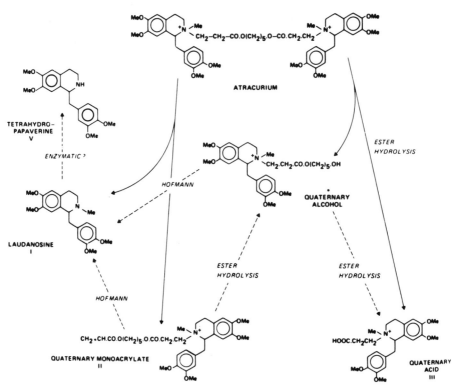

Figure 6-6. Proposed metabolic pathways for atracurium degradation. It is estimated that two-thirds of atracurium is degraded by ester hydrolysis. The quaternary alcohol is formed in significant concentrations in man.

The pharmacokinetics of atracurium have been studied in adults and children with acute liver failure.[13,14] Although the volume of distribution of atracurium was increased, its clearance and elimination half-life were normal. This is not surprising since the removal of atracurium is seemingly independent of the liver.[15] Severe liver disease may be associated with resistance to atracurium.[16] Some have speculated that this resistance is due to increased concentrations of alpha-1-glycoproteins (AAG).

Vecuronium

Vecuronium, the 16-β-monoquaternary analog of pancuronium, is more potent than pancuronium and has minimal, if any, cardiovascular side effects even at high multiples of the ED$_{95}$. The combination of a positively charged quaternary ammonium group at one end of the molecule and a polar ring at the opposite end favors the extensive heptobiliary uptake of vecuronium.[17] It has been estimated that as much as 75% of a dose of vecuronium may be excreted through the bile. Twenty-five percent is excreted as the 3-hydroxy (3-desacetyl) metabolite and 50% is excreted unchanged. In cats, exclusion of blood flow from the liver nearly doubles the duration of action of vecuronium and enhances its neuromuscular blockade.[18] Thus, of all the nondepolarizing relaxants, vecuronium is the most dependent on biliary excretion. The rapid uptake of vecuronium into the liver and subsequent metabolism may be responsible for its intermediate duration of action at several multiples of the ED$_{95}$. 3-Hydroxy vecuronium has 50–70% the neuromuscular blocking properties of vecuronium and has been shown to accumulate in humans after prolonged administration of vecuronium.[17,19] The kidney excretes both vecuronium and the 3-hydroxy metabolite.[20] Two other vecuronium metabolites (17-hydroxy vecuronium and 3,17-hydroxy vecuronium) are possible, although they are seemingly formed in minimal amounts, if at all, and have minimal neuromuscular blocking effects.[17,21,22] The elimination profile of vecuronium could be altered by administration of high doses (i.e., 0.4 mg/kg) or chronic administration in an intensive care setting.

Both increased sensitivity and tachyphylaxis have been reported.[19,23]

The pharmacodynamics and pharmacokinetics of vecuronium have been evaluated in patients with cirrhosis in several studies. Arden and coworkers noted that the onset time was prolonged in patients with liver disease (at 0.1 mg/kg) compared with control patients.[24] The recovery times, recovery index, and pharmacokinetics were unchanged by the liver disease. These dynamic data are consistent with other studies.[25,26] In contrast, Lebrault and colleagues showed a prolonged duration of action and a decrease in clearance when a larger dose of vecuronium (0.2 mg/kg) was administered to patients with hepatic cirrhosis.[27] The influence of liver disease on the dynamics and kinetics following relatively high doses of vecuronium (i.e., 0.4 mg/kg) is unknown. However, we have noted a markedly prolonged duration of blockade (i.e., 12–18 hours) after these high doses in patients having liver transplants.

Rocuronium (ORG 9426)

Rocuronium (ORG 9426) is a new, intermediate-acting steroidal relaxant without cardiovascular side effects. It is a derivative of vecuronium. Because of its lack of potency it has a relatively rapid onset rate in man. In cats, hepatic uptake and biliary excretion are the dominant mechanisms for its clearance.[28] Hepatobiliary clearance is about 75% and renal clearance is about 9%. It is thus anticipated that hepatic disorders alone or in association with impaired renal function will prolong the duration of action of rocuronium.

Relaxants of Long Duration

d-Tubocurarine

d-Tubocurarine has variable and complex routes of elimination. In normal patients 50–95% of *d*-tubocurarine is excreted unchanged in the urine and 5–18% in the bile.[29] Thus, although the differences are small, *d*-tubocurarine appears to be less dependent on the kidney for elimination than either metocurine or pancuronium. *d*-Tubocurarine diffuses passively into hepatocytes and is highly, actively concentrated in lysosomes.[30] Hepatic uptake and subsequent excretion appear to be an important alternative step in the elimination of *d*-tubocurarine.[31] This route is important in patients with severe renal disease. An increase in plasma level of bile acids, as seen in patients with cholestasis, inhibits the uptake of *d*-tubocurarine by the liver.[32] Resistance to *d*-tubocurarine has been reported in patients with liver disease.[33,34] This phenomenon has been attributed to increased binding of *d*-tubocurarine to gamma globulin.[35,36] The ratio of albumin to gamma globulin is frequently inverted in liver disease, and there is positive correlation between the gamma globulin level in the blood and the dose requirement of *d*-tubocurarine.[35–37] However, *d*-tubocurarine binds plasma protein to only a limited extent, and therefore, changes in plasma protein levels have minimal effect on its potency.[38,39] Moreover, several studies have shown that protein binding of drugs in cirrhotic patients is normal.[1,38,39] The most likely explanation for the resistance to *d*-tubocurarine in patients with liver disease is an increase in the drug's volume of distribution. Unfortunately, there are no studies on the pharmacokinetics of *d*-tubocurarine in these patients.

Pancuronium

Pancuronium, the biquaternary steroidal compound, is eliminated primarily by the kidney (70%) and also through hepatobiliary mechanisms. Hepatic biodegradation has been demonstrated for pancuronium in the following manner:[40] single deacetylation to 3-hydroxypancuronium (up to 25%) and to 17-hydroxypancuronium (<5%), and double deacetylation to 3,17-dihydroxypancuronium (<5%).[21,41,42] About 25% of pancuronium appears in the urine in the form of the 3-OH metabolite and less than 5% each in the form of the 17-OH and 3.17-dehydroxy metabolites.[41,42] Approximately 11% of pancuronium is excreted in the bile as the parent compound and its metabolites.[41]

Pancuronium has been studied extensively in patients with different types of hepatic dysfunction.[42–45] Several studies show prolonged elimination half-life and delayed recovery from pancuronium in patients with cholestasis.[42,44] Neuromuscular blockade lasts twice as long in patients with cholestasis compared with normal subjects.[42] The cause for the long duration of action may be related to a 50% reduction in plasma clearance of pancuronium[42] or an increase in its volume of distribution.[44] Regardless of the exact mechanism, the evidence is clear that in patients with biliary obstruction, the paralyzing effect of pancuronium is prolonged.

Duvaldestin and colleagues studied the pharmacokinetics of pancuronium in patients with cirrhosis and found an increased volume of distribution, a prolonged distribution half-life, a twofold increase in elimination half-life, and a 20% decrease in clearance.[43] These observations provide insight into the paradox of seeming resistance and increased sensitivity to pancuronium existing at the same time. The onset time of pancuronium would be prolonged because of the increase in the volume of distribution (i.e., resistance to the drug) and recovery would be delayed owing to prolonged elimination half-life, (i.e., increased sensitivity). Ward, Judge and Corall studied the pharmacokinetics of pancuronium in patients with hepatic failure and normal renal function.[45] The volume of distribution was normal, but the clearance was reduced by more than one-half, resulting in a threefold increase in elimination half-life. They noted that the dose required to produce paralysis was much larger than normal in these patients, implying that the neuromuscular junction was indeed resistant to the effects of pancuronium.

Pipecuronium

Pipecuronium is a new, long-acting steroidal relaxant without cardiovascular side effects. In humans about 25–30% of pipecuronium is excreted through the kidney and renal failure reduces its clearance.[3,46] Hepatic elimination and metabolic degradation are other possible mechanisms for clearance in humans. Metabolites have not been detected. In the rat there is only minimal hepatic elimination of pipecuronium, whereas in the pig significant hepatic elimination occurs.[3,47] Future studies are needed to resolve these issues.

Gallamine, Metocurine, and Doxacurium

Gallamine, metocurine, and doxacurium are eliminated largely unchanged in the urine. Liver disease, thus, appears to have no effect on the kinetics of these relaxants. The kidney is the sole pathway for gallamine elimination and 50–100% is excreted in 24 hours.[48–50] The dynamics and kinetics of gallamine have been studied in patients with extrahepatic cholestasis.[44,51] The onset, duration of action, and rate of recovery of neuromuscular transmission were normal; the pharmacokinetics were normal as well.

Metocurarine is second only to gallamine in its dependence on renal excretion and 40–60% is excreted unchanged in the urine.[29,52] Only 2% of a metocurine dose is found unchanged in the bile.[29]

Doxacurium, a new potent benzylisoquolinium relaxant, has a long duration of action and is devoid of cardiovascular and histamine-releasing side effects at clinically effective doses. Disposition studies in animals have shown that doxacurium is eliminated largely unchanged in the urine. In humans about 30% of doxacurium is excreted unchanged in the urine within 12 hours.[53,54] The pharmacodynamics and pharmacokinetics of doxacurium have been measured in normal patients and those with hepatic failure.[54] At equal doses of doxacurium (0.15 mg/kg) the patients with hepatic failure achieved a lesser and more variable degree of neuromuscular blockade than normal patients. The onset time and clinical duration tended to be longer in these patients. Hepatic failure had no effect on the clearance, volume of distribution, or mean residence time of doxacurium.

Summary

The role of the liver in the elimination of nondepolarizing muscle relaxants is reasonably well defined. This information can be used to predict the influence of severe end stage liver disease on the pharmacodynamics and pharmacokinetics of these relaxants.

References

1. Davis, P.J., Stiller, R.L., McGowan, F.X. et al. (1993) Decreased protein binding of alfentanil in plasma from children with kidney or liver failure. *Paediatric Anaesthesia* 3:19–22.
2. Rupp, S.M. (1987) Muscle relaxants and the patient with renal and/or hepatic failure. In *Muscle Relaxants* (Azar I., ed.). New York: Marcel Dekker, 149.
3. Caldwell, J.E., Canfell, P.C., Castagnoli, K.P., et al. (1989) The influence of renal failure on the pharmacokinetics and duration of action of pipecuronium bromide in patients anesthetized with halothane and nitrous oxide. *Anesthesiology* 70:7.
4. Magorian, T. and Lynam, D.P. Clinical use of muscle relaxants in patients with hepatic disease. In *Problems in Anaesthesia: Neuromuscular Relaxants* (S.M. Rupp, ed). Philadelphia: J.B. Lippincott, p. 500.
5. Phillips, B.J. and Hunter, J.M. (1992) Use of mivacurium chloride by constant infusion in the anephric patient. *British Journal of Anaesthesiology* 68:492.
6. Nigrovic, V. and Banoub, M. (1992) Pharmacokinetic modeling of a parent drug and its metabolite. *Clinical Pharmacokinetics* 22:396.

7. Stiller, R.L., Cook, D.R., and Chakravorti, S. (1985) In vitro degradation of atracurium in human plasma. *British Journal of Anaesthesiology* 57:1085.

8. Chapple, D.J., Miller, A.A., Ward, J.B. et al. (1987) Cardiovascular and neurological effects of laudanosine. *British Journal of Anaesthesiology* 59:218.

9. Al-Muhandis, W.M., Lauretti, G.R., and Pleuvry, B.J. (1991) Modification by drugs used in anaesthesia of CNS stimulation induced in mice by laudanosine and strychnine. *British Journal of Anaesthesiology* 67:608.

10. Katz, Y. and Gavish, M. (1989) Laudanosine does not displace receptor-specific ligands from the benzodiazepinergic or muscarinic receptors. *Anesthesiology* 70:109.

11. Pittet, J.F., Tassonyi, E., Schopfer, C., et al. (1990) Plasma concentrations of laudanosine, but not of atracurium, are increased during the anhepatic phase of orthotopic liver transplantation in pigs. *Anesthesiology* 72:145.

12. Ward, S., Boheimer, N., Weatherley, B.C., et al. (1987) Pharmacokinetics of atracurium and its metabolites in patients with normal renal function, and in patients in renal failure. *British Journal of Anaesthesiology* 59:697.

13. Ward, S. and Neill, E.A.M. (1983) Pharmacokinetics of atracurium in acute hepatic failure (with acute renal failure). *British Journal of Anaesthesiology* 55:1169.

14. Cook, D.R., Brandom, B.W., Stiller, R.L. et al. (1984) Pharmacokinetics of atracurium in normal and liver failure patients. *Anesthesiology* 61:A433.

15. O'Kelly, B., Jayais, P., Veroli, P., et al. (1991) Dose requirements of vecuronium, pancuronium, and atracurium during orthotopic liver transplantation. *Anesthesia and Analgesia* 73:794.

16. Gyasi, H.K. and Naguib, M. (1985) Atracurium and severe hepatic disease: A case report. *Canadian Anaesthetists Society Journal* 32:161.

17. Bencini, A., Scaf, A.H.J., Sohn, Y.J., Kersten, U., and Agoston, S. (1983) Clinical pharmacokinetics of vecuronium. In *Clinical Experiences with Norcuron* (Org NC 45 Vecuronium Bromide) (Agoston S., Bowman W.C., Miller R.D., Viby-Mogensen J., eds). Amsterdam: Excerpta Medica, p. 115.

18. Durant, N.N., Houwertjes, M.C., and Agoston, S. (1979) Hepatic elimination of Org NC 45 and pancuronium. *Anesthesiology* 51:S67.

19. Segredo, V., Matthay, M.A., Sharma, M.L. et al. (1990) Prolonged neuromuscular blockade after long-term administration of vecuronium in two critically ill patients. *Anesthesiology* 72:556.

20. Bencini, A.F., Houwertjes, M.C., and Agoston, S. (1985) Effects of hepatic uptake of vecuronium bromide and its putative metabolites on their neuromuscular blocking actions in the cat. *British Journal of Anaesthesiology* 57:789.

21. Miller, R.D., Agoston, S., Booij, L.H.D.J., Kersten, U.W., Crul, J.F., and Ham, J. (1978) The comparative potency and pharmacokinetics of pancuronium and its metabolites in anesthetized man. *Journal of Pharmacology and Experimental Therapeutics* 207:539.

22. Marshall, I.G., Gibb, A.J., and Durant, N.N. (1983) Neuromuscular and vagal blocking actions of pancuronium bromide, its metabolites, and vecuronium bromide (Org NC 45) and its potential metabolites in the anesthetized cat. *British Journal of Anaesthesiology* 55:703.

23. Agoston, S. (1991) Paralysis after long-term administration of vecuronium. *Anesthesiology* 74:792.

24. Arden, J.R., Lynam, D.P., Castagnoli, K.P., et al. (1988) Vecuronium in alcoholic liver disease: A pharmacokinetic and pharmacodynamic analysis. *Anesthesiology,* 68:771.

25. Bell, C.F., Hunter, J.M., Jones, R.S. et al. (1985) Use of atracurium and vecuronium in patients with oesophageal varices. *British Journal of Anaesthesiology* 57:160.

26. Hunter, J.M., Parker, C.J.R., Bell, C.F. et al. (1985) The use of different doses of vecuronium in patients with liver dysfunction. *British Journal of Anaesthesiology* 57:758.

27. Lebrault, C., Duvaldestin, P., Henzel, D. et al. (1986) Pharmacokinetics and pharmacodynamics of vecuronium in patients with cholestasis. *British Journal of Anaesthesiology* 58:983.

28. Khuenl-Brady, K., Castagnoli, K.P., Canfell, P.C. et al. (1990) The neuromuscular blocking effects and pharmacokinetics of ORG 9426 and ORG 9616 in the cat. *Anesthesiology* 72:669.

29. Meijer, D.K.F., Weitering, J.G., Vermeer, G.A., and Scaf, A.H.J. (1979) Comparative pharmacokinetics of *d*-tubocurarine and metocurine in man. *Anesthesiology* 51:402.

30. Weitering, J.G., Lammers, W., Meijer, D.K.F., and Mulder, G.J. (1977) Localization of *d*-tubocurarine in rat liver lysosomes: Lysosomal uptake, biliary excretion and displacement by quinacrine in vivo. *Naunyn-Schmiedebergs Archives of Pharmacology* 299:277.

31. Meijer, D.K.F., Scaf, A.J.H. (1968) Inhibition of the transport of *d*-tubocurarine from blood to bile by *k*-stropkantoside in the isolated perfused rat liver. *European Journal of Pharmacology* 4:343.

32. Vonk, R.J., Scholtens, E., Keulemans, G.T.P., and Meijer D.K.F. (1978) Choleresis and transport mechanisms: I.V. influence of bile salt choleresis on the hepatic transport of the organic cations *d*-tubocurarine and 4N-acetylprocaine ethobromide. *Naunyn-Schmiedebergs Archives of Pharmacology* 302:1.

33. Dundee, J.W. and Gray, T.C. (1953) Resistance to *d*-tubocurarine chloride in the presence of liver damage. *Lancet* 2:16.

34. El-Hakim, M.S. and Baraka, A. (1963) *d*-Tubocurarine in liver disease. *Kasr El-Aini Journal of Surgery.* 4:99.

35. Baraka, A. and Gabali, F. (1968) Correlation between tubocurarine requirements and plasma protein pattern. *British Journal of Anaesthesiology* 40:89.

36. Stovner, J., Theodorsen, L., and Bjelke, E. (1971) Sensitivity to tubocurarine and alcuronium with special reference to plasma protein pattern. *British Journal of Anaesthesiology* 43:385.

37. Thompson, J.M. (1976) Pancuronium binding by serum proteins. *Anaesthesia* 31:219.

38. Ghoneim, M.M., Kramer, Sr. E., Bannow, R., Pandya, H., and Routh, J.I. Binding of *d*-tubocurarine to plasma proteins in normal man and in patients with hepatic or renal disease. *Anesthesiology* 39:410.

39. Duvaldestin, P. and Henzel, D. (1982) Binding of tubocurarine, fazadinium, pancuronium and Org NC 45 to serum proteins in normal man and in patients with cirrhosis. *British Journal of Anaesthesiology* 54:513.

40. Savage, D.S., Sleigh, T., and Carlyle, I. (1980) The emergence of Org NC 45 from the pancuronium series. *British Journal of Anaesthesiology* 52:3S.

41. Agoston, S., Vermeer, G.A., Kersten, U.W., and Meijer, D.K.F. (1973) The fate of pancuronium bromide in man. *Acta Anaesthesia Scandia* 17:267.

42. Somogyi, A.A., Shanks, C.A., and Triggs, E.J. (1977) Disposition kinetics of pancuronium bromide in patients with total biliary obstruction. *British Journal of Anaesthesiology* 49:1103.

43. Duvaldestin, P., Agoston, S., Henzel, D., Kersten, U.W., and Desmonts, J.M. (1978) Pancuronium pharmacokinetics in patients with liver cirrhosis. *British Journal of Anaesthesiology* 50:1131.

44. Westra, P., Vermeer, G.A., deLange, A.R., Scaf, A.H.J., Meijer, D.K.F., and Wesseling, H. (1981) Hepatic and renal disposition of pancuronium and gallamine in patients with extrahepatic cholestasis. *British Journal of Anaesthesiology* 53:331.

45. Ward, S., Judge, S., Corall, I. (1982) Pharmacokinetics pancuronium bromide in liver failure. *British Journal of Anaesthesiology* 54:227P.

46. Ornstein, E., Matteo, R.S., Schwartz, A.E., et al. (1992) Pharmacokinetics and pharmacodynamics of pipecuronium bromide (Arduan) in elderly surgical patients. *Anesthesia and Analgesia* 74:841.

47. Pittet, J.F., Tassonyi, E., Schopfer, C., et al. (1990) Dose requirements and plasma concentrations of pipecuronium during bilateral renal exclusion and orthotopic liver transplantation in pigs. *British Journal of Anaesthesiology* 65:779.

48. Feldman, S.A., Cohen, E.N., and Golling, R.C. (1969) The excretion of gallamine in the dog. *Anesthesiology* 30:593.

49. Chagas, C. (1972) The Fate of Curare During Curarization: Ciba Foundation Symposium on Curare and Curare-like Agents (Reucks AVS, ed.). Boston: Little, Brown, p. 2.

50. Agoston, S., Vermeer, G.A., Kersten, U.W., and Scaf, A.H.J. (1978) A preliminary investigation of the renal and hepatic excretion of gallamine triethiodide in man. *British Journal of Anaesthesiology* 50:345.

51. Ramzan, M.I., Shanks, C.A., and Triggs, E.J. (1981) Pharmacokinetics and pharmacodynamics of gallamine triethiodide in patients with total biliary obstruction. *Anesthesia and Analgesia* 60:289.

52. Brotherton, W.P. and Matteo, R.S. (1981) Pharmacokinetics and pharmacodynamics of metocurine in humans with or without renal failure. *Anesthesiology* 55:273.

53. Dresner, D.L., Basta, S.J., Ali, H.A. et al. (1990) Pharmacokinetics and pharmacodynamics of doxacurium in young and elderly patients during isoflurane anesthesia. *Anesthesia and Analgesia* 71:498.

54. Cook, D.R., Freeman, J.A., Lai, A.A. et al. (1991) Pharmacokinetics and pharmacodynamics of doxacurium in normal patients and in those with hepatic or renal failure. *Anesthesia and Analgesia* 72:145.

THREE

Anesthetic Considerations

Chapter 7

Diagnostic Endoscopy, Sclerotherapy, and Biliary Procedures

Rosalind Ward and Julian Bion

This heterogeneous group of patients presents the anesthetist with a range of potential problems (Table 7–1) that need to be considered in relation to the periods before, during, and after anesthesia.

Preoperative Assessment and Preparation

The aim of preoperative assessment should be to identify physiological abnormalities that, if unrecognized or uncorrected, will lead to subsequent organ impairment and reduced postoperative survival.

Etiology of Disease

Most diagnostic endoscopies are performed under sedation and topical anesthesia, and anesthetists may be asked to provide a general anesthetic without time for preoperative assessment. The pathology

Table 7–1. Factors to be assessed.

Etiology of disease
Circulating volume
Clotting
Drug pharmacokinetics
Cerebral function
Renal function
Jaundice
Nutrition
Iatrogenic complications

may include acute or chronic obstruction of the esophagus, reflux esophagitis, peptic ulcer, carcinoma, and jaundice requiring endoscopic retrograde cholangiopancreatographic (ERCP) examination for diagnosis.

Sclerotherapy is performed for hemorrhage from esophageal or gastric varices resulting from cirrhosis and portal hypertension. The patient's alcohol consumption should be assessed; if high, it may necessitate increased dosage of some anesthetic agents (e.g., thiopentone, *d*-tubocurarine, pancuronium) because of cross-tolerance with alcohol and an increased volume of distribution. On the other hand, chronic alcohol abuse may have led to such severe hepatocellular damage that drug doses must be reduced because of decreased protein binding and prolonged elimination.[1] Patients with cirrhosis and edema may appear resistant to a first dose of muscle relaxant, because of the larger volume of distribution, yet show prolonged effects of the drug because of slow elimination.[2] Hepatitis B status must be established for patients with liver disease, and where positive, this requires measurement of antibody titers to hepatitis B core antigen. High titers indicate a high risk of infection, and full precautions must be taken by all hospital staff (Chapter 15). Patients with hemochromatosis may have impaired pancreatic and myocardial function as well as cirrhosis.[3] Blood glucose estimation determines the need for further investigation. Clinical examination, with cardiac ultrasound when indicated, gives a guide to left ventricular function.

Biliary surgery is performed in neonates for congenital abnormalities such as biliary atresia, but it is performed in adults for acquired disease, which in most cases is inflammatory or neoplastic. Disease of the gallbladder is common, including cholecystitis and gallstones; tumors include carcinoma of the head of the pancreas and, more rarely, carcinoma of the gallbladder or biliary tree. In longstanding biliary obstruction, ascending cholangitis and secondary hepatocellular damage may occur.

Circulating Volume

Clinical examination must concentrate on the capacity of the patient to maintain oxygen delivery to the tissues and therefore includes an assessment of cardiac output, respiratory reserve, and hemoglobin. The circulating blood volume may need to be restored to normal with either blood components or plasma substitutes. Patients who have suffered chronic blood loss (e.g., from an ulcer carcinoma) may need red cell replacement. Those with malnutrition or impaired liver synthetic function may be sufficiently hypoproteinemic to need albumin as well as red cells. Where nausea or vomiting has been prolonged, hypovolemia and hypokalemia may occur.

Recent acute bleeding in particular requires careful assessment because occult volume depletion can escape attention and needs correction before anesthesia can be induced. Accurate clinical assessment of circulating volume is difficult even in hematemeses,[4] although measurement of overt loss is important. Frequent measurement and recording of heart rate, blood loss, and central venous pressure indicate continuing loss, or adequate replacement, but it should be remembered that high venous tone will minimize the pressure changes on which the assessment of circulating volume is based.[5] Patients should be nursed in the lateral position to minimize the risk of aspiration of vomit. Colloid solutions may be given while awaiting the arrival of blood for transfusion, and modified gelatin solution will stay in the circulation for 4–5 hours; hetastarch provides plasma expansion for 12–48 hours and is then eliminated from the body at decreasing rates. The half-life is

17 days for the greater part of a dose, but 48 days for the last 10%.[6]

Temporary measures undertaken to control hemorrhage from varices before surgery include the use of splanchnic vasoconstrictors, such as vasopressin 0.4–0.8 units/minute, either alone or with glyceryl trinitrate;[7] glypressin or somatostatin;[8] or balloon compression using a Sengstaken-Blakemore tube. When in position, this tube may prevent the swallowing of saliva, which accumulates above the esophageal balloon unless a modified version with a suction port incorporated is used. Many of these patients have an impaired level of consciousness so they are at risk of aspiration pneumonia. Tracheal intubation may be necessary to ensure airway protection.

Clotting

Coagulation may be impaired because of the inability of a diseased liver to synthesize clotting factors, exacerbated in the presence of cholestasis by diminished vitamin K absorption, or due to abnormal consumption of clotting factors and platelets in disseminated intravascular coagulation. Laboratory estimations of prothrombin time (PT) and partial thromboplastin time, platelet count, fibrinogen levels, and fibrin degradation products will help to clarify the cause. The administration of fresh frozen plasma supplies clotting factors in the short term, and in the longer term vitamin K will help to return the PT toward normal in cholestasis. Platelet concentrates provide a brief elevation of platelet count, but a specific value below which they should be replenished has not been determined. Most clinicians provide platelet cover for surgery if the count is less than $50 \times 10^9/L$. Platelet function is as important as platelet count; moreover, platelets may be sequestered rapidly in splenomegaly.

Drugs

Patients with autoimmune liver disease may be taking steroids and other immunosuppressant drugs and are therefore vulnerable to infection. Particular attention must be given to aseptic techniques for vascular cannulation and to sterility of tracheal tubes. Steroids may need to be given parenterally during the perioperative period, but it is usually not necessary to restart steroids in patients who recently stopped the drug.[9]

A failing liver may be unable to metabolize the citrate present in large volumes of stored citrate-phosphate-dextrose blood or fresh frozen plasma. Low plasma levels of ionized calcium may result from chelation by the citrate. Ionized calcium levels should be measured and replaced with calcium chloride.

Cerebral Function

All central nervous system depressant drugs given to patients with hepatic encephalopathy have greatly enhanced effects. Sedative premedication is contraindicated, and narcotic analgesics should be given (when absolutely necessary) with great caution. Both hyponatremia and its rapid correction may worsen encephalopathy; and, in hyponatremia from other causes, pontine damage has been reported.[10] Cerebral perfusion must be maintained without increasing intracranial pressure; patients should be nursed in the head-up position to avoid the exacerbation of cerebral edema by venous congestion. If the patient's conscious level has deteriorated so that reflex protection of the airway is in doubt, particularly in the presence of vomiting, the traditional lateral head-down position cannot be used. In this situation tracheal intubation may be the best way to protect the airway. Mechanical hyperventilation to reduce $PaCO_2$ to 3–3.5 kPa reduces intracranial pressure only transiently, by reducing cerebral blood flow; this may not be advantageous.

Renal Function

Renal insufficiency associated with hepatic impairment is common and may form part of the hepatorenal syndrome. Acute renal failure may follow surgery to relieve obstructive jaundice. Until recent years this was invariably a fatal complication.[11] Renal dialysis has improved the outcome for many patients, but mortality is still extremely high.[12] Assessment of renal function is therefore an essential part of preoperative evaluation. Urine testing and measurement of blood urea, electrolytes, and crea-

tinine will indicate the need for further investigation of urine osmolality and electrolytes and creatinine clearance. Urinary sodium concentrations will help to distinguish between the hepatorenal syndrome (less than 10 mmol/L) and renal failure (more than 40 mmol/L). Preexisting renal impairment may be aggravated by anesthesia and surgery: hypoxemia, hypovolemia, and hypotension may result in impaired oxygen delivery to the kidneys.

Renal protection starts with an accurate assessment of circulating volume. Three specific measures are conventionally undertaken to preserve renal function: renal arterial vasodilators, loop diuretics, and mannitol. These agents should be started preoperatively rather than intraoperatively if renal function is deteriorating. The mode of action of these agents and their effect on outcome is not entirely clear, but animal work shows that dopamine in concentrations of less than 5 µg/kg/min increases renal blood flow; this has not yet been conclusively proven in humans, and its value is unknown. Frusemide reduces renal oxygen consumption[13] and together with mannitol increases tubular fluid flow, which may assist in the clearance of intraluminal debris and bilirubin.

Jaundice

The etiology of jaundice (prehepatic, hepatic, or posthepatic) will usually have been established before the patient is presented for anesthesia, although the detailed cause may not be known. Jaundice is significant because of the risks of bilirubin crystalluria and tubular obstruction. Bile salts may be important in binding endotoxin within the gut lumen, and obstructive jaundice may predispose to the development of endotoxinemia with an adverse effect on renal function;[14] this work has not been confirmed. Unrelieved biliary obstruction eventually causes hepatocellular damage, which affects the choice of anesthetic drugs and technique.

Nutrition

The nutritional state of these patients may be relatively normal, or it may reveal the malnutrition and vitamin deficiencies of the chronic alcoholic, the hypoproteinemia of liver failure, or the wasting and cachexia of carcinoma. By contrast, many patients with gallstones are obese, which may cause problems with venous access for the anesthetist and for the surgeon with the interpretation of abdominal signs. It also increases the risk of postoperative chest complications, which is already high for those patients with upper abdominal incisions.[15] Preoperative chest physiotherapy will assist those patients most at risk (e.g., smokers) to clear bronchial secretions.

Parenteral vitamin supplements and adequate calories should be provided when appropriate before non-urgent procedures.[16] For urgent cases, there may be time only for the addition of albumin to the intravenous regimen before the start of anesthesia. A solution of 5% albumin may be given to patients who require additional fluid as well as albumin and have low or normal serum sodium; 20% albumin solution (sodium content below 130 mmol/L) is preferable for patients with sodium retention or gross albumin depletion, as the amount of sodium given is small in relation to the amount of protein (13 mmol for every 20 g). Patients who have lost significant muscle bulk may have difficulty in establishing effective ventilation and clearing bronchial secretions after anesthesia.

Anesthetic Management

Premedication

Anxiety, heartburn, nausea, and pain are all problems that may need attention. Benzodiazepines are effective anxiolytics and can be given on the day of surgery, the previous night, or both. Patients with symptoms of esophageal reflux should be given an H_2 receptor antagonist (e.g., ranitidine) to reduce the volume and raise the pH of the gastric contents. Antiemetic drugs are inappropriate and ineffective for those patients whose nausea is caused by blood in the stomach; others may benefit from metoclopramide or a phenothiazine antiemetic (e.g., prochlorperazine or perphenazine). Some patients may need opioids for severe preoperative pain, but morphine is often avoided in patients with gallstones, as it may increase biliary tract pressure and cause spasm of the sphincter of Oddi. Pethidine is conventionally used in this situation, as these effects are less severe at equianalgesic doses.[17] This problem may be of more theoretical than practical sig-

nificance.[18] All sedative drugs should be avoided in patients with liver failure.

Anesthesia

Diagnostic Endoscopy

Patients with esophageal reflux or obstruction should be preoxygenated, then anesthetized with a rapid-sequence induction and cricoid pressure to minimize the risk of aspiration. Tracheal intubation is essential because of the shared airway with the surgeon. Hypnosis can be maintained either with a volatile agent added to the oxygen/nitrous oxide gas mixture or with increments of an intravenous (I.V.) induction agent. The use of intermittent positive pressure ventilation (IPPV) helps the surgeon, as instrumentation is easier (hence safer) in a paralysed patient; it also allows anesthesia to be maintained at a lighter plane than would otherwise be necessary, so that waking and recovery of reflexes occurs more rapidly. The choice of muscle relaxant for maintenance depends on the likely duration of the procedure. Increments of suxamethonium (following an anticholinergic given at induction; e.g., atropine or glycopyrrolate) may be the best choice if the anesthetic is expected to last less than 10 minutes. For longer procedures, atracurium or vercuronium are suitable, and small increments can be given which will last for only 5–10 minutes.

Patient monitoring should include ECG for heart rate and rhythm, noninvasive measurement of blood pressure, capnography and oxygen saturation. Tracheal extubation should be carried out (after satisfactory reversal of neuromuscular block) with the patient in a lateral position on a tipping trolley and able to obey simple commands.

Sclerotherapy

These patients will have suffered recent hemorrhage from varices, and stability of heart rate and blood pressure with adequate volume replacement should be achieved before induction of anesthesia. Rapid infusion of colloid may be needed during the anesthetic, so a wide-bore IV cannula must be in situ and a supply of blood, plasma, or a substitute available before the start. The choice of induction drug and dosage is made in the knowledge that these patients can easily be rendered hypotensive, and the presence of blood in the stomach demands a rapid-sequence induction with cricoid pressure following preoxygenation. IPPV should be employed to facilitate the surgical maneuvers and to avoid deep planes of anesthesia, which these sick patients tolerate badly. Isoflurane is the volatile agent of choice where liver function is compromised for two reasons: first, deleterious effects on function are unlikely;[19–21] second, total hepatic blood flow is well maintained.[22] The arterial fraction of this flow increases in dogs and pigs,[23–25] though not in humans.

Patients with compromised liver function may show delayed metabolism of all drugs handled by the liver, and these should be avoided where alternatives exist. For example, atracurium is the muscle relaxant of choice because its spontaneous (Hoffman) degradation will proceed regardless of hepatic function though clearance of its major metabolite, laundanosine, is significantly impaired in acute hepatic failure.[25a] Patients with long-standing disease have reduced cholinesterase synthesis, leading to slower hydrolysis of drugs such as suxamethonium and the local anesthetic esters cocaine, procaine, and amethocaine. However, liver disease alone is unlikely to prolong suxamethonium apnea beyond 30 minutes.[26] Diminished synthesis of plasma albumin means that some drugs that are significantly protein-bound will produce a higher free drug concentration from any given dose; for instance, the unbound fraction of thiopentone can increase by 75–90% and that of diazepam by 144%,[1] though binding of curare and pancuronium remains much the same in cirrhotic patients as in normal people.[27] Drug elimination is hampered in chronic liver disease by reductions in hepatic blood flow and intrinsic clearance, compounded by intra- and extrahepatic shunting in cirrhosis.[28]

Monitoring should include those features described for endoscopy. After satisfactory reversal of neuromuscular block, a good case can be made for tracheal extubation while the patient is still asleep (in a lateral, head-down position) to avoid coughing on the tracheal tube, which could precipitate fresh variceal bleeding.

Biliary Surgery

A balanced anesthetic technique with IPPV is most suitable for these patients. Hypotension and hypoxia are particularly hazardous to hepatic and renal blood flow when these organs are already at risk, as autoregulation may be impaired.

Volatile agents are not contraindicated in jaundiced patients, but their selection requires some consideration. Halothane can be used for biliary surgery if there has been no recent exposure to it; but given the rare incidence of hepatitis following its use and the elevation of liver enzymes that result from multiple exposures, it is probably best avoided. This may be particularly true for obese middle-aged women, who take up large amounts into fat depots from where it is slowly released over several days, leading to prolonged (and therefore increased) metabolism. Enflurane, while not normally nephrotoxic, does lead to the excretion of higher levels of inorganic fluoride than the other currently available agents, and may complicate matters in patients whose renal function is already at risk (i.e., those with obstructive jaundice undergoing surgery). Isoflurane, being only 0.2% metabolized, results in very low levels of organic or inorganic metabolites and is a good choice.

Obstructive jaundice impedes the elimination of any drugs that depend on biliary excretion to a significant extent. Pancuronium has an increased volume of distribution and prolonged elimination half-life,[29] and the same is likely to be true for vecuronium. While in theory renal excretion should increase to compensate, this may not be possible, especially since these very patients are prone to develop acute renal failure. It is prudent to avoid such drugs in these patients.

The scale of monitoring in these cases depends on the extent of the surgery as well as the condition of the patient. A fit patient having a routine cholecystectomy and common bile duct exploration requires a wide-bore cannula for rapid venous access, ECG, noninvasive blood pressure, and capnography and oxygen saturation displays. More extensive surgery in a sick patient requires central venous pressure measurement, and direct intra-arterial pressure monitoring is desirable if major hemodynamic changes are likely.

The high risk of acute renal failure after surgery for obstructive jaundice makes renal protective measures desirable. Maintenance of oxygen delivery to the tissues is crucial. Avoidance of hypotension, hypovolemia, and hypoxemia is paramount. The measures described for preoperative prophylaxis of renal function should be continued throughout the perioperative periods. These include mannitol 0.5 g/kg and frusemide 20–40 mg; if renal blood flow is impaired, then dopamine 3 μg/kg/min is an appropriate adjunct.

Postoperative Care

Immediate care includes observation of the airway, ventilation, and circulation as for any patient. Endoscopy patients are unlikely to need analgesia, but pain may occasionally be a sign of esophageal perforation. Frequent observations and inspection of the patient for surgical emphysema should be continued and a chest x-ray performed when this is suspected.

After sclerotherapy, patients with varices must be watched for signs of further bleeding, and urine output should be monitored for signs of hypovolemia or renal failure.

Biliary surgery commonly gives rise to postoperative nausea so antiemetics may be required. These operations are notorious for postoperative incision pain, which not only causes distress but also hinders deep breathing and coughing.[30] Postoperative chest physiotherapy helps patients clear bronchial secretions, but they will need adequate analgesia for this to be effective. Several methods are available.

The wound can be infiltrated with local anesthetic solution (e.g., 0.5% bupivacaine) by the surgeon during closure which can give good relief of incision pain,[31] though it will not help visceral pain. The same is true of intercostal nerve block, which can be useful for Kocher's incision provided sufficient segments are blocked; 3 mL bupivacaine 0.5% with adrenalin is injected at each space. The possibility of pneumothorax must be remembered and anticipated. Both these techniques can provide up to 8 hours of analgesia but then need to be repeated. Regional block by spinal or epidural injection of local anesthetics is not commonly used, as a high level block is needed, making hypotension a possibility. The patient needs to be nursed in a high-dependency unit with close observation of the blood pressure. However, such a block will give effective pain relief and improve postoperative lung function.[32,32a] It should not, of course, be performed if coagulation is abnormal. E.g., if prothrombin time or partial thromboplastin time are prolonged beyond normal range, or if platelet count is below 100×10^9/L. Opioids given by the intrathecal or extradural route can offer good analgesia without the risk of hypotension, since there is no sympathetic blockade.

The patient will still need high-dependency nursing because of the risk of delayed respiratory depression, which has been reported up to 24 hours after intrathecal opioids.

The traditional use of intramuscular opioids continues in the majority of cases and is only partially effective because of the difficulty in arranging for a repeat dose to be given before the previous one has completely worn off. The use of IV opioid infusions, either at a preset rate or on demand by the patient[33,34] seems to achieve a smoother result but requires close attention to the patient to provide optimal analgesia without significant respiratory depression.[35]

In the case of liver failure, opioids must be given extremely cautiously. A short-acting drug given by infusion (such as alfentanil) is very useful;[36] because of its potency, this should only be administered in a high-dependency unit. There has been one report of delayed alfentanil clearance following infusion in a critically ill patient.[37] Blood levels and therapeutic efficacy are difficult to predict clinically.[38]

The majority of these patients will present the anesthetist with few problems in the perioperative period, but, as both hepatic and renal impairment may coexist in a clinically covert state, assessment of the patient must be detailed and should include appropriate laboratory tests. The key is successful anesthesia is meticulous preoperative assessment.

References

1. Sear, J. W. (1987) Toxicity of I.V. anaesthetics. *British Journal of Anaesthesia* 59:24–45.
2. Hunter, J. M. (1987). Adverse effects of neuromuscular blocking drugs. *British Journal of Anaesthesia* 59:46–60.
3. Stoelting, R. K., Dierdorf, S. F., and McCammon, R. L. (1988a) *Anesthesia and Coexisting Disease,* 2nd edn. New York: Churchill Livingstone, p. 385.
4. Shippy, C. R., Appel, P. L. and Shoemaker, W. C. (1984) Reliability of clinical monitoring to assess blood volume in critically ill patients. *Critical Care Medicine* 12:107–12.
5. Weil, M. H., Shubin, H. and Rosoff, L. (1965) Fluid repletion in circulatory shock. *Journal of the American Medical Association* 192:668–74.
6. Hulse, J. D. and Yacobi, A. (1983) Hetastarch: an overview of the colloid and its metabolism. *Drug Intelligence and Clinical Pharmacy* 17:334–41.
7. Westaby, D. (1988) The management of active variceal bleeding. *Intensive Care Medicine* 14:100–05.
8. Triger, D. R. (1986) Management of bleeding oesophageal varices. *British Journal of Hospital Medicine* 35:96–105.

9. Plumpton, F. S., Besser, G. M. and Cole, P. V. (1969) Corticosteroid treatment and surgery. 2: the management of all steroid cover. *Anaesthesia* 24:12.

10. Sterns, R. H., Riggs, J. E. and Schochet, S. S. (1986) Osmotic demyelination syndrome following correction of hyponatraemia. *New England Journal of Medicine* 314:1535–42.

11. Dawson, J. L. (1965) The incidence of postoperative renal failure in obstructive jaundice. *British Journal of Surgery* 52:663–65.

12. Wilkinson, S. P., Moodie, H., Stamatakis, J. D., Kakker, V. V. and Williams, R. (1976) Endotoxaemia and renal failure in cirrhosis and obstructive jaundice. *British Medical Journal* 2:1415–18.

13. Brezis, M., Rosen, S., Silva, P. and Epstein, F. H. (1984) Renal ischaemia: a new perspective. *Kidney International* 26:375–83.

14. Cahill, C. J. (1983) Prevention of postoperative renal failure in patients with obstructive jaundice—the role of bile salts. *British Journal of Surgery* 70:590–95.

15. Diament, M. L. and Palmer, K. N. V. (1966) Postoperative changes in gas tensions of arterial blood in ventilatory function. *Lancet* i:180.

16. Grimes, C. J. C., Younathan, M. T. and Lee, W. C. (1987) The effect of preoperative total parenteral nutrition on surgery outcomes. *Journal of the American Diatetic Association* 87:1201–06.

17. Goodman, L. S. and Gilman, A. (1970) *The Pharmacological Basis of Therapeutics,* 4th edn. New York: Macmillan; pp. 246 and 257.

18. Chisholm, R. J., Davis, F. M., Billings, J. D. and Gibbs, J. M. (1983) Narcotics and spasm of the sphincter of Oddi. A retrospective study of operative cholangiograms. *Anaesthesia* 38:689–91.

19. McLaughlin, D. F. and Eger, E. I., II. (1984) Repeated Isoflurane anesthesia in a patient with hepatic dysfunction. *Anesthesia and Analgesia* 63:775–78.

20. Eger, E. I., II (1984) The pharmacology of Isoflurane. *British Journal of Anaesthesia* 56:712S–995S.

21. Hussey, A. J., Aldridge, L. M., Paul, D., Ray, D. C., Beckett, G. J. and Allan, L. G. (1988) Plasma glutathione s-transferase concentration as a measure of hepatocellular integrity following a single general anaesthetic with halothane, enflurane or isoflurane. *British Journal of Anesthesia* 60:130–35.

22. Payen, D., Gatecel, C., Dupuy, P., Caraco, J. J., Riche, F. and Valleur, P. (1988) Effects of isoflurane vs. halothane on human arterial hepatic blood flow and portal vein blood flow after surgical stress. *Anesthesiology* 69:A77.

23. Gelman, S., Fowler, K. C. and Smith, K. R. (1983) Liver circulation and function during Isoflurane anaesthesia in dogs. *Anesthesiology* 59:A224.

24. Gelman, S., Fowler, K. C. and Smith, L. R. (1984) Liver circulation and function during isoflurane and halothane anesthesia. *Anesthesiology* 61:726–730.

25. Gelman, S., Dillard, E., Bradley, E. L. (1987) Hepatic circulation during surgical stress and anesthesia with halothane, isoflurane, or fentanyl. *Anesthesia and Analgesia* 66:936–43.

25a. Bion, J.F., Bowden, M.I., Chow, B., Honisberger, L. and Weatherley, B.C. (1993) Atracurium infusions in patients with fulminant hepatic failure awaiting liver transplantation. *Intensive Care Medicine* 13:S94–S98.

26. Stoelting, R. K., Dierdorf, S. F. and McCammon, R. L. (1988b). *Anesthesia and Coexisting Disease,* 2nd edn. New York: Churchill Livingstone, p. 358.

27. Wood, M. (1986) Plasma drug binding: implications for anesthesiologists. *Anesthesia and Analgesia* 65: 786–804.

28. Williams R. L. (1983) Drug administration in hepatic disease. *New England Journal of Medicine* 309: 1616–22.

29. Westra, P., Vermeer, G. A., de Lange, A. R., Scaf, A. H. J., Meijer, D. K. F. and Wesseling, H. (1981) Hepatic and renal disposition of pancuronium and gallamine in patients with extrahepatic cholestasis. *British Journal of Anaesthesia* 53:331–38.

30. Spence, A. A. (1980) Postoperative pulmonary complications. In: *General Anaesthesia,* 4th edn. (Gray, T. C., Nunn, J. F. and Utting, J. E. eds). London: Butterworth, pp. 592–93.

31. Lewis, D. L. and Thompson, W. A. L. (1953) Reduction of postoperative pain. *British Medical Journal* 1:973–74.

32. Spence, A. A. and Smith, G. (1971) Postoperative analgesia and lung function: a comparison of morphine with extradural block. *British Journal of Anaesthesia* 43:144–48.

32a. Cushieri, R. J., Morran, C. G., Howie, J. C. and McArdle, C. S. (1985) Postoperative pain and pulmonary complications: comparison of three analgesic regimens. *British Journal of Surgery,* 72:495–498.

33. Chakravarty, K., Tucker, W., Rosen, M. and Vickers, M. D. (1979) Comparison of buprenorphine and pethidine given intravenously on demand to relieve postoperative pain. *British Medical Journal* 21:895–97.

34. Clyburn, P. A. and Rosen, M. (1988) Patient-controlled analgesia with a mixture of pethidine and doxapram hydrochloride. *Anaesthesia* 43:190–193.

35. Catling, J. A., Pinto, D. M., Jordan, C. and Jones, J. G. (1980) Respiratory effects of analgesia after cholecystectomy: comparison of continuous and intermittent papaveretum. *British Medical Journal* 281: 478–80.

36. Ferrier, E., Marty, J., Bouffard, Y., Haberer, J. P., Levron, J. C., Duvaldestin, P. (1985) Alfentanil pharmacokinetics in patients with cirrhosis. *Anesthesiology,* 62:480–84.

37. Yate, P. M., Thomas, D. and Short, S. M. (1986) Comparison of infusions of alfentanil or pethidine for sedation of ventilated patients on the ITU. *British Journal of Anaesthesia* 58:1091–99.

38. Lemmens, H. J. M., Bovill, J. G., Burm, A. G. L. and Hennis, P. J. (1988) Alfentanil infusion in the elderly. *Anaesthesia* 43:850–56.

Chapter 8
Major Hepatic Procedures

Andre M. De Wolf and Yoogoo Kang

Although patients with liver disease undergo many different surgical procedures, in this chapter emphasis is placed on the anesthetic management of partial hepatectomy for tumor, trauma of the liver, and portacaval shunt.

Detailed descriptions of anatomy, function, and circulation of the liver can be found in Part One of this book; however, a brief summary is warranted. The hepatic parenchymal cells secrete bile salts into the biliary tract, absorb digested material from the blood, and store and release carbohydrates, proteins, vitamins, and lipids. Approximately 10–15 g of albumin is produced by the liver each day, resulting in a serum albumin level of 3.5–5.5 g/dL to maintain about 80% of the colloid osmotic pressure of the plasma. Most clotting factors are synthesized in the liver. The hepatocytes detoxify and deactivate exogenous and endogenous compounds, including many drugs and hormones. The liver converts lipid-soluble drugs to more water-soluble and usually less active metabolites.

Hepatic blood flow is approximately 25% of cardiac output; about 75% is supplied by the portal vein, and 25% by the hepatic artery. Portal venous blood has a higher oxygen saturation than does systemic venous blood because of mesenteric shunting; therefore, temporary occlusion of the hepatic artery is usually well tolerated by the healthy liver. Portal venous blood flow is determined mainly by the arterioles in the preportal splanchnic organs (gastrointestinal tract and spleen), and presinusoidal sphincters determine the relatively uniform distribution of blood flow through the liver. However, the major site of venous resistance within the liver is at the postsinusoidal sphincters in the hepatic veins. Their caliber is regulated by the sympathetic nervous system through alpha-receptors. The major site of resistance in the arterial blood supply is at the arterioles. Hepatic arterial blood flow is controlled mainly by the hepatic arterial buffer response, a mechanism to maintain total hepatic flow relatively constant by buffering the impact of portal flow alterations.[1] A decrease in oxygen delivery (e.g., acute hemodilution to a hematocrit of 22%) does not increase hepatic arterial blood flow; hepatic oxygen consumption is maintained by an increase in oxygen extraction.[2] Autoregulation in the liver is less effective than in other organs, and compensatory vasodilation fails to maintain perfusion when systolic blood pressure is less than 70–80 mmHg. Adrenergic receptors influence hepatic blood flow; alpha stimulation decreases and beta stimulation increases hepatic blood flow. Mechanical ventilation, especially when combined with positive end-expiratory pressure (PEEP), diminishes hepatic blood flow, probably by raising central venous pressure. Hypercapnia increases total hepatic blood flow by increasing portal venous flow and slightly reducing hepatic arterial flow.[3] Hypocapnia has opposite effects.

All anesthetic techniques, in the absence of surgical stimulation, reduce hepatic blood flow by about 30%. This effect may result from decreased splanchnic blood flow, decreased hepatic arterial blood flow associated with reduced perfusion pressure or with selective hepatic arterial constriction, or a combination of these factors. During surgery, hepatic blood flow is further reduced as much as 70%, especially during major upper abdominal procedures, probably by stimulation of the sympathetic nervous system.[4] Traction and manipulation of the splanchnic organs also contribute to the diminished splanchnic blood flow. Thus, laparotomy reduces hepatic blood flow while anesthesia plays a modifying role.[5]

Plasma levels of hepatic enzymes are significantly elevated after major abdominal surgery but not after minor surgery.[5] Anesthetic technique does not influence the release of these enzymes. Thus, postoperative hepatic dysfunction is mainly a result of the operation per se, and major surgery in patients with liver disease can lead to clinically significant hepatic dysfunction. The perioperative death rate in patients with liver cirrhosis undergoing major surgery may be as high as 25%. Causes of death include uncontrolled bleeding, poor wound healing, infection, and hepatic failure.

Hepatic Resection for Tumor

Primary Liver Cancer

The incidence of primary hepatic cancer is high in Asia and Africa and is increasing in Western countries. Etiological factors include environmental conditions, chronic hepatitis B, alcoholic cirrhosis, and hemochromatosis. The three most common types of tumor are hepatocellular carcinoma (hepatoma), cholangiocellular carcinoma (cholangiocarcinoma), and a mixed form (hepatocholangioma). Hepatoma constitutes about 80% of primary hepatic cancers. In 70% of patients with hepatoma, the tumor has spread outside the liver when the diagnosis is made. Metastasis occurs frequently into the hilar and celic lymph nodes, lung, and peritoneal surface. The tumor can be highly vascularized and can invade the portal or hepatic veins and result in venous occlusion. Cholangiocarcinomas make up about 15% of primary liver cancers. They are usually well-differentiated adenocarcinomas that spread invasively into the hepatic parenchyma.

Extrahepatic metastases are the rule by the time the tumor is detected. The mixed tumors resemble hepatomas in their pathologic and clinical behavior. Angiosarcomas of the liver have been seen in workers exposed to vinyl chloride for a prolonged time.

The diagnosis of the neoplasms is often difficult. Initially, right upper quadrant pain and weight loss are the only symptoms. Hepatomegaly or a palpable mass are other symptoms. Serum bilirubin and alkaline phosphatase are increased in about one-third of the patients. The significance of these alterations is often difficult to assess, however, because 60–85% of these patients have cirrhosis.[6] Liver radionuclide scans, computerized tomography, ultrasound, and magnetic resonance imaging can be helpful in making the diagnosis. Angiography is useful in detecting small tumors. High concentrations of alpha-fetoprotein (AFP), an alpha-1 globulin normally present only in the fetal circulation, are found in the serum of about 80% of patients with primary hepatomas. Postoperative changes in AFP levels can be used as an index of the success of hepatic resection.

Primary hepatic cancers are resistant to chemotherapy, and resection of the tumor offers the only possibility of cure, yielding a mean 5-year survival rate of 20–30%.[6] To be resectable, the tumor must be confined to the liver, and the lesion must be entirely encompassed by local excision, lobectomy, or extended lobectomy. However, the presence of chronic liver disease in many patients with hepatocellular carcinoma[7] may preclude liver resection because immediate survival after resection depends mostly on the functional status of the remaining liver. Liver transplantation has become an option for the treatment of unresectable hepatocellular carcinoma confined to the liver, although recurrence of tumor is common.[8] Palliative treatment includes selective hepatic arterial infusion of chemotherapeutic agents (doxorubicin).[9]

Metastatic Neoplasms of the Liver

Metastatic cancer of the liver is much more common than primary liver tumors. Surgical resection of a metastatic tumor confined to the liver can offer a chance for long-term survival. The two-year survival rate is as high as 70% for patients with Wilms' tumor and colorectal carcinoma.[10,11] Other tumors that are amenable to resection include pancreatic islet cell carcinomas, renal cell carcinomas, and carcinoids. A carcinoid tumor has an endocrinologic origin and secretes hormonal substances, such as serotonin, bradykinin, substance P, and other tachykinins.[12] The clinical symptoms of the carcinoid syndrome may include flushing, diarrhea, hypotension, telangiectasia, cyanosis, pellagra, valvular lesions mostly of the right side of the heart, bronchoconstriction, and peripheral edema. Carcinoid symptoms usually are seen only after widespread metastases are present, especially in the liver.[12] Palliative treatment includes the administration of somatostatin and analogues to inhibit hormone secretion, and ketanserin, a serotonin antagonist. A debulking liver resection, sometimes performed in combination with hepatic artery ligation or embolization, may also provide palliation of the carcinoid syndrome. Curative therapy is possible in a few selected patients by en bloc resection of the tumor and surrounding organs, followed by orthotopic transplantation of the liver with or without the pancreas and duodenum ("cluster procedure"). Administration of ketanserin and somatostatin analogues before or during surgery has proved to be extremely helpful in preventing or treating a "carcinoid crisis."[13,14] Epinephrine is probably contraindicated in the treatment of hypotension because it can stimulate further release of hormones by the tumor.

Surgical Technique of Hepatic Resection

During major lobar resection, a lobe or segment is resected along with its vessels. Injury to vessels and bile ducts supplying the residual tissue should be avoided. Injury to vessels usually does not occur with wedge resections. An extended right hepatectomy (trisegmentectomy) removes all but 15–20% of the hepatic mass. Left lobectomy or left lateral hepatectomy usually can be performed through an abdominal incision, but procedures involving extirpation of the right lobe require a thoracoabdominal approach. Hilar vessels are divided before the dissection is begun to obtain satisfactory hemostasis. Major bleeding can be temporarily controlled by compression of the portal triad: the hepatic artery and portal vein can be occluded safely for up to 60 minutes.[15]

Preoperative Evaluation

Because hepatic function is compromised after major hepatic resection, the decision to perform such an operation must take into account the size and location of the tumor. The general condition of the patient and the preoperative functional status of the liver should be evaluated by the determination of plasma levels of albumin, bilirubin, coagulation factors, prothrombin time, and the presence of encephalopathy or ascites.[6,16] Cirrhosis is considered to be a relative contraindication for hepatic resection because the residual cirrhotic liver usually cannot meet the essential metabolic demands and has limited capacity for regeneration. However, small asymptomatic tumors found during systematic screening in high-risk patients can be resected in the presence of liver cirrhosis.[16] Active hepatocellular disease at the time of resection seriously lessens the chances of postoperative recovery. Therefore, markedly elevated hepatic enzyme levels or substantial inflammation in the liver biopsy specimen contraindicates hepatic resection until the active process subsides.

Cardiac function should be evaluated in patients who have received Adriamycin (doxorubicin) as part of their preoperative chemotherapy.

Anesthetic Management of Hepatic Resection

Although underlying cirrhosis is present in some patients undergoing resection, liver function is usually fairly normal. This is reflected by the normal preoperative coagulation status, metabolic function of the liver, and pharmacokinetics of anesthetics and other drugs. Therefore, intraoperative management is concentrated on maintenance of hemodynamic stability, including hepatic blood flow and metabolic support of the liver. Because major changes in hemodynamic variables and fluid balance commonly occur during surgery, optimal preparation and monitoring of the patient are required. An intra-arterial catheter is used for blood pressure monitoring and arterial blood sampling. Monitoring of the central venous pressure and/or pulmonary arterial pressures, cardiac output, and urine output are helpful in estimating intravascular blood volume and cardiac performance. Finally, body temperature and degree of neuromuscular blockade should be monitored, and a precordial Doppler may be useful to detect an air embolism.

Large-bore intravenous catheters (>14 gauge) are inserted, and some type of rapid-infusion system should be available.[17] The blood bank has to be prepared to supply enough blood products, including fresh frozen plasma, platelets, and cryoprecipitate. Autotransfusion is not recommended, except for a life-threatening situation, because collected blood may contain malignant cells. However, autotransfusion has been reported to be safe in some types of oncologic surgery.[18]

Many anesthetics have been used successfully for induction and maintenance of anesthesia during liver resection. An intravenous induction agent (sodium thiopental, ketamine, or etomidate) can be chosen according to the physical condition of the individual patient. Succinylcholine is frequently used to facilitate tracheal intubation. Isoflurane in an oxygen/air mixture, and narcotics and muscle relaxants (pancuronium, vecuronium, or atracurium) are usually used without complications. Halothane is avoided because it can decrease hepatic blood flow and hepatic function.[19] Nitrous oxide is avoided to minimize bowel distension and potential air emboli.

Intraoperative hemodynamic stability depends largely on maintaining effective intravascular volume, which may be affected by surgical blood loss and clamping or unclamping of major vessels. Intraoperative blood loss varies. Sometimes, blood loss can be as much as 20 times the blood volume, particularly in patients with a highly vascular tumor (hemangioma) or with previous abdominal surgery. The hemodynamic effects of acute clamping of the portal vein and hepatic artery have been studied in humans.[20] Cardiac filling pressures and cardiac output decreased somewhat, but arterial blood pressure increased because of a significant increase in systemic vascular resistance. The vascular clamping was tolerated well for periods up to one hour, and the release of the clamp resulted in normalization of all hemodynamic variables without cardiovascular collapse.

Hyperventilation is avoided, and PEEP is used when specifically indicated to avoid significant decreases in hepatic blood flow. Urine output, renal function, and acid–base state should be kept within the normal range.

Intraoperative fluid management consists of the administration of crystalloids, colloids (albumin or hetastarch), and blood products. When sudden blood loss occurs, crystalloid solution is usually effective in rapidly restoring intravascular volume and interstitial fluid deficits, and it is less expensive than colloid solution. However, administration of a large volume of crystalloid solution may result in

peripheral edema that can lead to impaired wound healing and nutrient transport[21] and possibly pulmonary edema. Colloid solution has been used frequently in an attempt to avoid peripheral and pulmonary edema caused by hypoalbuminemia.[22] Although albumin administration appears to reduce the incidence of peripheral edema, its effectiveness in preventing pulmonary edema is unclear.[23,24] The lung is very well protected against pulmonary edema by its ability to increase lymph drainage significantly.[25] Pulmonary edema is unavoidable, however, when this protective mechanism is overwhelmed or when capillary membrane permeability is altered, resulting in albumin leakage through the pulmonary capillary membrane. To complicate matters further, it is uncertain whether the gradient between colloid oncotic pressure and pulmonary artery occlusion pressure must be maintained to prevent pulmonary edema because many other factors in the Starling equation, such as capillary permeability, interstitial hydrostatic pressure, and interstitial colloid oncotic pressure, are unknown or may be changed during massive blood loss and resuscitation. Pulmonary and peripheral capillary permeability probably do not change early in the resuscitation, whereas diffuse capillary leakage can occur when complications such as sepsis are superimposed. Therefore, albumin is usually administered to decrease the incidence and severity of peripheral and possibly pulmonary edema and to avoid the potential for prolonged hypoalbuminemia postoperatively.

Massive blood transfusion can result in several other physiologic abnormalities. Myocardial depression caused by ionized hypocalcemia is a major concern when large amounts of citrated blood are transfused. It has been shown that ionized calcium levels stay within the normal range when liver function is normal, the blood transfusion rate does not exceed 30 mL/kg/h,[26] and an adequate circulating blood volume is maintained.[27] Ionized hypocalcemia occurs during more rapid transfusion, even in patients without hepatic dysfunction, but it recovers within 10 minutes when the transfusion rate decreases.[26] However, patients with inadequate citrate clearance (poor hepatic function, hypothermia, and inadequate urine output) are prone to develop citrate intoxication in a way similar to patients undergoing liver transplantation.[28] Because hepatic perfusion and function can be significantly reduced perioperatively, and transfusion requirements can exceed 30 mL/kg/h for a long period, ionized calcium levels should be monitored frequently and treated accordingly with calcium chloride or calcium gluconate.

Another major complication during massive blood transfusion is coagulopathy, with dilutional thrombocytopenia as the most frequent cause. The degree of coagulopathy depends on the preoperative platelet count, the amount of blood loss, and platelet function. Clinically significant thrombocytopenia may occur after the transfusion of about 1.5 times the blood volume, and traditionally platelets are transfused to maintain the platelet count above 50×10^9/L.[29] However, the disadvantage of measuring the platelet count is the time taken by the laboratory, which may limit its usefulness. Furthermore, it fails to measure platelet function. Thrombelastography has been used for the rapid analysis of overall coagulation function during liver transplantation[30] and major surgical procedures, including liver resection. The technique provides reliable information regarding the coagulation status and the need for platelets, coagulation factors (fresh frozen plasma and cryoprecipitate), or pharmacologic intervention with epsilon-amniocaproic acid.[31]

Inadvertent hypothermia should be minimized by warming all intravenous solutions and by using a warming blanket and a heated humidifier. Blood warmers may not be effective at high transfusion rates, and a rapid-infusion device with a heat exchanger (Rapid Infusion System, Haemonetics, MA, USA) should be available.

Postoperative Course

Patients require tracheal intubation and assisted ventilation in the early postoperative course, until intravascular volume status, hematocrit, electrolytes, acid–base balance, and temperature are within normal limits.

A patient can survive removal of as much as 80–85% of a normal liver. Rapid regeneration of the liver provides new functioning hepatocytes by the formation of new lobules and by expansion of residual lobules. Hepatotrophic factors (possibly including insulin and glucagon) may play a role in this process. Regeneration begins within 24 hours after surgery and continues until the original weight of the organ is restored, after approximately 4–5 weeks. When a large portion of the liver has been removed or when the residual liver has some degree of cirrhosis, liver function must be monitored closely for the first few postoperative weeks. Liver function is usually diminished for several weeks postoperatively, even in patients with relatively normal preoperative hepatic function: serum bilirubin level increases to 5–6 mg/100 mL (85–100 μmol/L) and returns to normal within 1–2 weeks. Metabolic support of the liver is essential and must continue in the postoperative period. Glucose-containing solutions are infused parenterally to prevent hypoglycemia. The serum albumin concentration decreases in many patients because of the depressed synthetic function of the residual liver; albumin is given by most clinicians. The concentrations of coagulation factors also decrease initially. Treatment including vitamin K and fresh frozen plasma may be necessary until the remaining liver recovers.

Severe postoperative complications may result in part from poor residual function of the liver. They include encephalopathy, hypoglycemia, acid–base abnormalities, hypoxia, renal failure, and intra-abdominal bleeding. In general, the incidence of postoperative complications correlates with intraoperative blood loss. Pulmonary atelectasis and pneumonitis of the right lung are common after partial hepatectomy, especially when a thoracoabdominal approach has been used. Many patients develop a fever from pulmonary complications or perihepatic abscess, but frequently no cause of fever can be identified. In about 5% of patients abscesses develop in or near the space created by the resection, requiring reexploration and drainage.[11]

Hepatic Trauma

In patients with abdominal trauma, the liver is the most commonly injured solid organ. Two-thirds of patients with hepatic wounds have additional injuries to other organs. Liver trauma can be classified as penetrating or blunt. In large cities, penetrating wounds are more frequent and in rural areas, blunt trauma has the higher incidence. Penetrating wounds are caused by bullets or knives lacerating the liver parenchyma and/or its blood vessels. Knife wounds produce a sharp, usually fairly superficial laceration. Gunshot wounds result in through-and-through perforations with contusion and sometimes stellate fractures, leading to a mortality that is four times higher than that from knife wounds. In addition, penetrating wounds usually are associated with injuries of the small bowel, colon, mesentery, and lung. Blunt trauma is caused by a direct blow to the upper abdomen or lower rib cage (e.g., motor vehicle accident) or can follow a sudden deceleration (fall from a great height). The injury to the liver ranges from small, subcapsular hematomas to large stellate fractures of an entire lobe. Usually explosive, bursting wounds with significant parenchymal destruction are seen. Injury to other organs frequently accompanies blunt trauma and contributes to morbidity and mortality: craniocervical trauma (50% of patients involved in motor vehicle accidents), splenic injury, and thoracic trauma (pulmonary or cardiac contusion, pneumothorax, hemothorax, and flail chest).

Resuscitation should start at the scene of the accident, where the airway should be secured, a shock suit applied, and the blood volume replaced with crystalloid solutions. When the liver injury is extremely severe, the patient dies before arrival at the hospital. About 5% of patients who arrive at the hospital alive die of exsanguination before surgery can be performed. However, once hemorrhage is controlled, the liver can support life even after severe injury. Early mortality is obviously related to the severity of accompanying injuries and the degree and duration of hemorrhagic shock, particularly in patients with shotgun and blunt trauma. Late mortality is also related to the occurrence and duration of shock, which can result in multiorgan failure and sepsis.

Diagnosis of Trauma Patients

The diagnosis of a penetrating abdominal wound is usually obvious on the basis of history, physical examination, and clinical signs (e.g., hypovolemic shock). In most cases, roentgenographic evaluation is of minor importance. Hepatomegaly may be evident on plain abdominal films, or the right diaphragm may be elevated. Fractured ribs over the liver should suggest liver injury. Computerized tomographic scans or angiography is rarely necessary, unless the patient is stable and only a minor injury is suspected. In severely traumatized patients, laparotomy is part of the diagnostic evaluation, especially when injury of the liver or other abdominal organs is suspected. Penetrating wounds entering the abdominal cavity always should be explored surgically. If the patient is in shock and does

not respond rapidly to intravenous fluid administration, surgery is usually the most critical resuscitative measure. Some surgeons perform thoracotomy before the laparotomy to control the greater vessels in case of excessive bleeding. The morbidity caused by waiting for diagnostic examination is far greater than that of a negative diagnostic laparotomy. When the abdomen is entered, all surfaces of the liver should be thoroughly inspected and palpated.

Surgical Management

The principal goals of surgery are to stop bleeding and debride devitalized liver tissue while preserving as much vital hepatic tissue as possible. Studies of large numbers of liver injuries indicate that all but a few are surgically manageable, although some degree of postoperative hepatic failure is common.

Obviously, operative management depends on the degree of liver injury. Most small liver injuries have stopped bleeding by the time the operation is performed. Minor superficial injuries require only hemostasis and drainage. Depending on the depth and location of the wound, however, bleeding may be difficult to control. Because subcapsular hematomas so often overlie an active bleeding site or parenchyma in need of debridement, they should be explored, even when the injury seems to be of limited severity and tamponade appears effective. Active bleeding from liver lacerations should be treated by direct suture of identifiable vessels and electrocautery of bleeding parenchyma.

Hepatotomy, or incision of the liver, is considered to be the technique of choice by many surgeons in treating severe hepatic injury and must be performed for all penetrating hepatic injuries. This technique enables inspection of the full extent of the wound and ligation of damaged vessels and biliary ducts,[32-34] and it allows preservation of as much liver tissue as possible. If bleeding is uncontrollable and obscures the field, temporary occlusion of the hepatic artery and portal vein (Pringle maneuver) may permit identification of the lesion.[35] This maneuver can be performed safely for up to one hour and can be repeated.[15] This safe time limit was determined in patients undergoing elective liver resection, and it was thought initially that patients suffering from posttraumatic hypovolemia or shock might not be able to tolerate similar ischemic periods. Recently, good results have been reported after use of the

Pringle maneuver for more than one hour in patients with liver trauma.[33] When bleeding is controlled, the liver should not be closed because good drainage probably decreases the incidence of local infection.

Lobar hepatic resection was popular several years ago. Most trauma surgeons now agree that this should be done only when an entire hepatic lobe is severely injured, because the procedure is associated with a high mortality (up to 50%). Lobectomy is acceptable only when there is substantial parenchymal destruction that cannot be controlled by hepatotomy. Thus, the proper use of hepatotomy should significantly lower the incidence of major lobar resection.[33]

Sometimes perihepatic packing can be used as a temporary measure to enable correction of the medical coagulopathy or to allow transport of the patient to a specialized center.[36] Ligation of the hepatic artery to achieve hemostasis is controversial, although this technique has some strong supporters.[37] Probably ligation should be performed only when arterial bleeding cannot be controlled otherwise.

Failure to control bleeding with a Pringle maneuver suggests the presence of an injury to the retrohepatic vena cava or major hepatic veins. Such injury presents a difficult problem. Temporary clamping of the inflow vessels may or may not slow blood loss enough to allow inspection and suture of the bleeding point. Occasionally, packs placed behind the liver for 20–30 minutes will stop the bleeding. For persistent bleeding from retrohepatic tears, the abdominal incision can be extended into a median sternotomy, and a shunt can be placed through the atrial appendage into the inferior vena cava, past the origin of the hepatic veins. In combination with hepatic inflow occlusion, this maneuver allows total isolation of the liver circulation without interruption of the venous blood return from the lower half of the body. Only after this is accomplished can correction of vascular injury be attempted.

Liver transplantation can be a useful approach when liver injury is so severe that it cannot be repaired or controlled.[38]

Anesthetic Management

It is obvious that one of the most important tasks for the anesthesiologist in the successful management of liver trauma is to restore and maintain intravascular blood volume. However, general aspects of emergent care are important as well: preexisting medical diseases, drug therapy, drug allergy, and associated injuries should not be overlooked.

Each trauma center should have a trauma operating room available at all times that is fully equipped with a state-of-the-art monitor, a rapid-infusion device, and a "resuscitation cart" (Table 8-1). On arrival in the operating room, the patient should be treated according to a prioritized protocol as listed in Table 8-2. Adequate oxygenation of the patient with early tracheal intubation is paramount.

Venous access should be obtained through veins above the diaphragm, because the inferior vena cava may be bleeding or may be clamped during the procedure to control bleeding. To accomplish this, several large-bore intravenous catheters are placed in the upper extremities, neck, or subclavian veins. Shock suits are deflated gradually while blood volume is being replaced to avoid frank hypovolemia.

Anesthesia should be induced with drugs that have the least depressing effects on the cardiovascular system, namely, etomidate or ketamine. Thiopental is used only in patients who are not hypovolemic and who are hemodynamically stable. After induction of anesthesia, all medications should be titrated carefully, since even minimal doses of anesthetics can be detrimental. Potent inhalation anesthetics frequently are not tolerated by trauma patients, and anesthesia relies on narcotics, muscle relaxants, and amnestic drugs, such as scopolamine and benzodiazepines. Nitrous oxide is avoided to minimize intestinal distension and myocardial depression and to allow the administration of high concentrations of oxygen. This light anesthesia technique in hemodynamically unstable patients, however, may cause recall of surgery.[39]

Table 8-1. Equipment for Trauma Operating Room

Anesthesia gas machine with ventilator with compressed air
Vital sign monitors with transducers
Pulse oximeter
Cardiac output computer
On-line mixed venous oximeter
Mass spectrometer or capnograph
Neuromuscular blockade monitor
Inspired gas humidifier
Cardiac defibrillator
Resuscitation cart
Rapid infusion device or blood pump with warmer
Autotransfusion system
Warming blanket
Stat laboratory for blood gas analysis

Table 8-2. Protocol for Anesthetic Management

1. Airway control, oxygenation, tracheal intubation, and ventilation
2. Monitoring of vital signs: blood pressure, ECG, pulse oximetry
3. Venous access
4. Blood sampling for type and crossmatch, hematocrit, and serum electrolytes
5. Blood transfusion (begin with type-specific blood, if necessary)
6. Insertion of intra-arterial catheter and analysis of arterial blood gas
7. Administration of anesthetics, if possible
8. Monitoring of temperature and neuromuscular blockade
9. Insertion of urinary catheter, central venous/pulmonary artery catheter

Arterial pressure should be monitored invasively through a radial artery catheter. Femoral arterial pressure monitoring is avoided because the abdominal aorta may be clamped during surgery. Other monitoring should include electrocardiography, temperature, capnography, pulse oximetry, urine output, and central venous pressure determination. A pulmonary artery catheter can be inserted after the acute crisis is over, particularly when the patient has a history of significant cardiac disease or when myocardial contusion is suspected.

Warmed crystalloid solution should be given to maintain normovolemia while waiting for, preferably, whole blood. If blood loss is massive and type-specific blood is not available, uncrossmatched type O, Rh negative blood can be given. Fluid replacement with crystalloid and colloid solutions and blood products must be guided by the serial determination of hematocrit, cardiac filling pressures, cardiac output, urine output, and the coagulation state. Fluid management is similar to that in patients undergoing liver resection. The use of fresh frozen plasma and platelets can be guided by coagulation tests such as thrombelastography. If this method is not available, platelets should be administered to maintain the platelet count above 50,000/mm³, and fresh frozen plasma is commonly used during massive transfusion because of dilution and decreased production by the liver. A rapid infusion system is helpful for the rapid administration of warmed blood products.

The use of an autotransfusion device is extremely helpful, especially when the blood bank is unprepared for massive transfusion. Blood is collected from the surgical field in a blood reservoir, and an anticoagulant (citrate) is added. The collected blood then is washed with one liter of saline or balanced electrolyte solution without calcium (Plasma-Lyte A), centrifuged to a hematocrit of 40%, and reinfused into the patient. The advantages of this technique are avoidance of hypovolemia, a reduced risk of transfusion-related disease transmission and immunologic incompatibility, and the ability to infuse fresh red blood cells without storage lesion. Overall, this system provides a safe and effective source of red blood cells.[40] Indications for autotransfusion include inability to crossmatch banked blood, exsanguination without available blood products, and religious beliefs preventing homologous transfusion. Drawbacks of autotransfusion include the delay between blood loss and blood reinfusion, and potential contamination with bowel contents (e.g., after penetrating abdominal injury). The washed blood reinfused into the patient does *not* contain coagulation factors. Therefore, coagulopathy is expected after autotransfusion of a large amount of blood, and it is not a direct result of autotransfusion per se.[40] In patients with multiple trauma undergoing emergent surgery, autotransfusion without washing and centrifugation has been used without significant complications.[40] When blood loss is very rapid, washing may be too time-consuming and is probably not required, as hemolysis is minimal.

Complications of Trauma

With current surgical techniques, hemorrhage from hepatic injury is rarely uncontrollable except with retrohepatic venous injuries. Patients may rebleed from the liver wound after initial hemostasis, and this is treated by reexploration and sometimes by lobectomy. Angiography and scintigraphy may provide useful diagnostic information in such patients. Hemobilia may be responsible for gastrointestinal bleeding in the postoperative period and can be diagnosed by selective angiography of the hepatic artery. Treatment consists of ligation of the artery supplying the bleeding vessel or, if that fails, segmental resection of the liver.

The most common postoperative complications are pulmonary complications and infection. Hepatic function is impaired in the immediate postoperative period, with resultant increases in hepatic enzymes serum glutamic oxalo—acetic transaminase [SGOT], serum glutamic pyruvic transaminase [SGPT], lactate dehydrogenase [LDH], alkaline phosphatase, and in total bilirubin, as well as decreases in total plasma protein levels and albumin levels. The latter are probably due to loss of protein from the wound combined with insufficient hepatic production and hemodilution. Hepatic function usually returns to normal in survivors.[41]

Prognosis

The mortality rate of 10–15% following hepatic trauma depends largely on the type of injury and the extent of associated injury to other organs. About one-third of patients admitted to the hospital in shock cannot be saved. Only 1% of penetrating wounds are lethal, whereas a 20% mortality attends blunt trauma. The death rate after blunt hepatic injury is only 10% when just the liver is injured. If three major organs are damaged, the death rate is close to 70%. Bleeding causes more than one-half of deaths.

Postoperative mortality is often caused by associated injuries such as brain injury, perihepatic abscess and sepsis, multiorgan failure including renal insufficiency, and respiratory failure.

Portacaval Shunt

The cause of portal hypertension may be prehepatic (thrombosis of portal vein or external compression of portal vein), hepatic (cirrhosis or fibrosis), or posthepatic (Budd-Chiari syndrome or increased central venous pressure) in origin. Portal hypertension leads to the development of a collateral circulation to the systemic veins, such as esophageal varices and sometimes hemorrhoidal varices. This results in two major clinical problems: the increased blood flow through collaterals may cause these vessels to burst, causing gastrointestinal bleeding; the toxins present in portal venous blood are not detoxified in the liver, causing hepatic encephalopathy. Esophageal varices can lead to massive hemorrhage, which carries a 50% mortality, not only because of the acute blood loss, but also because of the poor liver function and other systemic disease. Other complications of portal hypertension include ascites and splenomegaly.

The emergency treatment of massively bleeding esophageal varices consists of blood transfusion and prevention of further blood loss with intravenous vasopressin and balloon tamponade. Vasopressin reduces splanchnic blood flow by splanchnic vasoconstriction and therefore also reduces blood flow through the collaterals. Further therapy includes endoscopic sclerotherapy, which is now used more frequently than surgery.[42] Because it is associated with high morbidity and mortality, emergency surgery (portacaval shunt or esophageal stapling procedure) is indicated only if conservative therapy fails. Prevention of recurrent esophageal bleeding includes repeated endoscopy and sclerotherapy and the use of beta-adrenergic blocking agents (e.g., propranolol) to reduce cardiac output, splanchnic circulation, and, therefore, portal hypertension. Although propranolol decreases portal pressure, it is not clear if it lowers the incidence of variceal bleeding.[43] If esophageal varices continue to bleed despite repeated sclerotherapy, an elective portacaval shunt procedure should be performed.

The rationale behind the creation of a portacaval shunt is that a reduced portal pressure reduces the risk of esophageal variceal bleeding. However, the resulting decrease in hepatic blood flow after this shunting procedure can lead to further impairment of hepatic function and hepatic encephalopathy. Some patients, especially those with poor liver function, can be helped only by liver transplantation.

Emergency portacaval shunt procedures have a high success rate in stopping active esophageal bleeding. However, the probability of survival depends on the degree of liver disease: patients with poor hepatic function have a high perioperative death rate (approximately 50%). The perioperative survival rate of patients who undergo elective portacaval shunt is much better. Two main types of portacaval shunts can be differentiated: selective and nonselective. A shunt is nonselective if all portal blood is diverted from the liver, whereas with a selective shunt, portal venous blood flow is preserved to a certain degree. The nonselective type includes portacaval (end-to-side and side-to-side), mesocaval, and splenorenal shunts. The selective type consists of the coronary-caval and distal splenorenal shunts.[44]

The incidence of hepatic encephalopathy after the creation of a portasystemic shunt is 5–10% and is probably higher with nonselective total shunts compared with the distal splenorenal shunt.[45] The cause of the encephalopathy is directly related to the blood flow through the shunt, which prevents hepatic clearance of toxic substances. Liver perfusion, and therefore liver function, is better preserved with the distal splenorenal shunt.

Preoperative evaluation should include determination of liver function (levels of bilirubin, transaminases, and albumin; coagulation profile). Cardiac function should be evaluated as well, because many patients with Laennec's cirrhosis may have alcohol-induced cardiomyopathy. Before undergoing emergency portacaval shunt procedures, many patients receive intravenous vasopressin, and arterial blood pressure can be significantly elevated. In these patients, concomitant administration of a systemic vasodilator (e.g., sodium nitroprusside) can normalize the blood pressure without interfering with the effects of vasopressin on the splanchnic circulation. When vasopressin is discontinued, arterial blood pressure may decrease dramatically as the peripheral vasculature dilates.[46]

Intraoperative monitoring should include a radial arterial catheter for direct arterial blood pressure monitoring and blood sampling. A central venous catheter is useful to estimate intravascular blood volume. A pulmonary artery catheter probably is required in patients with cardiomyopathy. Anesthesia can be induced with thiopental or ketamine, and intubation facilitated with succinylcholine. Anesthesia usually is maintained with isoflurane in an oxygen-air mixture combined with the use of muscle relaxants (pancuronium, vecuronium, atracurium) and narcotics. The use of muscle relaxants should be guided by a peripheral nerve stimulator. All medications should be carefully titrated because of inadequate hepatic clearance in patients with liver disease.

The details of anesthetic management are similar to those for patients undergoing surgery for hepatic resection and hepatic trauma.

References

1. Lautt, W.W. (1985) Mechanism and role of intrinsic regulation of hepatic arterial blood flow: Hepatic arterial buffer response. *Am J Physiology* 249:G549–56.
2. Lautt, W.W. (1977) Control of hepatic and intestinal blood flow: Effect of isovolaemic haemodilution on blood flow and oxygen uptake in the intact liver and intestines. *Physiol (London)* 265:313–26.
3. Thompson, I.A., Fitch, W., Hughes, R.L., and Campbell, D. (1983) Effect of increased concentrations of carbon dioxide during halothane anaesthesia on liver blood flow and hepatic oxygen consumption. *Br J Anaesth* 55: 1231–37.
4. Gelman, S.I. (1976) Disturbances in hepatic blood flow during anesthesia and surgery. *Arch Surg* 111:881–83.
5. Harper, M.H., Collins, P., Johnson, B.H., Eger, E.I. II and Biava, C.G. (1982) Postanesthetic hepatic injury in rats: Influence of alterations in hepatic blood flow, surgery, and anesthesia time. *Anesth Analg* 61:79–82.
6. Di Bisceglie, A.M., Rustgi, V.K., Hoofnagle, J.H., Dusheiko, G.M. and Lotze, M.T. (1988) Hepatocellular carcinoma. *Ann Intern Med* 108:390–401.
7. Kanematsu, T., Takenaka, K., Matsumata, T., Furuta, T., Sugimachi, K. and Inokuchi, K. (1984) Limited hepatic resection effective for selected cirrhotic patients with primary liver cancer. *Ann Surg* 199:51–56.
8. Iwatsuki, S., Klintmalm, G.B.G. and Starzl, T.E. (1982) Total hepatectomy and liver replacement (orthotopic liver transplantation) for primary hepatic malignancy. *World J Surg* 6:81–85.
9. Lightdale, C.J. and Daly, J. (1987) Management of primary and metastatic cancer of the liver. In *Diseases of the Liver,* Schiff, L. and Schiff, E.R. (eds). Philadelphia: J. B. Lippincott, pp. 1159–70.
10. Morrow, C. E., Grage, T. B., Sutherland, D. E. and Najarian, J. S. (1982) Hepatic resection for secondary neoplasms. *Surgery* 92:610–14.
11. Ekberg, H., Tranberg, K. G., Anderson, R., et al. (1986) Determinants of survival in liver resection for colorectal secondaries. *Br J Surgery* 73:727–31.
12. Creutzfeldt, W. and Stockmann, F. (1987) Carcinoids and carcinoid syndrome. *Am J Med* 82 (suppl 5B):4–16.
13. Marsh, H.M., Martin, J.K., Kvols, L.K. et al. (1987) Carcinoid crisis during anesthesia: Successful treatment with a somatostatin analogue. *Anesthesiology* 66:89–91.
14. Roy, R.C., Carter, R.F. and Wright, P.D. (1987) Somatostatin, anaesthesia, and the carcinoid syndrome. Peri-operative administration of a somatostatin analogue to suppress carcinoid tumor activity. *Anaesthesia* 42:627–32.
15. Huguet, C., Nordlinger, B., Bloch, P., and Conard, J. (1978) Tolerance of the human liver to prolonged normothermic ischemia. A biological study of 20 patients submitted to extensive hepatectomy. *Arch Surg* 113: 1448–51.
16. Bismuth, H., Hiussin, D., Ornowski, J. and Meriggi, F. (1986) Liver resections in cirrhotic patients: A Western experience. *World J Surg* 10:311–17.
17. Sassano, J.J. (1986) The rapid infusion system. In *Hepatic Transplantation: Anesthetic and Perioperative Management,* Winter, P. M. and Kang, Y. G. (eds). New York: Praeger, pp. 120–34.
18. Klimberg, I., Sirois, R., Wajsman, Z. and Baker, J. (1986) Intraoperative autotransfusion in urologic oncology. *Arch Surg* 121:1326–29.

19. Gelman, S., Dillard, E. and Bradley, E.L. (1987) Hepatic circulation during surgical stress and anesthesia with halothane, isoflurane, or fentanyl. *Anesth Analg* 66: 936–43.

20. Delva, E., Camus, Y., Paugam, C., Parc, R., Huguet, C. and Lienhart, A. (1987) Haemodynamic effects of portal triad clamping in humans. *Anesth Analg* 66:864–68.

21. Hauser, C.J., Shoemaker, W.C., Turpin, I. and Goldberg, S.J. (1980) Oxygen transport responses to colloids and crystalloids in critically ill surgical patients. *Surg Gynecol Obstet* 150:811–16.

22. Coppa, G.F., Eng, K., Ranson, J.H.C., Gouge, T.H. and Localio, S.A. (1985) Hepatic resection for metastatic colon and rectal cancer. An evaluation of preoperative and postoperative factors. *Ann Surg* 202:203–8.

23. Virgilio, R.W., Rice, C.L., Smith, D.E. et al. (1979) Crystalloid vs. colloid resuscitation: Is one better? A randomized clinical study. *Surgery* 85:129–39.

24. Virgilio, R.W., Smith, D.E. and Zarins, C.K. (1979) Balanced electrolyte solutions: Experimental and clinical studies. *Crit Care Med* 7:98–106.

25. Brigham, K.L., Woolverton, W.C., Blake, L.H., and Staub, N.C. (1974) Increased sheep lung vascular permeability caused by pseudomonas bacteremia. *J Clin Invest* 54:792–804.

26. Abbott, T.R. (1983) Changes in serum calcium fraction and citrate concentrations during massive blood transfusions and cardiopulmonary bypass. *Br J Anaesth* 55:753–59.

27. Kahn, R.C., Jascott, D., Carlon G.C., Schweizer, O., Howland, W.S. and Goldiner, P.L. (1979) Massive blood replacement: Correlation of ionized calcium, citrate, and hydrogen ion concentration. *Anesth Analg* 58:274–78.

28. Marquez, J., Martin, D., Virji, M.A. et al. (1986) Cardiovascular depression secondary to ionic hypocalcemia during hepatic transplantation in humans. *Anesthesiology* 65:457–61.

29. Consensus Development Panel, Office of Medical Applications of Research, National Institutes of Health, Bethesda, MD (1987) Platelet transfusion therapy. *JAMA* 257:1777–80.

30. Kang, Y.G., Martin, D.J., Marquez, J. et al. (1985) Intraoperative changes in blood coagulation and thrombelastographic monitoring in liver transplantation. *Anesth Analg* 64:888–96.

31. Kang, Y., Lewis, J.H., Navalgund, A. et al. (1987) Epsilon aminocaproic acid for treatment of fibrinolysis during liver transplantation. *Anesthesiology* 66:766–73.

32. Pachter, H.L., Spencer, F.C., Hofstetter, S.R. and Coppa, G.F. (1983) Experience with the finger fracture technique to achieve intra-hepatic hemostasis in 75 patients with severe injuries to the liver. *Ann Surg* 197:771–78.

33. Feliciano, D.V., Mattox, K.L., Jordan, G.L., Burch, J.M., Bitondo, C.G. and Cruse, P.A. (1986) Management of 1000 consecutive cases of hepatic trauma (1979–1984). *Ann Surg* 204:438–45.

34. Pretre, R., Mentha, G., Huber, O., Meyer, P., Vogel, J. and Rohner, A. (1988) Hepatic trauma: Risk factors influencing outcome. *Br J Surgery* 75:520–24.

35. Pringle, J. H. (1908) Notes on the arrest of hepatic haemorrhage due to trauma. *Ann Surg* 48:541–48.

36. Calne, R.Y., McMaster, P. and Pentlow, B.D. (1979) The treatment of major liver trauma by primary packing with transfer of the patient for definite treatment. *Br J Surgery* 66:338–39.

37. Mays, E.T., Conti, S., Fallahzadeh, H. and Rosenblatt. M. (1979) Hepatic artery ligation. *Surgery* 86: 536–43.

38. Esquivel, C.O., Bernardos, A., Makowka, L., Iwatsuki, S., Gordon, R.D. and Starzl, T.E. (1987) Liver replacement after massive hepatic trauma. *J Trauma* 27:800–02.

39. Bogetz, M.S. and Katz, J.A. (1984) Recall of surgery for major trauma. *Anesthesiology* 61:6–9.

40. Hauer, J.M. and Thurer R.L. (1984) Controversies in autotransfusion. *Vox Sang* 46:8–12.

41. Kaku, N. (1987) Short-term and long-term changes in hepatic function in 60 patients with blunt liver injury. *J Trauma* 27:607–14.

42. Schiff, E.R. (1984) Nonsurgical management of emergency hemorrhage from esophageal varices. *World J Surg* 8:646–52.

43. Burroughs, A.K., Jenkins, W.J., Sherlock, S. et al. (1983) Controlled trial of propranolol for the prevention of recurrent variceal hemorrhage in patients with cirrhosis. *N Engl J Med* 309:1539–42.

44. Rossi, R.L., Jenkins, R.L. and Nielsen-Whitcomb, F.F. (1985) Management of complications of portal hypertension. *Surg Clin North Am* 65:231–62.

45. Henderson, J.M. and Warren W.D. (1983) Current status of the distal splenorenal shunt. *Semin Liv Dis* 3:251–53.

46. Shelly, M.P., Greatorex, R., Calne, R.Y. and Park, G.R. (1988) The physiological effects of vasopressin when used to control intra-abdominal bleeding. *Intens Care Med* 14:526–31.

Chapter 9
Liver Transplantation

John R. Klinck and John C. Berridge

Liver transplantation is now acknowledged to be the only effective treatment for most patients with end-stage hepatic disease. In most diagnostic groups 1-year survival is greater than 80%, mortality in subsequent years low, and the quality of life for long-term survivors excellent.[1,2] The indications for liver transplantation are increasing and the number of centers offering the procedure continues to grow.[3–5]

The anesthetic management of the liver transplant recipient presents a formidable challenge. Advanced hepatic failure produces complex pathophysiologic effects and is frequently associated with failure of other major organ systems. The surgical procedure is lengthy and often causes cardiovascular instability, intractable hemorrhage and significant electrolyte, acid–base and hemostatic disturbances. Knowledge of the pathophysiology of severe hepatic disease and of the potential pitfalls of the operation is essential. Good organization and technical support are also vital, as are careful and comprehensive monitoring, effective communication with surgical colleagues, and an aggressive approach to adverse physiologic trends.

Indications and Results

A large number of acute and chronic liver disorders have been managed by transplantation. In adults cirrhosis is the most common indication, comprising over 50% of patients, most suffering from chronic active hepatitis or primary biliary cirrhosis. Other common indications include sclerosing cholangitis, fulminant hepatitis, Budd-Chiari syndrome, and alcoholic cirrhosis. Fifty percent of children needing liver transplantation have congenital obstructive disorders, mainly extrahepatic biliary atresia, while a further 20% have metabolic disease, including alpha-1 antitrypsin deficiency and tyrosinosis. Other indications for both adults and children include drug-related hepatitides, Wilson's disease, vascular disorders, and tumors. Oxalosis, hemophilia, and congenital protein C deficiency, conditions with normal hepatic function, have also been treated successfully by transplantation.[6–8]

Transplantation is indicated when liver disease progresses to the point of major functional impairment and is likely to lead to death within one year.[9] Deciding on the timing of surgery may be difficult. In chronic conditions, poorer results associated with advanced disease must be weighed against the possible loss of months of relatively good health should complications follow an early operation. In fulminant cases recovery without transplantation may occur, yet delay can result in preventable death or permanent brain injury. As yet there are few published data to help the clinician with these important decisions, although in practice the timing of surgery is often determined by the availability of a donor organ. As this must, in all but the most desperate circumstances, be ABO compatible and of suitable size, a prospective recipient may wait weeks or even months once the decision to transplant has been made. Inevitably some die before an organ is found.

Long-term results of transplantation for hepatic malignancy and chronic hepatitis B infection are poor because the underlying disease usually recurs. Similarly, little impact has been made on the high mortality associated with halothane and most other drug-related hepatitides. Results of transplantation in fulminant non A-non B hepatitis and paracetamol overdose are at present poorer than those achieved in many chronic conditions (1-year survival 35–50%), although better than seen before the advent of transplantation. Outcome in other diagnostic groups does not vary widely, although age at operation is of some importance. Infants (<1 year) present major technical difficulties and have a poorer prognosis: 1-year survival is approximately 50%.[10] Teenagers tend to do well, with 90% survival at 1-year and little subsequent attrition.[11] Patients over 50 years of age, treated by Starzl, had survival figures similar to those of younger patients.[10] Those transplanted for alcoholic cirrhosis, providing they have been abstinent for at least 6 months and are free of malignancy, appear to do as well as other groups.[12]

Disease severity at the time of operation affects the likelihood of a successful outcome. Patients with advanced disease and severe nutritional impairment have poorer prospects than those who are relatively well at the time of transplantation,[13,14] and early surgery is increasingly favored. If all patients are included, current 1-year survival is in the range of 75–85%. Mortality beyond 1 year after transplantation is low in most diagnostic groups.

Preoperative Assessment and Preparation

Chronic liver disease is manifested by malnutrition, portal hypertension with ascites, impaired hepatic synthetic function, and peripheral and pulmonary microvascular shunting. Nutritional reserve is diminished by anorexia, malabsorption, and impaired protein synthesis[15] and is further depleted at the time of operation by the catabolic response to injury. This reduces resistance to infection[16] and impairs respiratory muscle function and wound healing. Dietary supplementation before surgery is important, although there is a need for low sodium intake when ascites is present and protein restriction in patients with encephalopathy.[17] Parenteral nutrition is needed when portal hypertension is associated with near-complete malabsorption, and preparations with a high proportion of branched chain amino acids may be particularly valuable in patients subject to encephalopthy. Vitamins, iron, and trace elements may also be beneficial and should be prescribed.

Portal hypertension may be associated with massive ascites, reduced lung volumes, and limited exercise tolerance. Ascites is often easily reduced with sodium restriction and diuretic therapy. This will improve pulmonary function and make most patients feel better. In intractable cases large volume paracenteses and infusions of albumin are effective.[18] Peritoneovenous shunting is also effective but makes subsequent transplantation more dangerous and should not be undertaken in potential transplant recipients.

Esophageal varices may be a source of significant bleeding before operation and portosystemic venous collaterals greatly increase blood loss during operation. Sclerotherapy not only helps prevent preoperative variceal bleeding but also reduces the risk of hemorrhage after transplantation, in the event of portal obstruction because of rejection or other pathological process.

Impaired synthetic function is reflected in reduced plasma concentrations of albumin and coagulation factors. Hypoalbuminemia aggravates ascites and peripheral edema and may be corrected by the infusion of 20% (salt-poor) human albumin solution. Coagulopathy, if uncorrected, is associated with gross operative hemorrhage, particularly in the presence of extensive venous collaterals and abdominal adhesions related to previous surgery or peritonitis. Most coagulation factors are synthesized only in the liver and will be depressed in advanced liver failure even with adequate provision of vitamin K. Platelet numbers and survival times are also frequently reduced, usually because of hypersplenism. It is essential to correct clotting defects by giving appropriate blood products immediately before surgery. This is discussed in detail below.

Preoperative laboratory investigations often reveal further abnormalities. Hemoglobin values are depressed in many patients. This may be related to malnutrition, gastrointestinal bleeding, or hypersplenism. Hyponatremia and hypokalemia are common, induced by diuretic therapy, secondary hyperaldosteronism, and other, poorly understood renal abnormalities. Preoperative correction of moderate hypokalemia (>3.0 mmol/L) is rarely necessary. Arrhythmias attributable to mild hypokalemia are infrequent,[19] and overzealous correction may enhance the risk of dangerous hyperkalemia when large amounts of potassium are introduced into the circulation by blood transfusion and graft reperfusion at operation. Hyponatremia, if severe (<120 mmol/L), increases the risk of disequilibrium myelinolysis after operation, particularly if operative blood loss is substantial and plasma sodium increases abruptly.[20] This syndrome, associated with protean and disabling neurological features, is well-recognized in liver transplant recipients and gradual correction before surgery is essential. Water restriction, albumin infusions, and a reduction of diuretic dosage can achieve this in most patients, although slow correction of refractory hyponatremia by hemofiltration has been described.[21]

Impaired metabolism of vitamin D may lead to osteomalacia and susceptibility to fractures. However, even in these patients, plasma concentrations of calcium, phosphorus, and magnesium are usually normal.

Hypoglycemia is an unusual finding in chronic hepatic failure, although it is common in patients with fulminant hepatic failure, in whom blood glucose should be measured frequently.

Renal function is well preserved in the majority of patients, although prerenal insufficiency is often seen because of tense ascites and excessive use of diuretics. Renal failure may be seen in patients with acute hepatic failure or severe sepsis. Alterations in renal handling of sodium and water are recognized in liver disease, but the mechanisms remain largely unexplained.[22] Renal microcirculatory changes may reduce the threshold for renal damage in many forms of chronic liver disease. However, evidence for this or any other specific causative mechanism in the "hepatorenal syndrome" remains inconclusive.[23] Impairment of renal function is reported to be a strong predictor of postoperative sepsis and mortality,[24,25] and measures to protect renal function during surgery should be part of routine practice. These are described in detail below.

Some uncommon renal disorders need simultaneous hepatic and renal transplantation.[7] These include tyrosinosis, characterized by aminoaciduria and type 2 renal tubular acidosis, and oxalosis, which presents as chronic renal failure.

In the absence of underlying cardiac disease, cardiovascular function is well maintained in all but the most advanced cases of hepatic decompensation. Studies in adults have shown that liver failure is characterized by a disturbance of microcirculatory function causing arteriovenous shunting, increased cardiac output and flow-dependent oxygen consumption.[27] Its degree appears to depend on the severity of the underlying hepatic disease, although it may occur in the presence of portal hypertension without significant jaundice and vice versa. Myocardial reserve in most patients is such that increased demand is not associated with left ventricular dilatation or pulmonary venous hypertension.

An exaggerated basal flow murmur is a common clinical finding, and echocardiography should be done when this or other features raise the possibility of a structural abnormality. Patients over 40 years of age may have occult or symptomatic coronary artery disease, and those with alcoholic cirrhosis, hemochromatosis, or Wilson's disease may have cardiomyopathy. In practice, evidence of heart failure is infrequently seen. The high output state characteristic of hepatic decompensation reveals significant left ventricular dysfunction early in the course of the disease, and this may affect mortality before transplantation is considered. Alternatively, liver disease may spare or even enhance myocardial function by unknown mechanisms. Nonetheless, any evidence of cardiac disease must be taken seriously in view of the major insults imposed during surgery and in the period after operation.

In the absence of published data quantifying cardiac risk during hepatic transplantation and given the rarity of primary cardiac deaths in the perioperative period, our approach is as follows. All patients are screened with a 12-lead electrocardiogram and chest x-ray. Those with overt coronary artery disease are considered for coronary angiography and possible coronary artery bypass grafting before transplantation, providing hepatic dysfunction is not severe. Left ventricular failure is associated with a high mortality in the context of any major vascular procedure and in most cases contraindicates liver transplantation. In our experience, mild valvular disease without significant ventricular dysfunction is not associated with increased perioperative mortality, and its investigation is usually limited to echocardiography. Patients with important risk factors, those in whom evidence of coronary disease is equivocal, or those in whom clinical assessment of ventricular function is difficult need radionuclide studies for further assessment. Ejection fraction at rest and during exercise may be determined by gated radionuclide ventriculography, which will also detect wall motion abnormalities suggestive of underlying coronary disease. Abnormal results in this investigation are associated with a high risk of intraoperative cardiovascular instability.[28] Thallium-dipyridamole scanning has been advocated as a sensitive test for occult coronary artery disease,[29] as has 24-hour ambulatory ST segment analysis. The impact of abnormal findings in these studies on perioperative management and mortality in patients receiving liver transplants remains to be determined.

The assessment of cardiac function in children presents fewer problems. These patients usually tolerate the transplant procedure without major cardiovascular instability, although there are some caveats. Children with biliary atresia have a high incidence of associated congenital abnormalities.[30] Systolic murmurs are heard in most children with advanced liver disease. Most are flow murmurs, but as in adults structural cardiac lesions should be excluded by echocardiography. Children with Alagille's syndrome (biliary hypoplasia, butterfly vertebrae, and tetralogy of Fallot) present a particular challenge. In the absence of a total correction of the tetralogy, pulmonary blood flow depends on the state of the palliative shunt. Both systemic oxygen delivery and myocardial reserve may be poor. Despite these difficulties transplantation has been successful in this condition.

Respiratory impairment in these patients has many potential causes. Reduced lung volumes and ventilation/perfusion imbalance associated with abdominal distension from ascites or hepatosplenomegaly account for the modest hypoxemia seen in many of these patients. Pulmonary arteriovenous shunting has been demonstrated[31,32] and in severe cases has been described as the "hepatopulmonary syndrome."[33] This is usually characterized by normocarbia or mild respiratory alkalosis. Noncardiogenic pulmonary edema is infrequently seen except in the setting of fulminant hepatic failure. It can be controlled by diuretic therapy and by cautious correction of hypoalbuminemia. A right-sided pleural effusion is common in patients with ascites and is usually managed in the same way. In some patients, however, it is necessary to drain the fluid to ensure satisfactory preoperative lung function. Aspiration

and pulmonary infection are less frequent causes of lung dysfunction and should be managed by appropriate antibiotic treatment and chest physiotherapy before transplantation is carried out. Because of the high incidence of chest infections after liver transplantation, any patient who smokes must be firmly advised to stop.

Immediately before surgery the correction of any coagulopathy present becomes the main consideration. Fresh frozen plasma in a dose of 10–30 mL/kg over 2–4 hours is given if the prothrombin time is prolonged. Cryoprecipitate should be added if the preoperative fibrinogen concentration is below 23.4 μmoL/L (0.8 g/dL): 1 unit per 5 kg increases the plasma concentration of fibrinogen by approximately 2.1 μmoL/L (0.075 g/dL).[36] Platelet concentrate should be given if the platelet count is less than 50×10^9/L. One donor unit per 10 kg may be expected to raise the platelet count by about 30×10^9/L.[37] Ten units of blood are routinely crossmatched, and the blood bank should ensure that at least 20 additional group-specific units are available if needed. Adequate supplies of fresh frozen plasma and platelets must also be available, whatever the preoperative coagulation values, because of the likelihood of dilutional or defibrination coagulopathy during surgery.

Special problems are encountered in patients with multisystem failure because of fulminant hepatitis or terminal decompensation in chronic liver failure. These patients usually have severe coagulopathy and encephalopathy with cerebral edema. Noncardiogenic pulmonary edema, renal insufficiency, and/or sepsis may also be present. Attempted correction of very severe coaguloapathy (prothrombin time (PT)>100 seconds) by simple infusion of clotting factors is difficult and possibly dangerous. Plasmapheresis allows fresh frozen plasma to be given without increasing plasma volume,[38] although this has not been shown to improve outcome. Raised intracranial pressure is commonly seen in fulminant hepatic failure with coma (grade III or IV encephalopathy). It may rapidly progress to fatal brain stem compression if untreated. Intracranial pressure monitoring is now widely advocated for this.[39] Elevated intracranial pressure should be treated by neuromuscular paralysis and hyperventilation, a 30-degree head-up tilt, and maintenance of modest hypertension and hemodilution. Noxious stimuli, which cause transient increases in intracranial pressure, should be minimized. Mannitol (0.25–0.5 g/kg/h) and thiopentone (2 mg/kg/h) are often used. The definitive treatment, providing brain stem activity remains intact, is urgent transplantation.

Renal failure is best managed by continuous arteriovenous or veno-venous hemofiltration. This technique is superior to intermittent hemodialysis because there is less cardiovascular instability and better control of intravascular volume. Correcting hyperkalemia before operation is particularly important as the inevitable, if transient, further increase in plasma concentration of potassium after graft reperfusion is potentially fatal. Hemofiltration also allows control of metabolic acidosis, maintenance of normal plasma sodium values, and appropriate adjustment of cardiac filling pressures. Extending its use into the operative period has also been advocated[40] and is undoubtedly useful in selected cases.

Sepsis may be difficult to diagnose in this setting as many of its clinical manifestations are mimicked in terminal hepatic decompensation. However, fever, hypotension, and dependence on vasopressors clearly suggest its presence, and the risks of proceeding with transplantation at this stage are prohibitive. Appropriate antimicrobial treatment and cardiovascular stability are needed before surgery can be considered. Unfortunately, many patients fail to respond to treatment once this state has been reached. In the absence of signs of infection, colonization with resistant organisms, common in cystic fibrosis and in patients previously immunosuppressed, does not appear to increase perioperative risk. Expert microbiological advice should always be sought regarding perioperative prophylaxis in these circumstances.

Surgical Technique

Knowledge of the surgical procedure is vital to the anesthetist because major cardiovascular and biochemical changes are directly related to operative events. The first part of the operation is the dissection phase, during which the liver and its vascular attachments are isolated from the surrounding tissues. The abdomen is opened through bilateral subcostal incisions with a midline extension to the xiphoid. The structures of the free edge of the lesser sac and porta hepatis are dissected out and the liver freed of its supporting ligamentous attachments.

The retrohepatic portion of the inferior vena cava is also mobilized and its branches ligated. Venous collaterals in the abdominal wall and mesentery may be extensive and will bleed heavily during this stage unless meticulous attention is paid to surgical hemostasis. Mesenteric adhesions from previous abdominal surgery may also cause major technical problems and substantially increase blood loss. This is particularly true when a portocaval shunt or esophageal transection has been performed, and the risk of fatal intraoperative hemorrhage is high in these circumstances. Previous porto-enterostomy in biliary atresia (Kasai procedure) is also a common source of difficulty. This initial phase of the procedure varies greatly in duration (about 1–6 hours) and difficulty.

The next stage is the anhepatic period. The bile duct, hepatic artery, portal vein, and infrahepatic inferior vena cava are divided and a clamp placed across the suprahepatic cava at the level of the diaphragm. This is divided and the diseased liver removed along with the hepatic veins and retrohepatic length of the inferior vena cava. The donor liver is removed from iced saline and placed in the hepatic fossa. Anastomosis of the suprahepatic cava is then performed, followed by the portal vein and infrahepatic cava. When the latter are nearly complete the new liver is perfused through a cannula in the portal vein, with an isotonic, potassium-free crystalloid or colloid solution. This washes out storage perfusate and air, which escape through the incomplete lower caval anastomosis. The final sutures are placed in the portal and infrahepatic caval anastomoses and the infra-and suprahepatic caval clamps released. After restoration of caval flow the portal vein is unclamped, beginning the final or "reperfusion" phase of the operation. The period immediately after graft reperfusion is associated with marked cardiovascular, biochemical, and hematological changes.

Hepatic artery and biliary anastomoses follow and are without major anesthetic difficulties. Biliary drainage may be accomplished by a donor-recipient end-to-end anastomosis, by use of the donor gallbladder as a conduit between donor and recipient bile ducts, or by a Roux-en-Y choledochojejunostomy, depending on the recipient's biliary anatomy.

Details of surgical technique vary between centers, particularly in the unclamping sequence of the three major anastomoses, the use and positioning of cannulas for veno-venous bypass (see below), and the use of in situ liver perfusion during the anhepatic phase. Duration of surgery also varies widely, from 3 to more than 12 hours depending on the patient and surgical team. Important recent departures from the conventional technique have been the transplantation of livers reduced in size by excision of the right lobe and the splitting of a single donor liver into two lobar grafts for separate recipients. These may be undertaken when size discrepancy would otherwise prevent transplantation in young children, for whom the availability of donor organs of appropriate size is a major problem.[41] Lobar grafts from living related donors have also been performed.

The Transplant Anesthesia Team

A consultant experienced in transplant anesthesia directs and takes responsibility for all members of the anesthesia team. An experienced registrar/resident provides assistance. In Cambridge two technicians prepare the operating theater and assist with induction of anesthesia. They also run infusion pumps, blood administration apparatus, and cell-saving equipment and maintain detailed records of infusions and losses. A third technician is needed when veno-venous bypass is used. A clinical measurement technician sets up and maintains monitoring equipment and performs routine measurements and blood sampling. Rapid access to biochemical and hematological laboratory facilities is essential. The results of routine studies, particularly arterial blood gases, hematocrit, plasma sodium, potassium, and ionized calcium must be available within minutes. The importance of well-organized and competent technical support cannot be overemphasized.

Anesthesia

Premedication is important in all age groups. Since intramuscular injections are best avoided in those with abnormal clotting, a short-acting oral benzodiazepine is the usual choice. Young children may be given low-dose ketamine (2 mg/kg) and atropine intravenously or intramuscularly to allow them to be placed on the operating table without causing them distress. Patients with encephalopathy or very marked abdominal distension may be vulnerable to respiratory depression and should be premedicated with due caution.

Venous access is usually easy, perhaps due to the low systemic vascular resistance and increased cardiac output that characterize advanced hepatic disease. Preoperative H_2-receptor blockade and pre-oxygenation followed by rapid sequence induction are recommended because portal hypertension and ascites may affect gastric emptying and lower esophageal sphincter function.

Any suitable induction agent may be used and suxamethonium in normal dosage permits prompt tracheal intubation. Clinical experience suggests that the effects of suxamethonium are little altered by the deficiency of plasma cholinesterase in liver disease. Orotracheal intubation may be followed in younger children by placement of a nasal tube, if clotting is near normal. This facilitates management after surgery, when mechanical ventilation for 24–48 hours may be needed. A nasogastric tube is passed, since gastric distension may interfere with surgical access, and postoperative ileus, occasionally with marked gastric dilation, occurs in all cases. These considerations outweigh the risks of traumatic bleeding from unidentified or untreated varices in patients with portal hypertension, although care must be taken.

The choice of agents for maintenance of anesthesia is determined chiefly by the need to preserve good myocardial function. Both preload and contractility may be dramatically altered during surgery and myocardial depression by anesthetic agents must be minimized. Fentanyl 10–20 µg/kg followed by increments or continuous infusion of 2–5 µg/kg/hour, given with air/oxygen/isoflurane, is a well-proven technique. Nitrous oxide is usually avoided for a number of practical and theoretical reasons. Bowel distension may interfere with abdominal closure, particularly when the transplanted liver is relatively large. Prolonged exposure may affect DNA synthesis and bone marrow function by oxidation of vitamin B_{12} and interference with folate metabolism.[42] Although nitrous oxide is known to produce myocardial depression in cardiac patients given morphine[43] and fentanyl,[44] this has not been seen in studies of healthy volunteers given nitrous oxide/oxygen/isoflurane,[45,46] and its effects in patients with hepatic disease are unknown. Animal work suggests that hepatic blood flow may be significantly reduced by nitrous oxide,[47] consistent with evidence that it causes sympathetically mediated vasoconstriction.[48,49] While of no consequence during the dissection phase, this is likely to be undesirable once the new liver is reperfused. The possibility of air embolism, a recognized hazard in liver transplantation[50,51] and probably more dangerous in the presence of nitrous oxide,[52] is a further reason not to use it.

Cardiovascular stability favors the use of isoflurane over halothane and enflurane.[45] A basal level of 1.3 minimum alveolar concentration (MAC) is a desirable minimum to ensure anesthesia, although reduction of vapor concentration is sometimes necessary during episodes of hypotension. Fentanyl and midazolam are added routinely to allay this concern. Although isoflurane may reduce hepatic blood flow, data from animal studies suggest that this is likely to be much less than occurs with other agents.[53–55] Techniques relying solely on high-dose opiates have been used in some centers, although variable hepatic function following grafting and the possibility of a washout effect related to massive blood replacement are theoretical disadvantages. A further reservation is that complete suppression of stress-related cardiovascular responses may not be advantageous in this clinical context. Nonetheless, in patients with evidence of coronary disease, high-dose fentanyl or sufentanil may indeed be safer than 1.3 MAC isoflurane, and practical difficulties with this technique have not been reported.

The choice of muscle relaxant presents less scope for controversy. Pancuronium has been used successfully for many years and its partial dependence on hepatic elimination has not proved clinically relevant. Atracurium lacks significant cardiovascular effects when given in appropriate dosage, and in contrast to other agents its half-life is not prolonged in patients with liver disease.[56] An increase in infusion dose requirements related to increases in volume of distribution and plasma clearance, and to rapid turnover of blood volume with operative hemorrhage, may be observed. However, the mean requirement reported in a group of adolescent and adult liver transplant patients of 0.38 mg/kg/h suggests that these effects are not clinically important.[57] The need for a period of postoperative mechanical ventilation, during which relaxants are rarely given, further diminishes the significance of relaxant kinetics.

Vascular Access

Large-bore intravenous access is vital. Placement of cannulas is facilitated by the high cardiac output of advanced liver disease, and in adult patients it is usually possible to insert 12G or larger cannulas pe-

ripherally. A Seldinger technique may be used if necessary. Intravenous cannulas must be placed in the upper extremities because caval clamping and the need in adults to spare the femoral or saphenous veins for veno-venous bypass make these vessels unusable. Two lines are dedicated to transfusion and a third is used for infusion of other blood products. A wire-guided double- or triple-lumen polyurethane catheter, preferably placed by the internal jugular route, is also essential. In adults a pulmonary artery catheter is used as well. It is our practice to place two 10FG cannulas (or 5FG catheters convertible to 10s) alongside the pulmonary artery catheter in the right internal jugular vein. These may be used as reserve volume-infusion lines or converted for use as part of a veno-venous bypass circuit (see below). When intracranial pressure is raised, the subclavian route is preferred because cannulation of the internal jugular veins may impair cerebral venous drainage. Subclavian cannulation is associated with a higher risk of local complications, however, and is usually avoided, particularly when clotting is abnormal.

Monitoring

Continuous direct monitoring of intravascular pressures is needed. Radial or femoral arterial cannulas and central venous catheters are essential, while pulmonary artery flotation catheters are used routinely in most centers.

Radial artery pressure monitoring may underestimate aortic pressure in hypotensive states and should be interpreted with caution. Pulmonary artery (PA) pressure and thermodilution cardiac output measurements assist in the assessment and management of hypotension, which may arise unpredictably because of changes in venous return, altered systemic vascular resistance, and cardiac or embolic events. A PA catheter that continuously measures mixed venous saturation is also useful for early detection of hypoperfusion and for measurement of oxygen consumption, thought to be an early indicator of graft function.[58,59]

Femoral venous pressure measurement allows prompt detection of caval occlusion during the dissection phase and gauges the efficacy of lower caval decompression during veno-venous bypass; renal perfusion pressure may thus be estimated.[60] The benefits of the technique must be balanced against risks: the authors have observed inadvertent femoral arterial puncture in a patient with coagulopathy needing surgical exploration for control of bleeding.

All transducers should be carefully zeroed, especially those used to measure cardiac filling pressures, as these must be maintained within a narrow range during rapid changes in circulating volume. Monitoring catheters must be securely fixed and easily accessible in the event of technical difficulties.

Cardiovascular monitoring may be further enhanced by the use of transesophageal echocardiography, which gives continuous information on ventricular function and an immediate diagnosis of embolization of air or thrombus.[61] Indirect measurement of gastric intramucosal pH assesses perfusion of the upper gut, although in our experience it is significantly influenced by other factors and is vulnerable to technical error.[62]

Temperature and oxygen saturation monitoring present few problems. The accuracy of pulse oximetry in patients with hyperbilirubinemia and potential inaccuracy of co-oximetry have been shown.[63] The decrease in cardiac index during the anhepatic phase rarely affects this monitor. Capnography gives a continuous measure of alveolar ventilation, although it is also influenced by changes in cardiac output and by the administration of sodium bicarbonate. Accurate monitoring of urine flow allows aggressive management of oliguria, and the tallying of shed blood aids the assessment of volume balance, since filling pressures do not always reflect changes in intravascular volume.

Measurement of arterial blood gases, sodium, potassium, glucose, ionized calcium, and hematocrit should be performed at frequent intervals, at least hourly during the initial and closing phases of the operation and more often during the anhepatic period. All are subject to rapid changes, to be discussed in detail below. Accurate measurement of ionized calcium is a significant recent advance in intraoperative monitoring, as this cannot be predicted from total calcium values. Citrate toxicity occurs readily in liver transplantation because of heavy blood transfusion and impaired hepatic metabolism of citrate. Cardiovascular stability is greatly enhanced by the rapid identification and treatment of ionic hypocalcemia.

The value of coagulation monitoring is also widely accepted.[64] Routine laboratory screening tests provide essential information, but results are often supplied too late to accurately reflect a changing situation. The problem of diagnostic delay may be overcome by the development of rapid bedside techniques for prothrombin time, partial thromboplastin time, and platelet count, although these have not yet been fully evaluated. Thromboelastography and the Sonoclot analyzer, sensitive bedside techniques quantifying the rate and quality of fibrin formation by measuring viscoelastic properties, provide excellent qualitative data and allow in vitro testing of potential corrective therapy with antifibrinolytics.[65,66] Clotting factor assays and laboratory evaluation of fibrinolysis (fibrin degradation products, euglobulin lysis time) are also advocated. However, no method of coagulation monitoring has been shown to reduce blood loss, and decisions about corrective therapy should always incorporate clinical factors. These include the patient's preoperative coagulation status, the presence or absence of generalized oozing and formed clot in the surgical field, and the likelihood of further surgical hemorrhage.

Blood Replacement and Fluid Management

Substantial operative hemorrhage is usual during hepatic transplantation. The amount of blood loss varies greatly, depending on the underlying disease, the state of the portal circulation, the presence of adhesions, and surgical technique. Early series described average adult blood replacement of 8–12 liters[67,68] and pediatric losses of 3.95 blood volumes (range 370 mL to 30 liters).[51] Transfusion requirements have shown a tendency to decrease with increasing surgical experience and better coagulation management. Adult patients in the Cambridge program from January 1988 to December 1991 had a median measured loss of 4.25 liters (range 0.34–128), while pediatric patients in the same period had a median loss of 1.16 blood volumes (range 0.03–25.9).

Measurement of blood loss is difficult and may be confounded by the inclusion of ascites. When bleeding is brisk, measured totals will lag far behind actual losses, and volume replacement should be guided by cardiac filling pressures. These should be maintained at the upper end of the normal range to allow a margin of safety should very rapid blood loss occur and to reduce the risk of air embolism.

A pressurized rapid infusion system for each of the two large-bore infusion lines is essential. The Hemonetics Rapid Infusion System[69] is valuable, if not essential in the management of major operative hemorrhage. This device incorporates a 3 liter reservoir, heat-exchange column, roller pump, 40-micron filter, and sensors for air, pressure, and temperature. It is capable of infusion rates of up to 1500 mL/minute, warms infused fluid to 39°C, and allows instantaneous and finely regulated control of transfusion. Its superior warming capacity permits body temperature to be well maintained during rapid bleeding; indeed, body temperature increases toward the infusate temperature if major hemorrhage is sustained. Disposable costs and priming deadspace are high, and because it can be set up in a few minutes, it should be used on a standby basis. For small children a volumetric infusion pump incorporating a bypass limb for rapid infusion is a useful innovation.[70]

Microfiltration of blood is advisable.[71] Twenty-micron depth filters have been advocated for maximum clearance of microaggregates but are prone to obstruction. Forty-micron screen filters are a more practical alternative. Filter replacement is needed after every 5–10 units of blood to avoid flow restriction.

Autotransfusion techniques have developed rapidly in recent years and may now reduce the use of bank blood by as much as 60%. In the Hemonetics system (Hemonetics Cell-Saver 4) red cells are salvaged through heparinized suction lines, then washed and centrifuged before reconstitution in a saline suspension with a hematocrit of about 55%. In practice, blood loss exceeding one liter is needed before processing can begin, and the rate of processing limits reinfusion to a maximum rate of 100–125 mL/minute, which is achieved through the use of a modified reinfusion bag system.[70] Reinfused cells must be diluted if high hematocrits are to be avoided and plasma proteins replenished from other sources. Cell-saving techniques are contraindicated in hepatic malignancy and in cases where bacterial soiling of the peritoneum has occurred.

The use of blood products to correct a coagulopathy before surgery and the intraoperative monitoring of coagulation were discussed above. Intraoperative replacement therapy is guided by cardiac filling pressures, clinical observation, and the results of regular monitoring of hematocrit, platelet count, and tests of coagulation. Increased concern about the risks associated with transfusion, particularly of infection, have affected transfusion practice in recent years. The use of whole blood in the initial management of major hemorrhage in preference to one-to-one administration of concentrated red cells and fresh frozen plasma, to reduce the number of donors to which the patient is exposed, has been advocated.[72] When stored in citrate-phosphate-dextrose, whole blood contains adequate levels of all coagulation factors except V and VIII for up to 35 days. Even these more rapidly depleted factors are relatively plentiful in blood stored for fewer than 5 days and are often present in concentrations high enough to sustain coagulation, although not to correct preexisting coagulopathy, in blood stored for much longer.[73–75] We use whole blood for the first 10 units replaced, in combination with fresh frozen plasma. The latter is given continuously at a rate of 1–2 units/hour, depending on coagulation screen results and rate of blood loss. Further losses need higher rates of fresh frozen plasma administration, and packed cells are then given. A packed cell volume of 30–35% is desirable once the new liver is reperfused, as this is thought to allow optimum oxygen transport and may reduce the risk of hepatic arterial thrombosis, a particular problem in children. In spite of the initial use of whole blood and fresh frozen plasma, hematocrits higher than this are sometimes seen and occasionally phlebotomy may be needed.

Fresh frozen plasma given before operation and continuously during the dissection phase is usually sufficient to prevent coagulopathy until hepatic reperfusion. At this stage an increased bleeding tendency is commonly seen. Dilutional changes may account for this in part and may be managed by further infusion of fresh frozen plasma and platelets. However, generalized bleeding in the operative field, unresponsive to efforts at surgical hemostasis and characterized by absence of clot formation in the wound, usually results from fibrinolysis. This may be a primary process in which fibrinolytic pathways are pathologically activated, destroying fibrin formed for physiologic hemostasis, or a secondary phenomenon triggered by disseminated intravascular coagulation. In some cases both processes may be present.[76] The best treatment remains to be established. Prophylactic infusion of aprotinin, a serine protease inhibitor acting on plasminogen to reduce formation of plasmin, appears to suppress this phenomenon and to reduce operative blood loss substantially.[77–79] Other antifibrinolytics (epsilon-aminocaproic acid, tranexamic acid) have also been successfully used, especially when given prophylactically. Therapy is safest when guided by specific tests of fibrinolysis, such as thromboelastography or euglobulin clot lysis times.[80] Cryoprecipitate is given, in addition to fresh frozen plasma, if fibrinogen levels are low.

In most cases fibrinolysis is short-lived, but when blood loss has already been substantial it may persist for many hours. If early graft function is impaired, clotting factor deficiencies will persist and correction of the coagulopathy may prove impossible. The management of intractable hemorrhage is discussed below. In all circumstances the rate of infusion and relative proportions of cellular and acellular blood products require titration against filling pressures and hematocrit.

Giving of platelet concentrates during the operation should also be guided by platelet counts and clinical observation. In the presence of normal coagulation before surgery, dilutional platelet deficiency is the most likely cause of coagulopathy associated with massive transfusion. However, platelet release from splenic and marrow reserves attenuates the predicted washout phenomenon.[81,82] In the presence of severe liver disease both platelet numbers and function may be affected and platelet concentrate may be indicated even when numbers are normal if microvascular oozing is apparent. The large donor pool to which the patient is exposed when standard platelet concentrates are used must be considered, and the increased use of pheresis packs, in which a single donor provides the equivalent of 6–8 units should be safer.

Citrate given in transfused blood and plasma depresses plasma ionized calcium, which must be maintained near normal levels if myocardial depression is to be avoided.[32] Calcium chloride is given, in doses that depend on the volume of blood products given and on the liver's ability to metabolize citrate. The latter depends in turn on body temperature, hepatic perfusion, and the severity of the underlying disease. Approximately 5 mmol of calcium ion per liter of citrated products should be given in patients with significant hepatic impairment, although frequent ionized calcium measurements are invaluable. Repeated intravenous bolus doses of 1–2 mmol/10 kg are well tolerated.

Losses of fluid other than blood must also be replaced. Respiratory evaporative losses can be minimized by humidifying inspired gases or the use of a heat and moisture exchanging device. Urinary and nasogastric losses may also be substantial. Probably more significant are evaporative and interstitial losses caused by prolonged exposure of and extensive trauma to the peritoneum, and possibly by global tissue ischemia during the anhepatic period.[83] Sodium and protein losses are adequately replaced when blood and colloid are infused, but water losses, especially in small children, must be replaced separately if hypernatremia is to be avoided.[84] The infusion of 4–6 mL/kg/hour of 0.18% sodium chloride in 4% dextrose throughout the procedure is adequate.

Management of Intractable Hemorrhage

In a minority of patients all efforts to obtain surgical hemostasis after reperfusion fail because of intractable coagulopathy and generalized small vessel oozing. There is no visible clot in the wound and coagulation testing shows persistent fibrinolysis. We give large quantities of clotting factors, based on measurement of prothrombin time, plasma concentration of fibrinogen, and platelet count. Hypothermia is corrected and tranexamic acid or aprotinin given. If these measures fail, a vasopressin infusion at 10 units per hour is started. The abdomen is closed and the patient placed in a pneumatic antishock garment. Intravesicle pressure is measured continuously and maintained at 30–35 mmHg, while mean arterial pressure is kept at 80 mmHg or higher to sustain a renal perfusion pressure above 50 mmHg. Care is taken to ensure that abdominal drains are not kinked and that the skin is adequately protected. The suit is left inflated for 24–48 hours. Oliguria is common with this regimen, but renal function recovers quickly when the garment is deflated.

Electrolyte and Acid-Base Changes

The infusion of large volumes of blood products and reperfusion of the donor liver cause marked changes in plasma biochemistry. In most patients blood glucose is normal before surgery but increases during the procedure because of administration acid-citrate-dextrose blood and stress-related insulin resistance. Hypoglycemia, occasionally seen before operation in infants and in those with fulminant hepatic failure, is not seen during operation even when normal hepatic glucose release is interrupted during the anhepatic and early reperfusion phases. A decrease in blood glucose concentration is seen once the new liver begins to function[51] but appears to depend in part on the use of insulin and of dextrose-free maintenance fluids. When insulin is not given, concentrations of glucose in excess of 15–20 mmol/L are common, but no harm appears to result and control is readily achieved soon after operation.

Plasma sodium also tends to increase and may, with glucose, contribute to moderate hyperosmolarity at the end of the procedure. Increases of more than 12 mmol/L in 24 hours have been associated with pontine myelinolysis and severe neurologic disability in both experimental animals and man. In susceptible patients this may happen with smaller increases.[85] Sodium citrate in blood products, sodium bicarbonate administration, and evaporative water loss all contribute. The use of a low sodium maintenance crystalloid solution appears to prevent hypernatremia and its use, especially in children, is advisable.[28]

Plasma potassium, low or normal initially, increases on reperfusion of the liver as blood from the obstructed portal system acquires extracellular potassium from the ischemic donor liver and rejoins the main circulation. Liver flush potassium values of over 100 mmol/L and arterial plasma levels as high as 11 mmol/L may be measured, and characteristic electrocardiographic changes are seen. In most patients redistribution follows within seconds and a progressive decrease is subsequently seen. Preexisting renal failure and residual beta-blockade in patients in whom portal hypertension has been treated with propranolol, however, may be associated with prolonged and life-threatening hyperkalemia. Administration of additional calcium chloride, dextrose-insulin, or beta-agonist may be of value until hepatic uptake becomes established or dialysis can be implemented. In contrast, intraoperative potassium supplementation is sometimes necessary late in the procedure when reuptake by the grafted liver may result in hypokalemia.

Metabolic acidosis is usually absent or minimal at first, but increases during the operation. It has many potential causes. Acidosis in arterial blood can sometimes be attributed to hyperlactatemia. Transfused blood introduces a substantial quantity of exogenous lactic acid into the circulation. Liver lactate and urea metabolism are impaired, as is renal function. Acid metabolites associated with venous stasis in the portal and lower body circulations, as well as those that accumulate in the new liver during transport and storage, are released into the general circulation on reperfusion, causing a further increase in acidosis.

Treatment of the acidosis includes modest hyperventilation and increasing cardiac output. The value of giving bicarbonate has been questioned. Evidence that global circulatory function is impaired by moderate metabolic acidosis is slight, while detrimental effects on oxygen delivery and intracellular pH associated with bicarbonate therapy have been shown.[86-88] Indeed, plasma lactate concentrations have been shown to increase and cardiac index to decrease after bicarbonate is given in animal models of hemorrhagic shock and hypoxic lactic acidosis and in patients with congestive heart failure.[89-91] Bicarbonate achieves its buffering effect by the production of carbon dioxide and combats acidosis in the tissues only if the CO_2 is efficiently cleared by the lungs. The presence of pulmonary arteriovenous shunting, well recognized in these patients, may inhibit this process and lead to increases in arterial CO_2 content. Experimental techniques measuring pH at cellular level will in the future guide therapy. Alternative buffers that produce less or no carbon dioxide may be of value but remain to be assessed.

If liver and cardiovascular function are adequate after reperfusion there is a tendency for metabolic acidosis to change to alkalosis. This may be related to the uptake of citrate ion by the new liver.[92] Hydrogen ions are taken up during the production of CO_2, which is then excreted, leading to a net loss of acid from the body. Lactic acid appears to be similarly cleared, while hypokalemia and steroids enhance alkalosis because of their renal effects. These mechanisms remain hypothetical, however, since no consistent relationship between blood replacement and postoperative alkalosis or between alkalosis and early graft function has been shown.

Hypomagnesemia has also been described during liver transplantation,[32] but the importance of this remains to be defined.

Cardiovascular Changes

Hypovolemia as a result of hemorrhage presents the greatest threat, and the ability to replace blood rapidly has been emphasized. Cardiac function may be impaired during the dissection phase by the sudden obstruction of venous return during surgical manipulation of the liver or by direct compression of the diaphragmatic surface of the heart. Some anesthetic agents and ionic hypocalcemia will amplify these effects. The responses to clamping of the inferior vena cava for hepatectomy and to un-clamping when the grafted liver is reperfused de-pend on several factors. The most important of these is whether or not veno-venous bypass, an ex-tracorporeal circuit designed to circumvent caval and portal obstruction, is used. This technique is discussed below.

In the absence of veno-venous bypass, clamping of the cava at hepatectomy produces a marked de-crease in venous pressure and cardiac output.[93,94] Systemic vascular resistance increases, but a de-crease in blood pressure is to be expected. Provided cardiac filling pressures and contractility are main-tained, frank hypotension (<80 mmHg systolic) is unusual. Lower filling pressures are accepted during the anhepatic phase as long as the lowest (presys-tolic) central venous pressure remains positive and arterial blood pressure is satisfactory. Overtransfu-sion at this stage may result in dangerously high fill-ing pressures following unclamping, with adverse effects on gas exchange and hepatic blood flow.

In patients in whom bypass is used the decrease in cardiac output is attenuated, reduced from 40–50% to 20–30%. Arterial pressure is well main-tained, although this depends on the flows obtained through the bypass circuit. Nonetheless, a progres-sive decline in cardiac output occurs during the an-hepatic phase and bypass falls short of maintaining a normal circulatory state.[95]

Reperfusion of the transplanted liver is usually associated with changes in heart rate, contractility, and peripheral vascular tone,[93,94] whether or not by-pass is used. Portal and caval unclamping allows acidic, desaturated blood from the obstructed portal circulation, which is cooled and made more acidic and potassium-rich by passage through the new liver, to perfuse the heart. Slowing of the heart is observed, as are electrocardiographic signs of acute hyperkalemia. These changes are usually mild and short-lived, but asystole and tachyarrhythmias, in-cluding ventricular fibrillation, are sometimes seen. Blood pressure decreases in almost all patients, and the magnitude of this appears to be greater in pa-tients in whom bypass is used,[96–98] possibly because compensatory peripheral vasoconstriction is less in-tense in these patients during the anhepatic phase. Hypotension occurs because of arteriolar vasodila-tion, with or without myocardial depression. These changes may be caused by inflammatory mediators from the ischemic liver, by peptides or other agents released during splanchnic stasis, or by reflex va-sodilation induced by hyperkalemia or a sudden in-crease in cardiac filling. Treatment just before revascularization with calcium chloride[99] and at-ropine[100] appears to modify these effects, and the use of small boluses of pressor agents when hypoten-sion is marked is common practice. In most patients blood pressure and cardiac output are restored to preclamping values within minutes. In a small num-ber of patients recovery takes longer and sustained vasopressor support is needed. Those undergoing urgent retransplantation for hepatic infarction may have circulatory failure before surgery. Hypoten-sion and acidosis after unclamping in these circum-stances may be progressive and irreversible.

The sequence in which the major venous clamps are removed as the transplanted liver is reperfused may also influence cardiovascular responses. An approach intended to achieve reoxygenation of the liver in the minimum time involves completion of the suprahepatic and portal anastomoses and restoration of portal flow before the infrahepatic caval anastomosis is started. Alternatively, all three venous anastomoses may be performed before reperfusion and the two caval clamps released first. The latter appears to be associated with less hy-potension and fewer arrhythmias, presumably be-cause vasoactive substances released from the donor liver enter a normal circulating volume and are diluted.[101] (Lai 1990).

Cardiovascular instability caused by air embo-lism has been described,[52,53] and the maintenance of a positive venous pressure is recommended. In one report high-frequency ventilation was associated with cerebral air embolization, raising the possibil-ity of air entering the circulation by the pulmonary route, possibly through abnormal arteriovenous channels. The use of positive end-expiratory pres-sure, while theoretically desirable for prevention of venous air embolism, must therefore be considered with caution.

Veno-Venous Bypass

Fatal hypotension caused by caval clamping during liver transplantation in the experimental animal ne-cessitated the development of shunting techniques to allow maintenance of venous return during the anhepatic phase. These techniques were difficult to apply in man because of the need for heparinization. Early attempts at bypass proved disastrous because of uncontrollable bleeding. The development of heparin-bonded tubing and nonocclusive pumps, which rely on centrifugal force created by a spinning conical device, allowed the safe use of pumped bypass in man without systemic heparinization.[67] Most centers use large-bore Bardic-type cannulas to shunt blood from the femoral and portal veins to the axillary vein at flows of 1.5–4L/minute. Advocates of bypass cite the substantial physiologic advantages it affords during the anhepatic period. These include decompression of the portal, lower caval, and renal venous systems and maintenance of cardiac output, preserving splanchnic, renal, and coronary blood flow. Control of bleeding, particularly when a large vein is torn, is also facilitated. The improved state of perfusion has allowed the anhepatic phase to be extended with little anxiety about renal and cardiac function.[102]

However, evidence that bypass improves results is lacking and a comprehensive evaluation of its complications has yet to be published. A number of units report good results without the use of bypass,[103,104] while others use it selectively for given medical and surgical indications. The most frequently cited account of the clinical use of bypass described a reduction in blood loss, better renal function after operation, and improved 30-day survival compared with historical controls in whom bypass was not used.[67] However, 90-day survival was not improved and blood losses were similar to those reported in patients treated in centers where bypass was not used.[68,104] Cardiovascular stability, advocated as a major advantage of the technique, is not uniform and hypotension on graft reperfusion is more profound than when bypass is not employed.[96–98] Intraoperative deaths caused by cardiac dysfunction have been no more frequent in our series of over 500 adult patients operated on without use of bypass (two patients) than have occurred in other large series during the bypass period, whereas fatal embolic events described in other series have not been seen. A beneficial effect on the incidence of renal failure, which is influenced by important variables other than the use of bypass, has also not been shown.

The most serious hazard of bypass is embolization of air or thrombus. This may occur when the portal cannula is dislodged and aspirates air or when thrombus forms in the bypass tubing during a period of occlusion or low flow. Pulmonary and systemic emboli have been demonstrated in a significant proportion of patients and fatalities have occurred.[61,105] Body temperature decreases during bypass, which in turn may affect coagulation and cardiovascular function. A decline of 0.5–1.5°C per hour of bypass is usual.[83] Local complications occur in a significant number of patients, including nerve injury, hematoma, lymphocoele, and infection.[67] An association between bypass use, which encourages longer anhepatic times and may thereby prolong warm ischemia, and primary nonfunction of the graft has not been investigated. Early graft failure is considerably less frequent in centers in which the technique is not routinely used.[103,104,106]

Thus, although the theoretical benefits of bypass are clear, a beneficial effect on morbidity and mortality remains unproved. It seems reasonable to balance potential benefit against risk, reserving the technique for patients most likely to gain from its use. Indications for veno-venous bypass in Cambridge include previous portocaval shunt, severe portal hypertension, renal or cardiac disease, metabolic acidosis, or vasopressor dependency, and an adverse response to trial clamping of the cava (systolic pressure <80 mmHg in the presence of adequate cardiac filling pressures. A modification of the widely used portofemoroaxillary technique is used, in which two 10FG or a single 20FG cannula are placed percutaneously in the internal jugular vein while 18–22FG Bardic cannulas are placed in the saphenous and mesenteric veins by the surgeon. Bypass flows of 1.5–4 L/minute are obtained, adequate for surgical decompression and circulatory support during an anhepatic period lasting 40–60 minutes.

Respiratory Function

Changes in respiratory function caused by liver disease are described above. Few primary respiratory problems are encountered intraoperatively. Rapid desaturation occurs easily after induction of anesthesia, even with preoxygenation, since functional residual capacity (FRC) is reduced in most of these patients and oxygen consumption increased. FRC decreases further with anesthesia, but appears to increase when the diseased liver is removed. Arterial oxygenation thus tends to improve during the anhepatic phase, although a 25% reduction in oxygen consumption related to removal of the liver may contribute.[108] Revascularization of the liver, by restoring oxygen uptake and reducing FRC, returns arterial oxygenation to preanhepatic values. Systemic and pulmonary vasodilators released from the liver and splanchnic circulation may also influence venous admixture.

Pulmonary edema presents a more important hazard. Overtransfusion occurs easily because of the highly variable rate of blood loss. Plasma oncotic pressure is often reduced and some patients appear to have abnormal vascular permeability, especially after reperfusion and if graft function is poor. Cardiac filling pressures should be observed continuously. Intraoperative atelectasis, pneumothorax, and pulmonary embolism have been described but are rare.

Renal Function

Significant changes in renal function are related to alterations in cardiac output and renal blood flow. Urine flow is diminished during the period of caval clamping as cardiac output is reduced and renal venous pressure acutely raised, although this response is attenuated when veno-venous bypass is used. Renal hypoperfusion is alleviated when caval blood flow is restored, but preexisting renal disease, prolonged hypotension and high transfusion volumes are associated with a high risk of postoperative renal failure. This is compounded by giving Cyclosporin A and aminoglycoside antibiotics intraoperatively and by abdominal tamponade after surgery if bleeding continues. Measures to prevent intraoperative renal damage include the use of a low-dose dopamine infusion (0.5–2 µg/kg/minute), mannitol (0.2 g/kg/h), and intermittent or continuous frusemide (0.1–0.5 mg/kg/h). Dopexamine, a dopaminergic agent with inotropic effects at low dosage, has also been used.[109] Evidence on the value of pharmacologic prophylaxis is conflicting,[110–112] and dopaminergic agents may increase bleeding during dissection by a splanchnic vasodilating action. Oliguria associated with hypotension during or following the anhepatic phase may respond to noradrenaline (0.05–0.5 µg/kg/minute) if systemic vascular resistance remains low.

Maintenance of Body Temperature

Core temperature invariably decreases during liver transplantation. Contributing factors include the poor nutritional state of most patients, the exposure of body surfaces during preparation for surgery, substantial evaporative heat loss from the large area of peritoneum exposed during the operation, the infusion of large volumes of fluids, the use of venovenous bypass,[97] and the placement in the abdomen of a donor liver stored at 2–4°C. Hypothermia impairs coagulation,[113] drug metabolism, renal function, and myocardial contractility and may alter the myocardial response to inotropes. Appropriate protective measures include the use of a warming mattress, humidification and warming of inspired gases, and warming of all infused fluids. Further reduction of heat loss is achieved by wrapping exposed areas in polyethylene or reflective sheeting, particularly important during the period after induction when monitoring and infusion catheters are inserted. Increasing the operating room temperature and using a radiant warmer are also of value during the preparation period, particularly in children.

With these measures core temperature can be usually be kept above 35.5°C until reperfusion of the donor liver, when a further decrease of one degree is usual. A gradual recovery then occurs as the operation is completed, although a subnormal core temperature or marked core-peripheral temperature gradient may persist for several hours.

Conclusion

The perioperative care of the liver transplant patient is complex and places great demands on the anesthetist. A sound understanding of the pathophysiology of hepatic failure and of the many hazards of the surgical procedure is essential. Equally vital are careful and comprehensive monitoring, good communication, and a well-organized team approach. The effort needed is substantial but yields substantial rewards: an increasing number of long-term, healthy survivors and experience that inevitably benefits a much wider group of critically ill surgical patients.

References

1. Zitelli, B.J., Gartner, J.C. Jr, Malatack, J.J. et al. (1987) Pediatric liver transplantation: Patient evaluation and selection, infectious complications and life style after transplantation. *Transplantation Proceedings* XIX: 3309–16.
2. Pennington, J.C. Jr (1989) Quality of life following liver transplantation. *Transplant Proceedings* xxi:3514.

3. Bismuth, H., Castaing, D., Ericzon, et al. (1987) Hepatic transplantation in Europe. *Lancet* ii:674–76.

4. Otte, J.B., de Ville, de Goyet J, de Hemptinne, B. et al. (1987) Liver transplantation in children: Report of two and a half years experience at the University of Louvain Medical School in Brussels. *Transplantation Proceedings* XIX:3289–302.

5. Starzl T.E., Demetris, A.J., and Van Thiel, D. (1989) Liver transplantation. *New England Journal of Medicine* 321:1014–22

6. Lewis, H.A. and Bontempo, F.A. (1985) Orthotopic liver transplantation in patients with hemophilia. *New England Journal of Medicine* 312:1189–1190.

7. Watts, R.W.E., Calne, R.Y., Rolles, K, et al. (1987) Successful treatment of primary hyperoxaluria type I by combined hepatic and renal transplantation. *Lancet* ii:474–75.

8. Casella, J.F., Lewis, J.F., Bontempo, F.A., Zitelli, B.J., Markel, H. and Starzl, T.E. (1988) Successful treatment of protein C deficiency by hepatic transplantation. *Lancet* i:435–37.

9. Neuberger, J. (1987) When should patients be referred for liver transplantation? *British Medical Journal* 295:565–66.

10. Starzl, T.E., Todo, S, Gordon, R. et al. (1987) Liver transplantation in older patients. *New England Journal of Medicine* 316:484–85.

11. Salt, A, Noble-Jamieson, G, Barnes, N.D. et al. (1992) Liver transplantation in 100 children: Cambridge and King's College Hospital series. *British Medical Journal* 304:416–21.

12. Bird, G.L., O'Grady, J.G., Calne, R.Y. and Williams, R. (1990) Liver transplantation in patients with alcoholic cirrhosis: Selection criteria and rates of survival and relapse. *British Medical Journal* 301:15–17.

13. Tizzard, E.J., Pett, S., Pelham, A.M. et al. (1987) Selection and assessment children for liver transplantation. In *Liver Transplantation,* (Calne, R.Y., ed). London: Grune and Stratton, pp. 119–129.

14. Van Thiel, D.H., Schade, R.R., Gavaler, J.S. et al. (1984) Medical aspects of orthotopic liver transplantation. *Hepatology* 4(suppl 1):79S–83S.

15. Hehir, D.J., Jenkins, R.L., Bistrian, B.R. et al. (1985) Nutrition in patients undergoing orthotopic liver transplantation. *Journal of Parenteral and Enteral Nutrition* 9:695–704.

16. Fredell, J., Takyi, Y., Gwenigale, et al. (1987) Fibronectin as a possible adjunct in treatment of severe malnutrition. *Lancet* ii:962.

17. Johnson, P.J., O'Grady, J., Calvey, H. et al. (1987) Nutritional management and assessment. In: *Liver Transplantation,* (Calne, R.Y., ed). London: Grune and Stratton, pp. 103–117.

18. Epstein, M. (1989) Treatment of refractory ascites (editorial). *New England Journal of Medicine* 321:1675–77.

19. Hirsch, I.A., Tomlinson, D.L., Slogoff, S. and Keats, A.S. (1988) The overstated risk of preoperative hypokalemia. *Anesthesia and Analgesia* 67:131–36.

20. Swales, J.D. (1987) Dangers in treating hyponatraemia. *British Medical Journal* 294:261–62.

21. Larner, A.J., Vickers, C.R. et al. (1988) Correction of severe hyponatraemia by continuous arteriovenous haemofiltration before liver transplantation. *British Medical Journal* 297:1514–15.

22. Epstein, M. (1986) The sodium retention of cirrhosis: A reappraisal. *Hepatology* 6:312–15.

23. Wilkinson, S.P. (1987) The hepatorenal syndrome revisited. *Intensive Care Medicine* 13:145–47.

24. Cuervas-Mons, Ve, Millan, I., Gaveler, J., Starzl, T.E. and Van Thiel, D.H. (1986) Prognostic value of preoperatively obtained clinical and laboratory data in predicting survival following orthotopic liver transplantation. *Hepatology* 6:922–27.

25. Adler, M., Gavaler, J.S. et al. (1988) Relationship between diagnosis, preoperative evaluation and prognosis after liver transplantation. *Annals of Surgery* 208: 196–202.

27. Bihari, D., Gimson, A.E.S., Waterson, M. and Williams, R. (1985) Tissue hypoxia during fulminant hepatic failure. *Critical Care Medicine.*

28. Berridge, J.C. and Klinck, J.R. (1989) Cardiovascular instability during hepatic transplantation: predictive value of exercise MUGA scanning. *European Journal of Anaesthesiology and Related Specialties* 1:25.

29. Cutler, B.S. and Leppo, J.A. (1987) Dipyridamole thallium 201 scintigraphy to detect coronary artery disease before abdominal aortic surgery. *Journal of Vascular Surgery* 1:91–100.

30. Miyomato, M. and Kajimoto, T. (1983) Associated anomalies in biliary atresia patients. In: Kasai, M. (ed), *Biliary Atresia and Its Related Disorders.* Amsterdam: Excerpta Medica, ics 627:13–14.

31. Keren, G., Boichis, H. et al. (1983) Pulmonary arteriovenous fistulae in hepatic cirrhosis. *Archives of Diseases of Childhood* 58:302–304.

32. Martin, D. (1986) Haemodynamic monitoring during liver transplantation. In: *Hepatic Transplantation,* (Winter, P.W. and Kang, Y.D. eds). New York: Praeger, pp. 95–102.

33. Eriksson, L.S. (1990) Hypoxaemia in cirrhotic patients. Presentation to Liver Intensive Care Group of Europe, Brussels.

36. Gordon, J.B., Bernstein, M.L., Oski, F.A. and Rogers, M.C. (1987) Hematologic disorders in the pediatric intensive care unit. In: Rogers, M.C. (ed), *Textbook of Pediatric Intensive Care.* Baltimore: Williams and Wilkins: 1181–1121.

37. Editorial. (1987) Platelet transfusion therapy. *Lancet* ii:490–91.

38. Munoz, F.D., Ballas, S.K., Moritz, M.M. et al. (1988) Perioperative management of fulminant and subfulminant hepatic failure with therapeutic plasmapheresis. Presentation to Third International Symposium on Perioperative Care in Liver Transplantation, Pittsburgh.

39. Potter, D., Peachey, T., Eason, J. et al. (1989) Intracranial pressure monitoring during orthotopic liver transplantation for acute liver failure. *Transplant Proceedings* xxi:3528.

40. Tuman, K.J., Spiess, B.D. et al. (1988) Effects of intraoperative arteriovenous hemofiltration during orthotopic liver transplantation. Presentation to Third

International Symposium on Perioperative Care in Liver Transplantation, Pittsburgh.

41. de Hemptinne, B., de Ville, de Goyet, J., Kestens, P.J. and Otte, J.B. (1987) Volume reduction of the liver graft before orthotopic liver transplantation: Report of clinical experience in 11 cases. *Transplantation Proceedings* XIX:3317–22.

42. Amess, J.A.L., Burman, J.F., Rees, G.M. Nancekievill, D.G. and Mollin, D.L. (1978) Megaloblastic haemopoeisis in patients receiving nitrous oxide. *Lancet* ii:339–42.

43. Lappas, D.G., Buckley, M.J., Laver, M.B. et al. (1975) Left ventricular performance and pulmonary circulation following addition of nitrous oxide to morphine during coronary artery surgery. *Anesthesiology* 43:61–69.

44. Lunn, J.F., Stanley, T.H., Eisele, J. et al. (1979) High dose fentanyl anaesthesia for coronary artery surgery: Plasma fentanyl concentrations and influence of nitrous oxide on cardiovascular responses. *Anesthesia and Analgesia* 58:390–95.

45. Stevens, W.C., Cromwell, T.H., Halsey, M.J. et al. (1971) The cardiovascular effects of a new inhalational agent, Forane, in human volunteers at constant carbon dioxide tension. *Anesthesiology* 35:8–16.

46. Dolan, W.M., Stevens, W.C., Eger, E. II et al. (1974) The cardiovascular and respiratory effects of isoflurane-nitrous oxide anaesthesia. *Canadian Anaesthetists' Society Journal* 21:557–68.

47. Seyde, W.C., Ellis, J.E. and Longnecker, D.E. (1986) The addition of nitrous oxide to halothane decreases renal and splanchnic flow and increases cerebral blood flow in rats. *British Journal of Anaesthesia* 58:63.

48. Smith, M.T., Eger, E., II, Stoelting, R.K. et al. (1970) The cardiovascular and sympathomimetic responses to the addition of nitrous oxide to halothane in man. *Anesthesiology* 32:410–21.

49. Eisele, J.H. and Smith, N.T.Y. (1972) Cardiovascular effects of 40% nitrous oxide in man. *Anesthesia and Analgesia* 51:956–61.

50. Mazzoni, G., Koep, L. and Starzl, T.E. (1979) Air embolus in liver transplantation. *Transplant Proceedings* xi:267–68.

51. Borland, L.M., Roule, M. and Cook, D.R. (1985) Anaesthesia for paediatric orthoptic liver transplantation. *Anesthesia and Analgesia* 64:117–-24.

52. Butler, B.D., Leiman, B.C. and Katz, J. (1987) Arterial air embolism of venous origin in dogs: Effect of nitrous oxide in combination with halothane and pentobarbitone. *Canadian Journal of Anaesthesia* 34:570–75.

53. Hursh, D.J., Gelman, S. and Bradley, E.L.J. (1987) Hepatic oxygen supply during halothane or isoflurane anaesthesia in guinea pigs. *Anesthesiology* 67:701–706.

54. Noldge, G, Kopp, K.H., Pelchen, T.H. and Geiger, K. (1989) Intraoperative oxygen supply and tissue oxygen pressure of the liver during volatile anaesthetics. *European Journal of Anaesthesiology and Related Specialties* 1:6.

55. Debaene, B., Goldfarb, G. et al. (1990) Effects of ketamine, halothane, enflurane and isoflurane on systemic and splanchnic hemodynamics in normovolemic and hypovolemic cirrhotic rats. *Anesthesiology* 73:119–24.

56. Ward, S. and Neill, E.A.M. (1983) Pharmacokinetics of atracurium in acute hepatic failure. *British Journal of Anaesthesia* 55:1169–1172.

57. Farman, J.V., Turner, J.M. and Blanloeil, Y. (1986) Atracurium infusion in liver transplantation. *British Journal of Anaesthesia* 58:96s–102s.

58. Spiess, B.D., Tuman, K.J. et al. (1988) Oxygen consumption and mixed venous oxygen saturation monitoring during liver transplantation. Presentation to Third International Symposium on Perioperative Care in Liver Transplantation, Pittsburgh.

59. Luebbe, N., Schaps, D. et al. (1989) Continuous monitoring of mixed venous oxygen saturation during liver transplantation. Presentation to Liver Intensive Care Group of Europe, Hannover.

60. Peachey, T., Eason, J. and Ginsburg, R. (1989) Effects of venovenous bypass on abdominal venous pressures during orthotopic liver transplantation in man. Presentation to Liver Intensive Care Group of Europe, Hannover.

61. Ellis, J., Lichtor, J. et al. (1989) Right heart dysfunction, pulmonary embolism, and paradoxical embolization during liver transplantation: A transesophageal two-dimensional echocardiographic study. *Anesthesia and Analgesia* 68:777–82.

62. Gutierrez, G., Palizas, F. and Doglio, G. (1992) Gastric intramucosal pH as a therapeutic index of tissue oxygenation in critically ill patients. *Lancet* 195–99.

63. Beall, S.N., and Moorhy, S.S. (1989) Jaundice, oximetry and spurious hemoglobin desaturation. *Anesthesia and Analgesia* 68:806–807.

64. Bontempo, F.A. (1987) Monitoring of coagulation during liver transplantation: How much is enough? *Mayo Clinic Proceedings* 62:848–849.

65. Kang, Y.G., Martin, D.J., Marquez, J. et al. (1985) Intraoperative changes in blood coagulation and thromboelastographic monitoring in liver transplantation. *Anesthesia and Analgesia* 64:888–96.

66. Owen, C.A., Rettke, S.R., Bowie, E.J.W. et al. (1987) Hemostatic evaluation of patients undergoing liver transplantation. *Mayo Clinic Proceedings* 62:678–84.

67. Shaw, B.W., Martin, D.J., Marquez, J.M. et al. (1984) Venous bypass in clinical liver transplantation. *Annals of Surgery* 200:524–34.

68. Wall, W.J., Grant, D.R. et al. (1987) Blood transfusion requirements and renal function in patients undergoing liver transplantation without venous bypass. *Transplant Proceedings* xix:17–20.

69. Sassano, J.J. (1986) The rapid infusion system. In *Hepatic transplantation: Anesthetic and Perioperative Management,* (Winter, P.M. and Kang, Y.G., eds). New York: Praeger.

70. Smith, M.F., Thomas, D.G. and Hesford, J.W. (1987) Perioperative support, monitoring and autotransfusion. In *Liver Transplantation,* (Calne, R.Y. ed). London: Grune and Stratton, pp. 179–196.

71. Derrington, M.C. (1985) The current status of blood filtration. *Anaesthesia* 40:334–37.

72. Gravlee, J.P. (1990) Optimal use of blood components. *International Anesthesiology Clinics* 28:216–23.

73. Counts, R.B., Haisch, C., Simon, T.L. et al. (1979) Haemostasis in massively transfused trauma patients. *Annals of Surgery* 190:91–99.

74. Harke, H. and Rahman, S. (1980) Haemostatic disorders in massive transfusion. *Bibliography of Haematology* 46:179–186.

75. Nilsson, L., Hedner, U., Nilsson, I.M. et al. (1983) Shelf life of bank blood and stored plasma with special reference to coagulation factors. *Transfusion* 23:377–81.

76. Harper, P., Luddington, R., Jennings, I., Seaman, M. and Carrell, R. (1989) Coagulation changes following hepatic reperfusion during liver transplantation. *European Journal of Anaesthesiology and Related Specialties* 1:20.

77. Neuhaus, P., Bechstein, W.O., Lefebre, B. et al. (1989) Effect of aprotinin on intraopertive bleeding and fibrinolysis in liver transplantation. *Lancet* ii:924–25.

78. Mallett, S.V., Cox, D., Burroughs, A.K. and Rolles, K. (1990) Aprotinin and reduction of blood loss and transfusion requirements in orthotopic liver transplantation. *Lancet* ii:886–887.

79. Grosse, H., Lobbes, W., Kobusch, K. et al. (1990) Is accelerated fibrinolysis during liver transplantation an indication for aprotinin? *European Journal of Anaesthesiology and Related Specialties* 2:8.

80. Kang, Y.G., Lewis, J.H., Navaglund, M.V. et al. (1987) Epsilon-aminocaproic acid for treatment of fibrinolysis during liver transplantation. *Anesthesiology* 66:766–73.

81. Collins, J.A. (1987) Recent developments in the area of massive transfusion. *World Journal of Surgery* 11:75–81.

82. Myllyla, G. (1988) New transfusion practice and haemostasis. *Acta Anaesthesiologica Scandinavica* 32 suppl 89:76–80.

83. Paulsen, A.W., Whitten, C.W. et al. (1989) Considerations for anesthetic management during veno-venous bypass in adult hepatic transplantation. *Anesthesia and Analgesia* 68:489–96.

84. Dyer, P.M., Blanloeil, Y.G. and Farman, J.V. (1987) Liver transplantation in children. Blood transfusion and metabolic disorders. *Annales Francaises d'Anaesthesie et Reanimation* 6:163–68.

85. Laureno, R. and Karp, B.I. (1988) Pontine and extrapontine myelinolysis following rapid correction of hyponatraemia. *Lancet* ii:1439–41.

86. Graf, H. and Arieff, A.I. (1986) Sodium bicarbonate in the therapy of organic acidosis. *Intensive Care Medicine* 12:285–88.

87. Bishop, R.L. and Weisfeldt, M.L. (1976) Sodium bicarbonate administration during cardiac arrest. Effect on arterial pH, pCO_2 and osmolality. *Journal of the American Medical Association* 235:506.

88. Mattar, J.A., Weil, M.H., Shubin, H. et al. (1974) Cardiac arrest in the critically ill. II: Hyperosmolal states following cardiac arrest. *American Journal of Medicine* 56:162.

89. Graf, H., Leach, W. and Arieff, A.I. (1985) Metabolic effects of sodium bicarbonate in hypoxic lactic acidosis in dogs. *American Journal of Physiology* 249:F630.

90. Makisalo, H.J., Soini, H.O. and Nordin, A.J. (1989) Effects of bicarbonate therapy on tissue oxygenation during resuscitation from hemorrhagic shock. *Critical Care Medicine* 17:1170–74.

91. Bersin, R., Chatterjee, K. and Arieff, A.I. (1986) Metabolic and systemic effects of bicarbonate in hypoxic patients with heart failure. *Kidney International* 29:180.

92. Driscoll, D.F., Bistrian, B.R., Jenkins, R.L. et al. (1987) Development of metabolic alkalosis after massive transfusion during orthotopic liver transplantation. *Critical Care Medicine* 15:905–908.

93. Carmichael, F.J., Lindop, M.J. and Farman, J.V. (1985) Anaesthesia for hepatic transplantation: Cardiovascular and metabolic alterations and their management. *Anesthesia and Analgesia* 64:108–16.

94. Marquez, J.M. Jr and Martin, D. (1986) Anaesthesia for liver transplantation. In: *Hepatic Transplantation* (Winter, P.W. and Kang, Y.D., eds). New York: Praeger, pp. 44–57.

95. Paulsen, A.W., Valek, T.R. et al. (1989) Determination of an adequate flush volume for removal of preservation fluid prior to revascularisation of donor liver. *Transplant Proceedings* xxi:2349–50.

96. Van Obbergh, L.J., Carlier, M. et al. (1988) Haemodynamic variations in patients with veno-venous bypass. Presentation to Liver Intensive Care Group of Europe, Cambridge.

97. Aggarwal, S., Kang, Y., Freeman, J.A. et al. (1987) Postreperfusion syndrome: Cardiovascular collapse following hepatic reperfusion during liver transplantation. *Transplant Proceedings* xix (suppl. 3):54–55.

98. Estrin, J.A. and Bellani, K.G. (1988) Is there a reperfusion syndrome? Presentation to Third International Symposium on Perioperative Care in Liver Transplantation, Pittsburgh.

99. Martin, D.J., Marquez, J.M., Kang, Y.D. et al. (1984) Liver transplantation: Hemodynamic and electrolyte changes seen immediately following revascularisation. *Anesthesia and Analgesia* 63:246(S).

100. Paulsen, A.W., Valek, T.R. et al. (1989) Effects of atropine pre-treatment on the revascularisation syndrome. *Transplant Proceedings* xxi:2341–42.

101. Lai, F.O. and Klinck, J.R. (1990) Influence of unclamping sequence of blood pressure during graft reperfusion in liver transplantation. Presentation to Liver Intensive Care Group of Europe, Brussels 1990.

102. Shaw, B.W. (1987) Some further notes on venous bypass for orthotopic transplantation of the liver. *Transplant Proceedings* xix (suppl. 3):13–16.

103. Wall, W.J., Grant, D.R., Duff, J.H. et al. (1987) Liver transplantation without venous bypass. *Transplantation* 43:56–61.

104. Stock, P.G., Payne, W.D. et al. (1989) Rapid infusion technique as a safe alternative to veno-venous bypass in orthotopic liver transplantation. *Transplant Proceedings* xxi:2322–25.

105. Plevak, D.J., Akasmit, A.J. et al. (1988) Cerebrovascular complications following liver transplantation. *Transplant Proceedings* xxi:3528.

106. Busuttil, R.W., Colonna, J.O. II et al. (1987) The first 100 liver transplants at UCLA. *Annals of Surgery* 206:387–402.

107. Friend, P.J., Lim, S. et al. (1989) Liver transplantation in the Cambridge/King's College Hospital series— the first 400 patients. *Transplant Proceedings* xxi:2397–98.

108. Burchett, K.R., Smith, M.F. and Park, G.R. (1990) Changes in alveolar-arterial oxygen partial pressure difference during orthotopic liver transplantation. *British Journal of Anaesthesia* 64:42–44.

109. Burns, A.M., Gray, P.A., Bodenham, A.R. and Park, G.R. (1990) Dopexamine: Studies in the general intensive care unit and after liver transplantation. *Journal of Autonomic Physiology* 10 (suppl 1):S109–14.

110. Swygert, T.H., Roberts, L.C., Valek, T.R. et al. (1991) Effect of intraoperative low-dose dopamine on renal function in liver transplant recipients. *Anesthesiology* 75:571–576.

111. Polson, R.J., Park, G.R., Lindop, M.J. et al. (1987) The prevention of renal impairment in patients undergoing orthotopic liver grafting by infusion of low dose dopamine. *Anesthesia* 42:15–19.

112. Salem, M.G., Crooke, J.W., McLoughlin, G.A. et al. (1988) The effect of dopamine on renal function during aortic cross clamping. *Annals of the Royal College of Surgeons of England* 70:9–12.

113. Valeri, R.C., Cassidy, G. et al. (1987) Hypothermia-induced reversible platelet dysfunction. *Annals of Surgery* 205:175–81.

Chapter 10

Coagulation in Liver Disease and Massive Blood Transfusion

Yoogoo Kang

The liver plays a central role in hemostasis by producing coagulation factors and inhibitors and by clearing activated factors. Therefore, patients with liver and biliary tract disease frequently have imbalances between activators and inhibitors and between coagulation and fibrinolysis, causing a tendency to bleed. Changes in the coagulation system vary with the type of disease. For example, patients with neoplasms may have relatively normal coagulation. Patients with cholestatic liver disease may have a vitamin K–related factor deficiency, whereas patients with severe hepatocellular damage have significant generalized coagulopathy. This chapter describes the changes in coagulation that occur in patients with liver and biliary tract disease, the methods of monitoring coagulation and treating coagulopathies, and the modes and complications of blood transfusion.

Coagulation in Patients with Liver Disease

Vitamin K Deficiency-Related Coagulopathy

Hepatic synthesis of coagulation factors II, VII, IX, and X depends on vitamin K, a cofactor for post-translational carboxylation.[1] Vitamin K, a lipid-soluble vitamin, is either obtained directly from dietary intake or produced from a precursor by the action of intestinal flora. Intestinal absorption of vitamin K requires bile salts. Deficiencies of vitamin K–related coagulation factors result from a poor diet, inadequate production or excretion of bile salts, or suppression of normal intestinal flora by antibiotics. Drugs such as cholestyramine resin bind to bile salts and thus inhibit the absorption of vitamin K.[2]

Vitamin K levels can be either normal or increased for several days after acute obstruction of the biliary tract. Persistent cholestatic disease causes decreased vitamin K levels, associated with a prolonged prothrombin time (PT) and tendency to bleed. In patients with severe hepatocellular disease, the administration of vitamin K_1 is ineffective because of either an inadequate amount of coagulation factor precursors or incomplete carboxylation.[3]

Decreased Hepatic Synthesis of Coagulation Factors

The liver is the major site for production of fibrinogen; prothrombin; prekallikrein; high-molecular-weight kininogen; factors V, VII, IX, X, XI, XII, and XIII; plasminogen; alpha-2-antiplasmin; and antithrombin III. Factor VIII is produced by both the liver and the vascular endothelium.

Fibrinogen

Fibrinogen is produced by the hepatocytes.[4] Levels of fibrinogen can be normal or increased in patients with advanced hepatocellular,[5] cholestatic,[6] and neoplastic diseases.[7] Hypofibrinogenemia can develop during fulminant hepatitis from inadequate hepatic synthesis, disseminated intravascular coagulation (DIC), fibrinogenolysis, and a dilutional effect.[8] Dysfibrinogenemia has been seen in cirrhotic patients. This appears to be related to the abnormal polymerization of fibrin caused by incorporation of excess amounts of sialic acid into the molecule,[9] as evidenced by the reduction of thrombin time after the removal of sialic acid from the fibrinogen. This abnormal fibrinogen delays the aggregation of fibrin monomers, but its clinical significance is unknown.

Factor V (Proaccelerin)

Factor V is synthesized in the reticuloendothelial cells of the liver.[10] Its level is reduced in patients with hepatocellular disease but can be normal or increased in those with cholestatic or neoplastic disease. A low factor V level is caused by either decreased hepatic synthesis, DIC, or destruction by plasmin. A deficiency of factor V and the vitamin K–dependent factors prolongs PT and increases the bleeding tendency. In hepatocellular disease, hepatic synthesis of factor V is decreased; thus, an assay of factor V (half-life, 5 hours) is considered to be a highly sensitive indicator of hepatocellular damage.

Surface-Mediated Clotting Factors

All factors initiating coagulation, such as Hageman factor, plasma prekallikrein (Fletcher factor), high-molecular-weight kininogen, and plasma thromboplastin precursors (plasma thromboplastin antecedent factor, factor XI), are produced by the liver. The level of Hageman factor is generally high in patients with cholestatic or neoplastic disease. A low level of prekallikrein is associated with initial activation and subsequent inactivation by the Hageman factor.[11] The clinical significance of a deficiency of these factors is unclear.

Factor VIII

Factor VIII is a complex of factors VIII R:Ag, VIII R:vW, and VIII:C. Factors VIII R:Ag and VIII R:vW, produced by the vascular endothelium, interact with platelets and vascular walls, whereas factor VIII:C, produced by the liver, participates in the coagulation cascade.[12] Many patients with liver cirrhosis and neoplasms have supernormal levels of factor VIII.[13] This increase may be associated with the stress response, an increased vascular surface, or decreased catabolism.[14] Increased levels of factor VIII have an unknown clinical significance.

Factor XIII

Factor XIII is produced by the liver and is diminished in patients with hepatocellular disease.[15] It promotes cross-linkage between fibrin monomers and linkage between fibrin and alpha-2-plasmin inhibitor, both of which decrease susceptibility to fibrinolysis.

Inhibitors of Coagulation and Fibrinolysis

Inhibitors affect the hemostatic process by inhibiting either coagulation (antithrombin III) or fibrinolysis (alpha-2-antiplasmin and alpha-2-macroglobulin). Antithrombin III is synthesized by the liver, and its level is reduced in those with liver disease.[16] Alpha-2-antiplasmin, a major plasmin inhibitor, is low in cirrhotic patients.[17] Alpha-2-macroglobulin, produced by the macrophages, inhibits thrombin and plasmin,[18] and its level is somewhat increased in hepatocellular disease.[19] Normal or increased levels of alpha-1-antitrypsin, a plasma protease inhibitor that is produced in both the liver and monocytes, are found in patients with liver disease.

Platelets

Thrombocytopenia (platelet count <100,000/mm³) occurs in 30% of people with cirrhosis and in 70% of patients with advanced liver disease.[20] Bone marrow aspirates contain a normal or increased number of megakaryocytes, indicative of normal platelet production, but the life span of the platelets appears to be reduced.[21] Thrombocytopenia is caused primarily by splenomegaly associated with portal hypertension. About 30% of platelets are trapped in the spleen under normal circumstances, and the enlarged spleen may sequester a much larger fraction of platelets, although no relation has been found between the size of the spleen and the platelet count. Splenectomy is rarely indicated for thrombocytopenia. Creation of a portacaval shunt without splenectomy increases platelet count in one-third of patients.[22] In patients with acute viral or chemical hepatitis, thrombocytopenia may be caused by intravascular coagulation or the presence of autoantibodies against platelets.

Although platelets play a major role in hemostasis, platelet count does not correlate with bleeding time in many patients,[23] possibly because of defective platelet function.[24,25] Platelet dysfunction causes diminished clot retraction; impaired aggregation of platelets by adenosine diphosphate, collagen, or thrombin; and reduced agglutination after the administration of ristocetin. This impaired aggregation of platelets appears to be related to either the preponderance of small hypofunctional platelets[26] or a deficiency of folic acid. Abnormal platelet function in patients with severe hepatorenal syndrome is caused by dialyzable or nondialyzable plasma factors. Thrombocytosis occasionally occurs, and its cause is unclear.

Abnormal Fibrinolytic Activity

Accelerated fibrinolysis, or the digestion of fibrin by plasmin, is frequently observed in patients with cirrhosis.[27] It may result from the delayed removal of circulating plasminogen activator or from decreased synthesis of fibrinolysis inhibitors. Plasminogen is released from vascular endothelium or monocytes in response to stress or vasoactive substances. It is activated to form plasmin by kallikrein, tissue plasminogen activator, or Hageman factor. Plasmin, in turn, stimulates fibrinolysis and breaks down fibrinogen, factor V, and factor VIII. The products of fibrinolysis, fibrin degradation products (FDP), are increased in patients with liver disease, and they inhibit the formation of thrombin and the polymerization of fibrin monomers. Plasminogen titers are often decreased in cirrhotic patients,[28] however, because of decreased hepatic synthesis or increased consumption during intravascular coagulation. The levels of inhibitors, such as alpha-2-antiplasmin and histidine-rich glycoprotein, are also decreased in patients with liver disease. The reason for the existence of fibrinolysis in the presence of decreased levels of plasminogen inhibitors is unclear. The clinical importance of fibrinolysis also is

uncertain, but in patients who undergo surgery, generalized bleeding associated with fibrinolysis appears to be clinically significant.

Disseminated Intravascular Coagulation

The frequent occurrence of DIC in patients with chronic liver disease has been suggested.[29] Whether this abnormal coagulation state is actually due to DIC, or whether the changes can be explained on the basis of liver disease per se or primary fibrinolysis remains unsolved. Evidence for the existence of DIC as a separate entity is based on the following observations. The coagulation profile of patients with liver disease is similar to that of patients with DIC: thrombocytopenia, low levels of prothrombin and plasminogen, shorter half-life of fibrinogen, and presence of FDP.[30] In addition, the abnormal coagulation state does not improve with the administration of either fresh frozen plasma (FFP) or antifibrinolytic agents, but it is reversed by heparin.[31] The suggested etiology of DIC includes the release of necrotic hepatocytes or intestinal endotoxin, defective hepatic clearance of activated clotting factors, and decreased titers of coagulation inhibitors.[32]

This abnormal coagulation state may be attributable to liver disease, however. Generally, levels of fibrinogen and factor VIII are supernormal in patients with chronic liver disease, whereas they are low in patients with DIC. When hypofibrinogenemia occurs in patients with liver disease, it may be associated with an increased loss of fibrinogen by extravasation, transudation, exudation, or bleeding; rapid destruction of fibrinogen by plasmin and other proteases; or rapid clearance of fibrinogen due to altered flow characteristics or abnormal molecular structure. Thrombocytopenia may be associated with hypersplenism, increased FDP with reabsorption of extravascular fibrins or decreased hepatic clearance of FDP, shortened euglobulin lysis time with inadequate clearance of plasminogen activators, or a lower level of antithrombin III with decreased hepatic synthesis. Although FDP levels may be positive in patients with liver disease, differential measurements of the degradation products of fibrinogen and fibrin have not been performed in most studies. Furthermore, the administration of heparin alone or heparin with FFP improved coagulation defects in some patients,[33] but the treatment did not improve the outcome of patients with toxic hepatic necrosis.[34] Microemboli in major organs, a characteristic finding in patients with DIC, are rarely seen at autopsy in patients with acute or chronic liver disease.[35] Therefore, DIC appears to play a relatively minor role, if any, in patients with liver disease.

Coagulation in Various Disease States

Acute Hepatitis

The coagulation profile is relatively normal in most patients with acute hepatitis, whereas marked abnormalities develop in patients with subacute hepatitis. Factor VII level is reduced in the early stage of hepatitis, and its recovery to normal is associated with the recovery of hepatic function. Severe fulminant hepatitis is often associated with marked abnormalities, consisting of generalized decreases in coagulation factor levels, including fibrinogen and factor VIII. DIC may occur in fulminant hepatitis resulting from the release of necrotic hepatic tissues or intestinal toxins, impaired removal of activated coagulation factors, and decreased synthesis of antithrombin III. Coagulation abnormalities described above also occur in chronic hepatocellular disease.

Cholestatic Disease

Coagulation disturbances are not as severe in patients with cholestatic disease as in those with hepatocellular diseases, although similar changes may be seen in end-stage cholestatic liver disease. Bilirubin glucuronides exert an antithrombin action and could contribute to the hemostatic defect.

Neoplasms

The coagulation profile may be normal in patients with uncomplicated neoplasms. Levels of fibrinogen and factors V and VIII may increase, however, and fibrinolytic activity may be impaired by a nonspecific increase of glycoproteins in response to the neoplasm. Necrosis of a tumor may trigger DIC.

Other Diseases

Patients with congenital metabolic disorders such as Dubin-Johnson syndrome, Gilbert's syndrome, and Rotor syndrome have low titers of factor VII.

When the level decreases to less than 20% of the normal value, a tendency to bleed is likely.[36,37] Patients with familial antithrombin deficiency, a rare autosomal-dominant genetic disease, are prone to developing thromboembolism. They are resistant to heparin, and administration of FFP may increase the antithrombin III level.

Laboratory Tests and Monitoring

Coagulation Tests

A number of tests are performed to evaluate the coagulation system or to assess the prognosis of the patient with liver disease. Generally, a simple coagulation profile is determined to assess coagulation in surgical patients. It includes bleeding time, PT, activated partial thromboplastin time (aPTT), and platelet count. The bleeding time reflects the interaction of the platelet with the wall of the blood vessel and the subsequent formation of a hemostatic plug. It is prolonged when the function of platelets, von Willebrand's factor, fibrinogen, factor V, or the vessel wall is defective. PT is a measure of coagulation activity initiated by the extrinsic system, particularly the level of factor VII. It is also prolonged when factors VIII, IX, XI, and XIII, prekallikrein, and kininogen are deficient. aPTT represents the intrinsic coagulation system and is prolonged when there is a generalized decrease in coagulation factors and vitamin K deficiency. Platelet count is one of the most important coagulation tests, because thrombocytopenia frequently causes a tendency to bleed. Additional information is obtained by more specific tests.

Platelet function tests determine the adhesion and aggregation of platelets, the release reaction, and coagulant activity. The tests are influenced by many variables, however, and results of in vitro tests may not reflect platelet function in vivo. Thrombin time frequently is prolonged in patients with hypofibrinogenemia, dysfibrinogenemia, or an increased level of FDP. Results of both thrombin time and reptilase time differentiate a heparin effect from acquired dysfibrinogenemia associated with liver disease; both are increased with dysfibrinogenemia, whereas only thrombin time is increased by heparin. Measurement of degradation products of fibrin and fibrinogen aids in the differential diagnosis of primary and secondary fibrinolysis; degradation products of fibrinogen (A, B, C, or H) are frequently seen in primary fibrinolysis and those of fibrin (D dimer) in DIC.

Attempts have been made to correlate coagulation test results with clinical coagulation states. In general, blood coagulability cannot be predicted solely on the basis of the coagulation test results. Relations between prothrombin level and clinical bleeding[38] and between gastrointestinal bleeding and abnormal fibrin polymerization[39] have been reported. The level of factor VII has no prognostic value in fulminant hepatitis,[40] and determinations of factor XIII and plasminogen appear to have a limited clinical prognostic value.[41] On the other hand, patients with a low coagulation abnormality score appear to require more transfused blood during liver transplantation.[42]

Thrombelastographic Coagulation Monitoring

Because of the severe coagulopathy that occurs in patients with liver disease, particularly perioperatively, continual monitoring of coagulation is essential. Conventional coagulation tests have been used to assess the hemostatic function, but they have several drawbacks for clinical use. PT and aPTT are sensitive tests for abnormal hepatic synthetic function and the effectiveness of anticoagulation therapy. PT and aPTT are prolonged in most patients with liver disease, and their normalization may be difficult. Platelet count does not provide qualitative information, and platelet function tests are unreliable in patients with thrombocytopenia (platelet count $< 50,000/mm^3$). Euglobulin lysis time measures only plasminogen activity, and not antiplasmin activity. The presence of FDP is not uncommon during major surgery and results from localized intravascular coagulation and reabsorption of extravascular FDP. The coagulation profile must be performed in the laboratory, results may not be available readily, and the tests ignore cellular and humoral effects on coagulation.

Thrombelastography (TEG) has proved to be an extremely valuable monitoring technique for guiding replacement and pharmacologic therapy during liver transplantation.[20,43] TEG monitors the coagulability of whole blood, including coagulation and fibrinolysis, and provides clinically useful information within 30 minutes.[44] The apparatus consists of a small cup containing 0.36 mL of whole blood and a freely suspended pin that is lowered into a blood specimen.[45] The cup is kept at 37°C and swivels at a 4.5-degree angle. When fibrin strands adhere to the surface of the cup and pin, the cup and pin are coupled, and thus the shear elasticity of the blood clot is recorded on thermal paper.

Recording generally begins 4 minutes after blood sampling. The variables measured by TEG are shown in Figure 10-1. Reaction time (r) is the interval from the start of recording to an amplitude of 2 mm. It is the time taken to generate initial fibrin strands, a function of the intrinsic coagulation system. Maximum amplitude (MA), the largest amplitude reached, is a function of platelets primarily and fibrinogen secondarily. Clot formation rate (alpha), the speed with which a solid clot forms, is a function of fibrinogen primarily and platelets secondarily. The time interval between maximum amplitude and subsequent zero amplitude is the whole blood clot lysis time (F), which is a function of fibrinolysis. A_{60} is the amplitude 60 minutes after maximum amplitude, and fibrinolysis is indicated when the fibrinolysis index ($A_{60}/MA \cdot 100$) is less than 80%.

Typical TEG patterns in normal and diseased states are shown in Figure 10-2. Hemophilia and a heparin effect are characterized by a prolonged reaction time and a slow clot formation rate, with normal maximum amplitude. Thrombocytopenia is represented by a small amplitude and prolonged reaction time, owing to the insufficient platelet effects on the coagulation cascade. Fibrinolysis is seen as a rapid decrease in amplitude after maximum amplitude. A prolonged reaction time and decreased maximum amplitude are also seen, resulting from the net decrease in the number of fibrin strands formed. A hypercoagulable state is shown as a very short reaction time, an accelerated clot-formation rate, and a large maximum amplitude. TEG also measures the effects of physiologic changes such as hypothermia and hypocalcemia on coagulation; ionized hypocalcemia (< 0.6 mmol/L) and hypothermia ($< 34°C$) are associated with poor clot formation.[46]

TEG is an excellent clinical technique for monitoring the functional status of the coagulation cascade, fibrinogen, and platelets, although it is not a diagnostic tool that assesses specific abnormalities in coagulation. The use of TEG to guide replacement therapy and pharmacologic therapy during liver transplantation has been well documented.[20,47,48] Briefly, 2 units of FFP are transfused when reaction time is greater than 15 minutes, 10 units of platelets when maximum amplitude is less

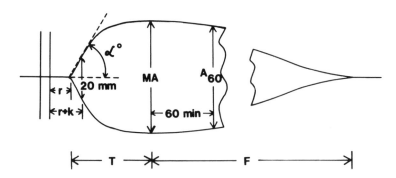

Figure 10-1. Variables and normal values measured by thrombelastography. From Kang, Y.G., Martin, D.J., Marquez, J. et al. Intraoperative changes in blood coagulation and thrombelastographic monitoring in liver transplantation. Anesthesia and Analgesia 64:888–96 (1985) by the permission of the International Anesthesia Research Society.

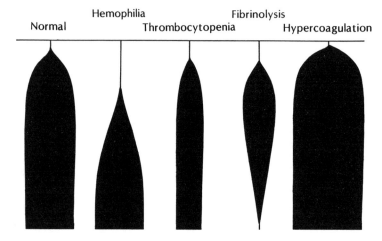

Figure 10-2. TEG patterns of normal and disease states. From Kang, Y.G. (1986) Monitoring and treatment of coagulation. In *Hepatic Transplantation: Anesthetic and Perioperative Management,* edited by P.M. Winter and Y.G. Kang, pp. 151–73. New York: Praeger. By permission of the publisher.

than 40 mm, and 6 units of cryoprecipitate when alpha angle is less than 40°. In cases of severe fibrinolysis (F < 60 min), a single dose (1 g) of epsilon-aminocaproic acid has been effective, without complication, during liver transplantation.

Treatment of Coagulopathy

The therapeutic approach to a coagulopathy should be tailored to the specific clinical circumstances, such as the degree of coagulation defects and the nature or location of bleeding. Treatment of coagulation includes administration of vitamin K, FFP, prothrombin complex, platelets, cryoprecipitate, protamine sulfate, and antifibrinolytic agents and plasmapheresis.

Vitamin K

For a mild form of vitamin K deficiency, oral administration of vitamin K and bile salts is a sufficient treatment. Intramuscular or intravenous ad-

ministration of vitamin K_1 (5 mg/day) is effective in correcting PT within 24–48 hours. Repeated administration of vitamin K_1 and coagulation factors is usually adequate to remedy the tendency to bleed in surgical patients with obstructive jaundice. Vitamin K is ineffective in patients with severe hepatocellular disease, but it may be used in an attempt to evaluate the effectiveness of vitamin K therapy in these patients (10 mg/day for 3 days). When surgery is indicated, additional FFP may be given to lessen the factor deficiency. The administration of concentrated vitamin K–dependent factors has been suggested, but it is only partially successful, may transmit hepatitis, and may cause thrombotic complications.[3]

Fresh Frozen Plasma

FFP is the most suitable agent for the correction of multiple coagulation defects in patients with liver disease because it contains all coagulation factors and inhibitors present in the blood. However, FFP improves coagulation only temporarily in patients with hemorrhagic symptoms, and the large volume required may cause fluid overloading.

Prothrombin Complex

Prothrombin complex is available commercially and contains high concentrations of factors II, VII, IX, and X. It has been used successfully in patients undergoing liver biopsy.[49,50] Its complications, however, are transmission of blood-borne disease, risk of a thromboembolic episode such as a deep venous thrombosis or a pulmonary embolism, and potential DIC. The embolic phenomenon appears to be associated with inadequate clearance of activated coagulation factors in the concentrate or low levels of antithrombin III.[51,52] Its incidence was reported to be lower when FFP (6–8 mL/kg) containing antithrombin III was administered concomitantly.[49] Therefore, this regimen is reserved for those who require surgery and do not respond to any other form of therapy. Also, patients receiving such therapy should be observed closely to detect any signs of excessive activation of coagulation.

Platelets

Platelet transfusion is required for severe thrombocytopenia. Platelet transfusion is only temporarily effective in patients with liver disease, however, because transfused platelets are removed rapidly from the circulation by the spleen and liver. Clinically, a tendency to bleed is not seen when the platelet count is greater than 100,000/mm³, but satisfactory hemostasis can be obtained with lesser platelet counts (> 50,000/mm³), if platelet function is normal. Platelets express class I HLA antigens, and specific alloimmunization to these antigens may cause refractoriness to platelet transfusion[53] as seen in highly sensitized patients, who required two times more platelet transfusion during liver transplantation.[54] These patients may benefit from transfusion of type-specific platelets.

Cryoprecipitate

Cryoprecipitate contains fibrinogen and factors VIII and XIII. Because of a high level of factor VIII

in patients with liver disease, transfusion of cryoprecipitate is indicated when hypofibrinogenemia occurs. One unit of cryoprecipitate contains 300 mg of fibrinogen. Transfusion of one unit of cryoprecipitate increases the fibrinogen level about 10 mg/dL in a patient weighing 60 kg. The half-life of the fibrinogen is about 3–4 days, and repeated transfusion of cryoprecipitate is necessary to supplement the loss.

Anticoagulation Therapy

Anticoagulation therapy is used rarely in patients with hepatocellular disease. When it is indicated, careful titration is required because the response to the oral anticoagulants is unpredictable. Heparin can cause thrombocytopenia, and its effect may be exaggerated in the presence of thrombocytopenia. Therefore, the clinical use of heparin is not recommended, although a subcutaneous injection of a small dose appears to be acceptable.[55] The role of heparin in patients with liver disease is controversial.

Antifibrinolytic Agents

Antifibrinolytic agents stabilize fragile hemostatic plugs in localized bleeding, such as a gastric mucosal ulcer or bleeding esophageal varices. In addition, these agents may decrease the bleeding tendency in patients without signs of fibrinolysis, although epsilon-aminocaproic acid is ineffective in improving coagulopathy in patients with liver disease.[56] During liver transplantation, trans-p-aminomethyl-cyclohexanecarboxylic acid has been used without documentable complication, and epsilon-aminocaproic acid has proved to be very effective in treating fibrinolysis without causing thrombotic complications.[43]

Treatment of Disseminated Intravascular Coagulation

The treatment of DIC is controversial, mainly because of difficulty in diagnosis and its complex clinical picture. Transfusion of vitamin K–dependent factors has been shown to augment DIC.[57] Cryoprecipitate can be given to increase the fibrinogen level, but it may further promote coagulation. The use of heparin with additional administration of antithrombin III-containing FFP appears to be effective.[33] However, heparin is not recommended unless a definite diagnosis has been made because it can exaggerate bleeding. Generally, replacement therapy using FFP and platelets, with or without the judicious use of heparin (< 5,000 units), is accepted by most clinicians while the underlying disease is being treated.

Plasmapheresis

For the severe coagulopathy that occurs in patients with acute fulminant hepatitis, plasmapheresis in combination with replacement therapy may improve the coagulation state and decrease hepatic encephalopathy by removing filterable humoral elements and coagulation inhibitors. Plasmapheresis of 36.8 mL/kg of blood reportedly has shortened PT from 28.3 to 17.7 seconds and aPTT from 64.8 to 43.3 seconds in patients awaiting liver transplantation.[58]

Blood Transfusion

In addition to severe coagulopathy, cirrhotic patients invariably have hypochromic microcytic or macrocytic anemia (hemoglobin < 10 g/dL) from malabsorption of iron and folic acid, frequent variceal bleeding, and hypersplenism. The reduction in red blood cell survival results from changes in lipid metabolism. Also, the intravascular volume frequently becomes depleted from continuous formation of ascites and diuretic therapy, although blood volume is increased by 10–20% of the normal value. Therefore, most patients receive blood transfusions to restore oxygen-carrying capacity, coagulation, and intravascular blood volume, particularly when they undergo surgery. This section describes modes and complications of massive blood transfusion in patients with acute variceal bleeding or those undergoing major operations.

Blood Component Therapy

Hematocrit is maintained at 26–28% to optimize circulatory rheology and reduce the loss of red blood cells. The volume of blood transfusion is guided by monitoring hemodynamic variables and urine output because blood loss is very difficult to estimate. Hemodynamic monitoring with the use of a pulmonary artery catheter is essential, and monitoring mixed venous hemoglobin oxygen saturation is helpful in estimating preload, assuming that oxygen-carrying capacity, myocardial contractility, and oxygen consumption are relatively constant. The administration of a coagulation factor-rich solution (FFP or fresh whole blood) is required to maintain blood coagulability, and colloid solution (albumin) may be given as well to maintain oncotic pressure. Loss of free water to the interstitial space is corrected by the administration of a balanced salt solution. A fluid mixture of 200 mL of red blood cells, 300 mL of FFP and 250 mL of Plasma-Lyte A meets these criteria and has been used successfully during liver transplantation.[20] A calcium- and glucose-free isotonic electrolyte solution (Plasma-Lyte) is chosen to avoid both clot formation in the fluid mixture and hyperglycemia. This fluid mixture yields a hematocrit of 26–28% and coagulation factors greater than 30% of the normal value, except for factor V (10%), which are adequate for hemostasis. Levels of electrolytes in the mixture are relatively normal, except for a low ionized calcium level and a high potassium level. Administration of this fluid mixture maintains adequate intravascular volume without postoperative weight gain.

Additional FFP, platelets, and cryoprecipitate may be given according to TEG monitoring, as described earlier, because dilutional coagulopathy is a common complication during massive blood transfusion. When TEG is unavailable, a simplified coagulation profile is used for guidance: platelet count > 50,000/mm³, fibrinogen > 100 mg/dL, and PT and aPTT less than two times the control value.

Transfusion Systems

Generally, a pressurized blood transfusion device with a blood-warming element is available for massive blood transfusion. However, a rapid-infusion system (Haemonetics, Braintree, MA) has been very effective[59] for the massive transfusions common during hepatic resection or liver transplantation (up to 500 mL/min or 300 units of red blood cells in 12 hours). The system consists of a reservoir, a heat exchanger, a roller pump, blood filters, and air detectors; it provides rapid, controllable delivery of prewarmed and premixed blood. Four large spikes rapidly transfer blood and fluids to a cardiotomy reservoir, where they are mixed. The cardiotomy reservoir (2.5 L capacity) is lined with a 170-micron filter and is connected to a heat exchanger that can increase blood temperature from 0–4°C to greater than 33°C in one pass. A roller pump delivers blood at a rate of up to 1.5 L/minute with a line pressure of less than 300 mmHg when two large-bore tubings are connected to two 8.5-French catheters. The transfusion rate can be adjusted according to clinical need: a continuous infusion mode with a variable rate, or a 100 mL or 500 mL bolus fluid challenge mode with a speed of 400 mL/minute. A micropore filter (40 micron), a line pressure sensor, two air detectors, and a fluid level sensor are installed in the circuit to prevent the transfusion of aggregates, overpressurization, and air embolism. Overtransfusion and air emboli are possible, although unlikely to occur because of the fluid level sensor and two air sensors.

Autotransfusion

An autotransfusion system has been used during liver transplantation.[60] The system salvages up to 30–40% of lost red blood cells, thereby reducing the need for banked blood. When the scavenged blood has been anticoagulated with a citrate solution (6 mL/min) and washed with Plasma-Lyte (1 L), the effects of autotransfusion on coagulation, electrolyte balance, and plasma-free hemoglobin have been clinically satisfactory.[61] Bacterial contamination has been detected in up to 30% of the processed blood, but the quantity of the bacteria was clinically negligible and no bacteria culture was positive after autotransfusion.[61] Autotransfusion is not recommended in patients with intra-abdominal neoplasms, a positive hepatitis B antigen, or possible intraperitoneal infection.

Complications of Blood Transfusion

Recent advances in screening and preserving blood products using citrate-phosphate-dextrose-adenine have prolonged the survival of red blood cells. However, homologous blood transfusion has several drawbacks. Transmission of blood-borne disease is significant, and banked blood suffers from some degree of degradation during storage: decreased levels of 2,3-diphosphoglycerate (2,3-DPG), altered hemoglobin–oxygen affinity, hemolysis, hyperkalemia, acidosis, increased carbon dioxide tension, decreased factors V and VIII, thrombocytopenia, microaggregates, and denatured proteins.

Generally, most of the storage lesion of banked blood is reversible. A decrease in the 2,3-DPG level shifts the hemoglobin–oxygen dissociation curve leftward, but this is countered by a rightward shift caused by the blood's acidity. Additionally, transfused red blood cells regain their normal 2,3-DPG level after transfusion. Intravascular hemolysis can occur when relatively old banked blood is transfused. However, complications induced by intravascular hemolysis are relatively uncommon and mild except for those of mismatched blood transfusion. Inadvertent hypothermia occurs during massive blood transfusion if the capacity of the blood-warming device is insufficient. Hypothermia should be avoided because it may increase irritability of the heart, decrease myocardial contractility, and affect blood coagulability. Transient but significant hyperkalemia occurs during massive blood transfusion. The degree of hyperkalemia has a strong correlation with the rate of transfusion, particularly when relatively old stored blood is transfused into patients with impaired renal function. Hyperkalemia manifests as a tall peaked T wave on the electrocardiogram and bradycardia progressing to sinus arrest. Hyperkalemia can be prevented by administration of glucose (25 g) with regular insulin (10 units), transfusion of washed red blood cells prepared by the blood bank,[62] or autotransfusion.[63] The administration of calcium chloride and sodium bicarbonate treats hyperkalemia symptomatically. Hypokalemia may occur after blood transfusion as a result of reuptake of potassium by the transfused red blood cells. A potassium supplement may be required.

Ionized hypocalcemia (citrate intoxication) is a major concern in cirrhotic patients who require a massive transfusion of blood stored in citrate anticoagulant. Inadequate hepatic clearance of the citrate-calcium complex leads to severe ionized hypocalcemia, as demonstrated during the anhepatic stage of liver transplantation.[64] The serum citrate level has an inverse relation to the serum ionized calcium level and reaches the level present in the banked blood during the anhepatic stage. Severe myocardial depression has occurred when the serum ionized calcium level decreased below 0.56 mmol/L; this low level also adversely affects coagulation. Therefore, monitoring and normalization of the ionized calcium level are mandatory. For the treatment of hypocalcemia, calcium chloride has been preferred, because calcium gluconate requires hepatic metabolism to liberate Ca^{++}. However, a recent study showed that equimolar doses of calcium chloride and calcium gluconate are equally effective in correcting ionized hypocalcemia in patients undergoing liver transplantation.[65] Citrate also binds with magnesium to cause hypomagnesemia, which may lead to tachycardia, hypotension, seizures, a prolonged Q-T interval, myocardial depression, and possible sudden death. A deficiency of magnesium should be considered in patients with persistent hemodynamic instability, and magnesium chloride may be given.

Progressive metabolic acidosis and an increase in the lactate level occur as a result of an increased acid load from the transfused blood and inadequate hepatic clearance. Therefore, metabolic acidosis should be treated more aggressively in patients with liver disease by administration of sodium bicarbonate to maintain hemodynamic stability. Liberal use of sodium bicarbonate in combination with hepatic metabolism of citrate may precipitate postoperative metabolic alkalosis. However, postoperative metabolic alkalosis following liver transplantation did not correlate with the volume of blood products administered or the dose of sodium bicarbonate.[66] When hyperosmolality and hypernatremia are of concern, tromethamine may be used to prevent these complications and possibly the development of central pontine myelinolysis.

The increased glucose load from the stored blood and inadequate glycogenesis can lead to hyperglycemia. Insulin (5–10 units) may be given to maintain blood glucose levels of less than 200 mg/dL.

Transmission of blood-borne diseases, particularly viral hepatitis and the acquired immunodeficiency syndrome (AIDS), is a serious complication of blood transfusion. The incidence of posttransfusion viral hepatitis was reported to be 1% per unit of transfusion[67] and 5–21% in a period between 1974 and 1981.[68] It decreased about 70% between 1985 and 1987, mainly from the use of volunteer blood donors and better serologic screening. However, this high incidence remains. Among 58,000 viral hepatitis cases that occurred in the United States in 1984, 11.9% of non-A, non-B hepatitis, 3.1% of hepatitis B, and 2.5% of hepatitis A occurred after blood transfusion.[69] Transmission of non-A, non-B hepatitis is a particular concern considering that the incidence of transfusion-related hepatitis A and B is similar to that in hospitalized patients without blood transfusion (2.2%).[70] The recent introduction of a serologic test for non-A, non-B hepatitis (hepatitis C) should be able to reduce the transmission of non-A, non-B (C) hepatitis.

Another fatal disease is AIDS. U.S. Public Health Services projects that 179,000 cumulative deaths will occur in 270,000 cumulative AIDS cases by 1991.[71] Surprisingly, transfusion of human immunodeficiency virus (HIV)-containing blood was the cause of AIDS in more than 10% of patients in 1987.[72] This incidence has been decreasing since the introduction of a serologic test for HIV.

Other rare and less significant infectious diseases transmitted by transfusion include malaria, syphilis, cytomegalovirus and Epstein-Barr virus infection, babesiosis, Lyme disease, trypanosomiasis, leishmaniasis, toxoplasmosis, filariasis, and various bacterial infections.[73] To prevent these infectious diseases, volunteer blood donors are preferred, proper serologic screening is performed, blood transfusion is minimized, and exposure to multiple blood donors is minimized by transfusing whole blood instead of packed red blood cells and FFP from multiple donors.

Coagulation Defects Associated with Hepatic Surgery

LeVeen Shunt

The use of the LeVeen shunt to treat intractable ascites is associated with a DIC phenomenon, and severe hemorrhage and death have been reported.[74,75] DIC appears to be more severe when the shunt is patent and functional, with improvement when the shunt is nonfunctional.[76] This phenomenon appears to be related to direct systemic introduction of endotoxin in the ascitic fluid or to the cellular component of ascites.[77,78] Ligation of the shunt has been recommended when clinically significant DIC occurs.[76]

Major Hepatic Surgery

Intraoperative changes in coagulation during major hepatic surgery depend on the patient's preoperative coagulation state, the level of function of the remaining liver, and the degree of dilution caused by bleeding. When a prolonged anhepatic state is encountered, coagulation factors with a short half-life, such as factors V, VII, VIII, IX, and X, decrease to low levels. Fibrinolysis may also occur, resulting from the decrease in hepatic clearance of activated coagulation factors and fibrinolytic activators that are released during surgical trauma.[79,80] Extensive hepatic resection is associated with a transient decrease in vitamin K–dependent factors.

Liver Transplantation

During the preanhepatic stage, dilutional coagulopathy superimposes on the coagulopathy associated with poor hepatic synthetic function, quantitative and qualitative defects in platelets, and fibrinolysis. The deficiency in coagulation factors is corrected by administration of FFP. The decrease in platelet function, indicated by a decrease in the maximum amplitude on the TEG, is corrected by transfusion of platelets. Transfusion of 10 units of platelets increases the platelet count by 40,000–50,000/mm³.[46] Because of high levels of fibrinogen and factor VIII, it is rarely necessary to administer cryoprecipitate containing fibrinogen, factor VIII, and factor XIII during this period. FFP contains relatively small amounts of factor V but enough to maintain blood coagulability. A heparin effect is observed at the onset of veno-venous bypass when a small dose of heparin (1000–2000 units) is added in the bypass cannula to prevent thrombosis during preparation. This heparin effect may last for 30–60 minutes and is not usually detectable at the end of the anhepatic stage. The dilutional coagulopathy may continue, although surgical bleeding is less severe than in the preanhepatic stage. Fibrinolysis can occur at this time possibly by a progressive increase in the level of tissue plasminogen activator uncleared by the liver.[81] During the anhepatic stage when an unheparinized veno-veno bypass is used, administration of platelets and epsilon-aminocaproic acid is reserved only for severe cases of thrombocytopenia and fibrinolysis to avoid potential thromboembolism.

Reperfusion of the grafted liver is associated with severe coagulopathy: dilutional coagulopathy from the influx of preservation solution, a heparin effect from the release of heparin or a heparin-like substance from the donor hepatocytes, explosive fibrinolysis from the release of tissue plasminogen activator from the donor liver, and inhibition of coagulation by unknown substances.[20,82] The cause of this pathologic coagulation on reperfusion can be determined by comparing the TEGs of whole blood, blood plus protamine sulfate, and blood plus epsilon-aminocaproic acid.[43] If a heparin effect persists 30 minutes after reperfusion, it is treated with 50 mg of protamine sulfate. Epsilon-aminocaproic acid (20 mg/kg, single dose) is administered to treat severe fibrinolysis (fibrinolysis time < 60 min). In a series of patients, this treatment was necessary in 20% of recipients and was effective without complications.[48] It is controversial whether the fibrinolysis on reperfusion of the grafted liver is primary fibrinolysis or secondary to DIC. However, the primary fibrinolysis theory is gaining support from several findings: an association of fibrinolysis with a selective decrease in levels of fibrinogen and factors V and VIII,[83] demonstration of an "explosive" increase in tissue plasminogen activator,[84] and successful use of epsilon-aminocaproic acid without thrombotic complications.[43] On the other hand, administration of antithrombin III was recommended because of a gradual increase in the thrombin-antithrombin complex level resulting from DIC,[85] although the antithrombin III level appears to be steady during liver transplantation.[86] A recent clinical trial of aprotinin, a protease inhibitor, demonstrated a reduced blood loss during liver transplantation.[87] However, generalized inhibition of coagulation and fibrinolysis seen in an in vitro study[61] suggests that patients receiving aprotinin should be monitored closely. Severe coagulopathy improves gradually during the neohepatic stage unless major surgical bleeding continues. Poor graft function resulting from ischemic insult or poor hepatic perfusion leads to coagulopathy.[82,88]

The hypercoagulable state seen in patients with the Budd-Chiari syndrome and neoplasms becomes normalized or hypocoagulable because of surgical bleeding and other coagulation changes in liver transplantation. When bleeding is minimal, however, a small dose of heparin (1000–2000 units) can be administered during the anhepatic stage and in the postoperative period. For patients with hemophilia A or hemophilia B, deficient coagulation factors are administered to raise their level to 50% of the normal value during the preanhepatic and anhepatic stages. Additional treatment is unnecessary once the graft liver begins to function.[89] Patients with protein C deficiency are prone to developing thromboembolism, and anticoagulation therapy is continued into the immediate preoperative period. Heparin may be given while coagulation is monitored until the grafted liver begins to produce protein C. Administration of FFP is usually adequate to raise the antithrombin III level in patients with familial antithrombin III deficiency, and the disease is cured by liver transplantation.

Children undergoing liver transplantation appear to have coagulation abnormalities similar to those of adult patients. Then coagulopathy appears to be less severe, however, possibly because they have a greater prevalence of cholestatic disease, a shorter duration of disease, and better-functioning donor organs.[48]

Heterotopic Liver Transplantation

In heterotopic liver transplantation, the donor liver is placed in the paravertebral gutter or in the pelvis without removing the diseased liver. The coagulation changes that occur are similar to those in orthotopic liver transplantation but less severe.[90] In heterotopic liver transplantation, surgical bleeding associated with hilar dissection is less likely, a completely anhepatic state is avoided, and the reperfusion coagulation syndrome is less severe because coagulation inhibitors and activators are cleared by the diseased but functioning native liver.

References

1. Stenflo, J., Fernlund, P., Egan, W. and Roepstorff, P. (1974) Vitamin K dependent modifications of glutamic acid residues in prothrombin. *Proceedings of the National Academy of Science (USA)* 71:2730–3.
2. Gross, L. and Brotman, M. (1970) Hypoprothrombinemia and hemorrhage associated with cholestyramine therapy. *Annals of Internal Medicine* 72:95–6.
3. Blanchard, R.A., Furie, B.C., Jorgensen, M. et al. (1981) Acquired vitamin K-dependent carboxylation deficiency in liver disease. *New England Journal of Medicine* 305:242–8.
4. Straub, P.W. (1963) A study of fibrinogen production by human liver slices in vitro by an immunoprecipitin method. *Journal of Clinical Investigations* 42:130–6.
5. Grun, M., Liehr, H., Brunswig, D. and Thiel, H. (1974) Regulation of fibrinogen synthesis in portal hypertension. *Thromb. Diath. Haemorrh.* 32:292–305.
6. Walls, W.D. and Losowsky, M.J. (1971) The hemostatic defect of liver disease. *Gastroenterology* 60:108–9.
7. Rubin, R.N., Kies, M.S. and Posch, J.J. Jr. (1978) Coagulation profiles in patients with metastatic liver disease. *Blood* 52(suppl 1):193.
8. Jacobson, R.J., Wagner, S., Weinberg, R. and Bjornsson, S. (1971) Bleeding complications in fulminant hepatitis. *Lancet* 2:14266.
9. Martinez, J., Palascak, J.E. and Kwasniak, D. (1978) Abnormal sialic acid content of the dysfibrinogenemia associated with liver disease. *Journal of Clinical Investigations* 61:535–8.
10. Olson, J.P., Miller, L.L. and Troup, S.B. (1966) Synthesis of clotting factors by the isolated perfused rat liver. *Journal of Clinical Investigations* 45:690–701.
11. Vliet, A.C.M., van Vliet, H.H.D.M., van Džolijić-Danilović, G., and Wilson, J.H.P. (1981) Plasma prekallikrein and endotoxemia in liver cirrhosis. *Thromb. Haemost.* 45:65–7.
12. Shaw, E., Giddings, J.C., Peake, I.R. and Bloom, A.L. (1979) Synthesis of procoagulant factor VIII, factor VIII related antigen, and other coagulation factors by the isolated perfused rat liver. *British Journal of Haematology* 41:585–91.
13. Meili, E.O. and Straub, P.W. (1970) Elevation of factor VIII in acute fatal liver necrosis. *Thromb. Diath. Haemorrh.* 24:161–74.
14. Green, A. J. and Ratnoff, O.D. (1974) Elevated antihemophilic factor (AHF, factor VIII) procoagulant activity and AHF-like antigen in alcoholic cirrhosis of the liver. *Journal of Laboratory and Clinical Medicine* 83:189–97.
15. Lechner, K., Niessner, H. and Thaler, E. (1977) Coagulation abnormalities in liver disease. *Semin. Thromb. Hemost.* 4:40–56.
16. Hensen, A. and Loeliger, E.A. (1963) Antithrombin III: Its metabolism and its function in blood coagulation. *Thromb. Diath. Haemorrh.* 9(suppl 1):1–84.
17. Aoki, N. and Yamanaka, T. (1978) The alpha 2-plasmin inhibitor levels in liver diseases. *Clin Chim. Acta* 84:99–105.
18. Hovi, T., Mosher, D. and Vaheri A. (1977) Cultured human monocytes synthesize and secrete alpha2-macroglobulin. *J. Exp. Med.* 145:1580–9.
19. Murray-Lyon, I.M., Clarke, H.G.M., McPherson, K. and Williams, R. (1972) Quantitative immunoelectrophoresis of serum proteins in cryptogenic cirrhosis, alcoholic cirrhosis and active chronic hepatitis. *Clin. Chim. Acta* 39:215–20.
20. Kang, Y.G., Martin D.J., Marquez, J. et al. (1985) Intraoperative changes in blood coagulation and thrombelas-

tographic monitoring in liver transplantation. *Anesthesia and Analgesia* 64:888–96.

21. Aster, R.H. (1966) Pooling of platelets in the spleen: Role in the pathogenesis of "hypersplenic" thrombocytopenia. *Journal of Clinical Investigations* 45:645–57.

22. Sullivan, B.H. Jr. and Tumen, H.J. (1961) The effect of portacaval shunt on thrombocytopenia associated with portal hypertension. *Annals of Internal Medicine* 55:598–603.

23. Ballard, H.S. and Marcus, A.J. (1976) Platelet aggregation in portal cirrhosis. *Archives of Internal Medicine* 136:316–9.

24. Thomas, D.P., Ream, V.J. and Stuart, R.K. (1967) Platelet aggregation in patients with Laennec's cirrhosis of the liver. *New England Journal of Medicine* 276: 1344–8.

25. Rubin, M.H., Weston, M.J., Bullock, G. et al. (1977) Abnormal platelet function and ultrastructure in fulminant hepatic failure. *Quarterly Journal of Medicine* 46:339–52.

26. Karpatkin, K.S. and Freedman, M.L. (1978) Hypersplenic thrombocytopenia differentiated from increased peripheral destruction by platelet volume. *Annals of Internal Medicine* 89:200.

27. Kwaan, H.C., McFadzean, A.J.S. and Cook, J. (1956) Plasma fibrinolytic activity in cirrhosis of the liver. *Lancet* 1:132–6.

28. Mowat, N.A.G., Brunt, P.W. and Ogston, D. (1974) The fibrinolytic enzyme system in acute and chronic liver injury. *Acta Haematol.* 52:289–93.

29. Rake, M.O., Flute, P.T., Parnell, G. and Williams, R. (1970) Intravascular coagulation in acute hepatic necrosis. *Lancet* 1:533–7.

30. Tytgat, G.N., Collen, D. and Verstraete, M. (1971) Metabolism of fibrinogen in cirrhosis of the liver. *Journal of Clinical Investigations* 50:1690–701.

31. Straub, P.W. (1977) Diffuse intravascular coagulation in liver disease. *Semin. Thromb. Hemost.* 4:29–39.

32. Verstraete, M., Vermeylen, J. and Collen, D. (1974) Intravascular coagulation in liver disease. *Ann. Rev. Med.* 25:447–55.

33. Rake, M.O., Shilkin, K.B., Winch, J. et al. (1971) Early and intensive therapy of intravascular coagulation in acute liver failure. *Lancet* 2:1215–8.

34. Gazzard, B.G., Clarke, R., Borirakchanyavat, V. and Williams, R. (1974) A controlled trial of heparin therapy in the coagulation defect of paracetamol-induced hepatic necrosis. *Gut* 15:89–93.

35. Oka, K. and Tanaka, K. (1979) Intravascular coagulation in autopsy cases with liver diseases. *Thromb. Haemost.* 42:564–70.

36. Seligsohn, U., Shani, M., Ramot, B. et al. (1970) Dubin-Johnson syndrome in Israel. II. Association with factor-VII deficiency. *Q. J. Med.* 39:569–84.

37. Seligsohn, U., Shani, M. and Ramot, B. (1970) Gilbert syndrome and factor VII deficiency (letter). *Lancet* 1:1398.

38. Donald, A.C., Hunter, R.B., Tudhope, G.R. et al. (1954) Prothrombin and haemorrhage. *British Medical Journal* 2:961–3.

39. Green, G., Thomson, J.M., Dymock, I.W. and Poller, L. (1976) Abnormal fibrin polymerization in liver disease. *British Journal of Haematology* 34:427–39.

40. Green, G., Poller, L., Thomson, J. M. and Dymock, I.W. (1976) Factor VII as marker of hepatocellular synthetic function in liver disease. *Journal of Clinical Pathology* 29:971–5.

41. Biland, L., Duckert, F., Prisender, S. and Nyman, D. (1978) Quantitative estimation of coagulation factors in liver disease. The diagnostic and prognostic value of factor VIII, factor V and plasminogen. *Thromb. Haemost.* 39:646–56.

42. Bontempo, F.A., Lewis, J.H., Ragni, M.V. and Starzl, T. E. (1986) The preoperative coagulation pattern in liver transplant patients. In *Hepatic Transplantation: Anesthetic and Perioperative Management* (Winter, P.M. and Kang, Y.G., eds). New York:Praeger, pp. 135–46.

43. Kang, Y., Lewis, J.H., Navalgund, A. et al. (1987) Epsilon-aminocaproic acid for treatment of fibrinolysis during liver transplantation. *Anesthesiology* 66:766–73.

44. Zuckerman, L., Cohen, L., Vagher, J.P. et al. (1981) Comparison of thrombelastography with common coagulation tests. *Thromb. Haemost.* 46:752–6.

45. De Nicola, P. (1957) *Thrombelastography.* Springfield, IL:Charles C. Thomas, pp. 5–27.

46. Kang, Y.G. (1986) Monitoring and treatment of coagulation. In *Hepatic Transplantation: Anesthetic and Perioperative Management* (Winter, P.M. and Kang, Y.G., eds) New York: Praeger, pp. 151–73.

47. Kang, Y. and Gelman, S. (1986) Liver transplantation. In *Anesthesia and Organ Transplantation* (Gelman, S., ed) Philadelphia:W. B. Saunders, pp. 139–86.

48. Kang, Y., Borland, L.M., Picone, J. and Martin, K.K. (1989) Intraoperative coagulation changes in children undergoing liver transplantation. *Anesthesiology* 71:44–7.

49. Mannucci, P.M., Franchi, F. and Dioguardi, N. (1976) Correction of abnormal coagulation in chronic liver disease by combined use of fresh-frozen plasma and prothrombin complex concentrates. *Lancet* 2:542–5.

50. Gazzard, B.G., Henderson, J.M. and Williams, R. (1975) The use of fresh frozen plasma or a concentrate of factor IX as replacement therapy before liver biopsy. *Gut* 16:621–5.

51. Kasper, C.K. (1973) Postoperative thrombosis in hemophilia B. *New England Journal of Medicine* 289:160.

52. Gazzard, B.G., Lewis, M.L., Ash, G. et al. (1974) Coagulation factor concentrate in the treatment of the hemorrhagic diathesis of fulminant hepatic failure. *Gut* 15:993–8.

53. Dutcher, J. P., Schiffer, C.A., Aisner, J. and Wiernik, P.H. (1981) Alloimmunization following platelet transfusion: The absence of a dose-response relationship. *Blood* 57:395–8.

54. Weber, T., Marino, I.R., Kang, Y.G. et al. (1989) Intraoperative blood transfusions in highly immunized patients undergoing orthotopic liver transplantation. *Transplantation* 47:797–801.

55. Coleman, M., Finlayson, N., Bettigole, R.I. et al. (1975) Fibrinogen survival in cirrhosis: Improvement by low dose heparin. *Annals of Internal Medicine* 83:79.

56. Lewis, J.H. and Doyle, A.P. (1964) Effect of epsilon aminocaproic acid on coagulation and fibrinolytic mechanism. *Journal of the American Medical Association* 188:56–63.

57. Hiller, E.J., Hegemann, F. and Possinger, K. (1981) Hypercoagulability in acute esophageal variceal bleeding. *Thromb. Res.* 22:243–51.

58. Munoz, S.J., Ballas, B.E., Moritz, M.M. et al. (1989) Perioperative management of fulminant and subfulminant hepatic failure with therapeutic plasmapheresis. *Transplantation Proceedings* 21:3535–6.

59. Sassano J.J. (1986) The rapid infusion system. In *Hepatic Transplantation: Anesthetic and Perioperative Management* (Winter, P.M. and Kang, Y.G., eds) New York:Praeger, pp. 120–34.

60. Smith, M.F., Thomas, D.G. and Hesford, J.W. (1987) Perioperative support, monitoring and autotransfusion. In *Liver Transplantation* (Calne, R., ed) London:Grune Stratton, pp. 179–97.

61. Kang, Y.G., Aggarwal, S., Virji, M. et al. (1991) Clinical evaluation of autotransfusion during liver transplantation. *Anesthesia and Analgesia* 72:94–100.

62. Belani, K.G. and Estrin, J.A. (1987) Biochemical, metabolic and hematologic effects of intraoperative processing of CPDA-1 and AS-1 packed red cells (Abstract). *Anesthesiology* 67:A156.

63. Brown, M.R., Ramsay, M.A.E. and Swygert, T.H. (1989) Exchange autotransfusion using the cell saver during liver transplantation (letter). *Anesthesiology* 70:168–9.

64. Marquez, J., Martin, D., Kang, Y. et al. (1986) Cardiovascular depression secondary to citrate intoxication during hepatic transplantation in man. *Anesthesiology* 65:457–61.

65. Martin, T., Kang, Y., Marquez, J.M. et al. (1990) Pharmacokinetics and hemodynamic effects of calcium chloride and calcium gluconate during liver transplantation. *Anesthesiology* 73:62–5.

66. Fortunato, F.L., Jr., Kang, Y., Aggarwal, S. et al. (1987) Acid–base status during and after orthotopic liver transplantation. *Transplantation Proceedings* 19 (suppl 3):59–60.

67. Conrad, J.M. (1981) Diseases transmissible by blood transfusion. Viral hepatitis and other infectious disorders. *Seminars in Hematology* 18:122–46.

68. Bove, J.R. (1987). Transfusion-associated hepatitis and AIDS (letter). *New England Journal of Medicine* 317:242–5.

69. Centers for Disease Control: Hepatitis surveillance report number 50 (1986). U.S. Public Health Service Centers for Disease Control. Atlanta.

70. Aach, R.D., Lander, J.J. and Sherman, L.A. (1978) Transfusion transmitted viruses: Interim analysis of hepatitis among tranfused and nontransfused patients. In *Viral Hepatitis* (Vyas, G.N., Cohen, S.N., and Schmid, R., eds) Philadelphia:Franklin Institute Press, p. 383.

71. Morgan, W.M. and Curran, J.W. (1986). Acquired immunodeficiency syndrome: Current and future trends. *Public Health Rep.* 101:459–65.

72. Centers for Disease Control: AIDS weekly surveillance report (1987). U.S. Public Health Service Centers for Disease Control. Atlanta.

73. Barker, L.F. and Dodd, R.Y. (1989) Viral hepatitis, acquired immunodeficiency syndrome, and other infections transmitted by transfusion. In *Clinical Practice of Transfusion Medicine* (Petz, L.D. and Swisher, S.N. eds) New York:Churchill Livingstone, pp. 667–712.

74. LeVeen, H.H., Wapnick, S., Grosberg, S. and Kinney, M.J. (1976) Further experience with peritoneo-venous shunt for ascites. *Annals of Surgery* 184:574–81.

75. Matseshe, J.W., Beart, R.W. Jr. Bartholomew, L.G. and Baldus, W.P. (1978) Fatal disseminated intravascular coagulation after peritoneovenous shunt for intractable ascites. *Mayo Clinic Proceedings* 53:526–8.

76. Harmon, D.C., Demirjian, Z., Ellman, L. and Fischer, J.E. (1979) Disseminated intravascular coagulation with the peritoneovenous shunt. *Annals of Internal Medicine* 90:774–6.

77. Lerner, R.G., Nelson, J.C., Corines, P. and del Guercio L.R.M. (1978) Disseminated intravascular coagulation. Complication of peritoneovenous shunts. *Journal of the American Medical Association* 240:2064–6.

78. Phillips, L.L. and Rodgers, J.B. (1979) Procoagulant activity of ascitic fluid in hepatic cirrhosis: In vivo and in vitro. *Surgery* 86:714–21.

79. Walt, A.J. (1964) The surgical management of hepatic trauma and its complications. *Ann. R. Coll. Surg. Engl.* 45:319–39.

80. Rö, J.S. (1973) Hemostatic problems in liver surgery. *Scandinavian Journal of Gastroenterology* 8(suppl) 19:71–81.

81. Virji, M.A., Aggarwal, S. and Kang, Y. (1989) Alterations in plasminogen activator and plasminogen activator inhibitor levels during liver transplantation. *Transplantation Proceedings* 21(suppl 3):3540–1.

82. Groth, C.G., Pechet, L. and Starzl, T.E. (1969) Coagulation during and after orthotopic transplantation of the human liver. *Archives of Surgery* 98:31–4.

83. Lewis, J.H., Bontempo, F.A., Awad, S.A. et al. (1989) Liver transplantation: Intraoperative changes in coagulation factors in 100 first transplants. *Hepatology* 9:710–4.

84. Porte, R.J., Bontempo, F.A., Knot, E.A. et al. (1989) Systemic effects of tissue plasminogen activator-associated fibrinolysis and its relation to thrombin generation in orthotopic liver transplantation. *Transplantation* 47:978–84.

85. Kratzer, M.A.A., Dieterich, J., Denecke, H. and Knedel, M. (1991) Hemostatic variables and blood loss during

orthotopic human liver transplantation. *Transplantation Proceedings* 23:1906–11.

86. Lewis, J.H., Bontempo, F.A., Ragni, M.V. and Starzl, T.E. (1989) Antithrombin III during liver transplantation. *Transplantation Proceedings* 21:3543–4.

87. Mallett, S.V., Cox, D., Burroughs, A.K. and Rolles, K. (1990) Aprotinin and reduction of blood loss and transfusion requirements in orthotopic liver transplantation (letter). *Lancet* 336:886–7.

88. Flute, P.T., Rake, M.O., Williams, R. et al. (1969) Liver transplantation in man—IV, Haemorrhage and thrombosis. *British Medical Journal* 3:20–3.

89. Bontempo, F.A., Lewis, J.H., Gorenc, T.J. et al. (1987) Liver transplantation in hemophilia A. *Blood* 69:1721–4.

90. Porte, R.J., Knot, E.A.R. and De Maat, M.P.M. et al. (1988) Fibrinolysis detected by thrombelastography in heterotopic, auxillary liver transplantation: Effect of tissue type plasminogen activator. *Fibrinolysis* 2(suppl 3): 67–73.

11

Anesthesia for the Pediatric Patient Requiring Hepatic Surgery

Peter J. Davis and D. Ryan Cook

Various forms of liver disease, with a wide range of causes, occur throughout childhood. Some occur in an obstructive or cholestatic form, while others mainly affect hepatocellular function. Although it is convenient to classify the diseases as either obstructive or hepatocellular, most hepatic disease entities begin with one form and either slowly or rapidly progress to the other. Thus, liver disease is an inhomogeneous grouping of disorders with a wide range of underlying pathophysiologic implications.

Because the liver is the major site of drug metabolism, liver disease frequently results in variable and unpredictable drug pharmacology. In addition to the effects of disease, growth and development can influence drug disposition and elimination. Rapid growth, development, and maturation of organ function occur within the first few years of life. Pediatric anesthesiology involves the anesthetic management of patients during this period of development. Consequently, knowledge of the pathophysiologic basis of disease as well as an understanding of the normal developmental changes that occur with growth and maturation are essential for a rational anesthetic approach to the infant or child undergoing hepatic surgery.

This chapter focuses on anesthetic management in five major types of pediatric surgical liver disease. These five diseases have been grouped into three areas:

1. obstructive or cholestatic diseases; that is, biliary atresia and choledochal cysts
2. surgical hepatocellular disease; namely, hepatic tumors and abscesses
3. portal hypertension

In all three parts, the discussion of anesthetic management includes the pathophysiologic implications of the underlying disease as well as the basic considerations of pediatric anesthesia.

Biliary Disease

Biliary atresia is characterized by grossly impatent extrahepatic bile ducts and is a major cause of obstructive jaundice in the newborn period. The incidence of biliary atresia is about one in 15,000 live births[1] (Figure 11-1) Between 10% and 15% of patients with biliary atresia have other associated abnormalities of embryologic development, such as polysplenia with abdominal heterotaxia, levocardia, and intra-abdominal vascular anomalies.[2] Biliary atresia is often classified in two forms: a "correctable" type, in which the proximal extrahepatic bile ducts are patent and the distal ducts occluded and a "noncorrectable" type, in which both proximal and distal ducts are occluded. Although biliary atresia is often thought of as a congenital lesion, it has dynamic properties as well. Evidence that it is an ongoing disease process is supported by

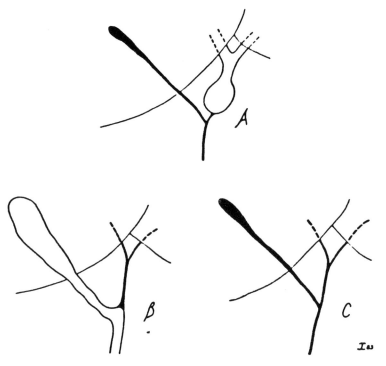

Figure 11-1. Drawing of the three most common expressions of biliary atresia. (A) Correctable biliary atresia. The proximal bile ducts are patent although hypoplastic. (B) Variant (15%) of noncorrectable biliary atresia, in which the gallbladder, cystic duct, and common bile duct are patent but the proximal bile ducts are occluded. (C) Most common type of noncorrectable biliary atresia, in which the entire extrahepatic bile ducts are nonpatent. (Courtesy of Dr. Jack Chang.)

studies in which serial microscopic evaluations were made. Nietgen and others studied the histological and immunohistochemical characteristics of the liver in 44 children with extrahepatic biliary atresia from specimens taken during three time periods: Kasai operation, relaparotomy, and hepatectomy for liver transplant. These biopsies showed a progressive loss of intrahepatic bile ducts over time.[3] Other evidence suggesting the dynamic nature of the disease is that the success rate for the palliative procedure (Kasai) has been reported to be 80% in infants operated on under 10 weeks of age and 50% when performed before the patient is 4 months old. When postoperative biliary drainage is not sufficient to clear the jaundice, 80% of infants die by their third birthday. In addition to the patient's age at the time of the procedure, precise surgical dissection, prevention of postoperative cholangitis, and early reoperation when clinically indicated are all factors which have improved operative results.[4]

Clinically, onset of the disease occurs in the first 6 weeks of infancy. About 50% of these infants are anicteric until the second or third week of life. The diagnosis of biliary atresia is often suspected from technetium-99m iminodiacetic acid (IDA) scans and ultrasound examination. Alpha-1-antitrypsin phenotyping also must be performed[5] because IDA and ultrasound studies of patients with biliary atresia, and α-1-antitrypsin deficiency may be similar. The diagnosis of biliary atresia, however, is confirmed by liver biopsy. Ductal proliferation in the wide portal space with hepatic fibrosis is the most characteristic histologic finding of biliary atresia.

The surgical procedure or repair depends on the anatomy of the underlying defect. In correctable forms of biliary atresia, a Roux-en-Y anastomosis is performed to the normal remnant of ductal tissue. In the noncorrectable form, the Kasai procedure is used.[6] In this operation, the extrahepatic ducts are removed, and an intestinal jejunal conduit is sewn to the transected duct at the level of the liver hilum. Some surgeons prefer to lower the intraluminal pressure of the conduit and consequently lower the hepatic secretory pressure gradient by exteriorizing the conduit. After 3–6 months when biliary flow has reached a steady state, the conduit is closed, and intestinal continuity is achieved.[7,8]

In patients (roughly 15%) who have a patent gallbladder, cystic duct, and distal common duct, the jejunal Roux-en-Y anastomosis is omitted, and the hilum is anastomosed to the gallbladder. Because of the high incidence of biliary leaks and biliary obstruction, a temporary catheter is often used

CHOLEDOCHAL CYSTS
'Todani Classification'

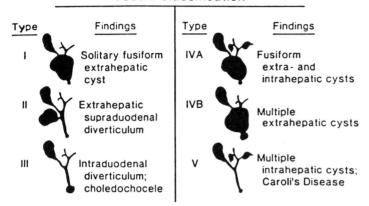

Type	Findings	Type	Findings
I	Solitary fusiform extrahepatic cyst	IVA	Fusiform extra- and intrahepatic cysts
II	Extrahepatic supraduodenal diverticulum	IVB	Multiple extrahepatic cysts
III	Intraduodenal diverticulum; choledochocele	V	Multiple intrahepatic cysts; Caroli's Disease

Figure 11-2. Classification of choledochal cysts.

to decompress the gallbladder.[9,10] The catheter is removed after the anastomosis has healed and the biliary ducts have dilated.

Complications of the surgical repair and the underlying disease state include cholangitis, portal hypertension, and fat-soluble vitamin deficiency.[11,12] Complications after surgery for biliary atresia appear early and late. Early complications (cholangitis) occur within 7 months after surgery and are usually related to obstruction of the hepatic duct. Late complications usually occur 4 years after surgery and are related to end-stage liver disease. Factors associated with late complications include cholangitis soon after the operation, high portal pressures at the initial operation, advanced age at the time of operation, a history of reoperation, and a long interval before the disappearance of jaundice and the surgical procedure.[13] Long-term follow-up in patients with biliary atresia has been reported in several studies. In the long-term outcome study by Laurent and others, in 72 of the 82 patients who died within 10 years of surgery, the cause of death was a complication from underlying liver disease; in the remaining 10 patients, death was secondary to refractory cholangitis. Forty of the 122 patients (32%) were alive 10 years after their surgery.[14] In a survey spanning 25 years, Engelskirchen and others reported on 90 patients with biliary atresia.[15] In patients who did not undergo a biliary drainage procedure, mortality was 65% compared with 75% in patients undergoing biliary drainage procedures. Kasai and others have reported 10- and 20-year survival rates after hepatoporto-jejunostomy of 26% and 13%, respectively.[16] Of the patients who were

alive for at least 10 years, there was no correlation of survival with the age at operation.[14,15] Long-term outcome results may be further modified in that patients with failed Kasai procedures are now being referred for liver transplantation.[15,17–19]

Choledochal cysts are congenital cystic dilations of the common bile duct. They are commonly categorized into five types (Figure 11-2).[20] Almost 90% of all choledochal cysts are type 1.[20] Clinically, choledochal cysts become evident at two different age spans. Infants have a clinical presentation similar to those of patients with biliary atresia, obstructive jaundice, and acholic stools (beginning at 2–3 months of age). The later-onset form (adult type) generally begins after 2 years of age with the signs of pain, intermittent jaundice, and a mass. For most lesions (type I), surgical treatment involves cholecysteotomy, cyst excision and Roux-en-Y anastomosis, and hepaticojejunostomy. However, for the remaining types of choledochal cysts, surgical treatment depends on the anatomy. Intrahepatic cysts (types IV and V) that are inaccessible for drainage are treated by hepatic resection. Diverticula of the extrahepatic bile ducts (type II) are excised or drained into the duodenum.[20–22]

Anesthetic Management

Because anesthetic considerations for biliary atresia and choledochal cysts are similar, biliary atresia will be used as the model for anesthetic management. The anesthetic management for a Kasai procedure is founded on basic principles of infant

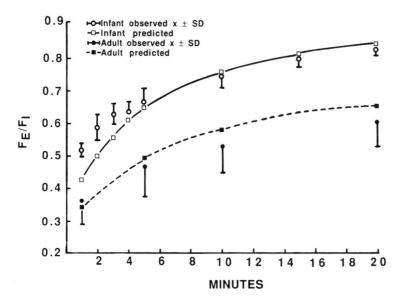

Figure 11-3. Predicted versus observed F_EF_I for halothane in infants and children. (Reprinted with permission from Brandom, B.W., Brandom, R.B. and Cook, D.R. (1983). Uptake and distribution of halothane in infants: In vivo measurements and computer simulations. *Anesthesia Analgesia* 62:404–410).

anesthesia. In infants in whom venous access is present before the onset of anesthesia, anesthesia is induced with a short-acting barbiturate (thiopental sodium, 7 mg/kg), and a muscle relaxant (e.g., atracurium besylate, 0.5 μg/kg) is used to facilitate tracheal intubation and surgical relaxation. In infants without an intravenous catheter in place, inhalation anesthesia is induced with oxygen, nitrous oxide, halothane, or isoflurane. Once the child is adequately anesthetized, an intravenous catheter is inserted and a muscle relaxant is administered to facilitate tracheal intubation and to decrease the concentration of the potent inhalation anesthetic.

It must be remembered that the incidence of bradycardia, hypotension, and cardiac arrest during the induction of inhalation anesthesia is higher in infants and small children than in adults.[23,23a,24] This greater incidence of untoward effects from potent agents can be attributed to age-related differences in uptake, anesthetic requirements, and sensitivity of the cardiovascular system. The uptake of inhalation anesthetics is more rapid in infants and small children than in adults because of major differences in blood–gas solubility coefficients, blood–tissue solubility coefficients, body composition, alveolar ventilation, and the distribution of cardiac output.[25–31] Thus, early in the induction of anesthesia, the infant has higher tissue concentrations of anesthetic than an adult would have (e.g., in brain, heart, muscle) (Figure 11-3).[32]

The anesthetic requirements for various inhalation agents (e.g., halothane, isoflurane, enflurane,

desflurane) are generally inversely related to age.[33–37] Thus, higher inspired concentrations are often used early in induction to compensate for age-related differences.

Infants have heart-rate–related changes in cardiac output, and bradycardia reduces cardiac output and results in hypotension. Anesthetic agents also blunt the baroreceptor reflexes[38–41] in a concentration-dependent manner to a greater degree in infants than in older patients. Consequently, in infants, atropine is administered intravenously immediately after venous access has been achieved. After induction, anesthesia is maintained with an air, oxygen, isoflurane mixture; nitrous oxide is avoided because of its tendency further to distend the bowel.

Anesthesia monitoring for the patient undergoing a Kasai procedure is similar to that used for other surgical procedures in infants. Although the advent of more sophisticated monitoring equipment enables moment-to-moment monitoring of blood pressure, electrocardiogram, oxygen saturation, temperature, central venous pressure, and end-tidal gases, the esophageal or precordial stethoscope remains the patient's lifeline to the anesthesiologist. This monitor, though simple, can detect subtle changes in the quality of the heart tones as well as changes in heart rate.

Blood pressure can be measured by the oscillometric method, by electronic instruments that use Doppler ultrasound to detect Korotkoff sounds, or by electronic oscillometrics to detect pulsating oscillation. Arterial cannulation and central venous pressure monitors to detect moment-to-moment changes in blood pressure and cardiac filling pressures are rarely used. They generally are reserved for patients with other coexisting problems such as sepsis, pneumonia, cholangitis, or severe cirrhosis. In general, hemodynamic stability is maintained, and the need for intraoperative vasoactive agents is rare. However, sometimes the surgical approach involves dividing the triangular and coronary ligaments and displacing the whole liver anteriorly. Although this technique may facilitate exposure, it may compress the inferior vena cava and thereby result in hypotension by decreasing venous return. Ventilation is controlled, and end-tidal gases are monitored for carbon dioxide, nitrogen, and volatile anesthetic agents. The adequacy of oxygenation is monitored by the pulse oximeter, which enables continuous beat-to-beat monitoring of arterial saturation.

Kasai procedures tend to be lengthy, but major blood loss generally does not occur. Perioperative fluid therapy may involve the initiation of fluid management or, alternatively, may be a continuation of established fluid therapy. It can be as simple as replacing the deficits arising from preoperative fluid restriction and providing maintenance fluids or as complex as correcting abnormal preoperative electrolyte and water deficits, perioperative translocated fluids, and variable blood loss, in addition to providing maintenance fluids. The "third-space" fluid loss of surgical trauma is associated with isotonic transfer of fluids from the extracellular fluid compartment and, to a lesser extent, from the intracellular compartment to a nonfunctional interstitial compartment.[42–46] In infants, estimated third-space loss during the Kasai operation varies from 6–10 mL/kg/h. Because fluid shifts can occur in association with third-space loss and because massive blood loss is a potential, although infrequent, complication, we usually insert two intravenous catheters for administering fluids.

Various calculations involving body weight, surface area, or caloric expenditure have been used to determine maintenance fluid requirements for infants and children (e.g., Holliday and Segar, 1957; Roy and Sinclair, 1975; Bell and Oh, 1979).[47–49] Infants weighing 1–10 kg need 100 mL of water/kg/day; or approximately 4 mL/kg/h maintenance fluids. Quarter-normal saline in 5% dextrose is used for maintenance fluid, while lactated Ringer's solution is used to restore third-space losses. Although third-space fluid losses are estimated, the end point of third-space replacement therapy is titrated to an age-appropriate blood pressure as well as adequate tissue perfusion and urine volume.

Classically, infants who need a Kasai procedure undergo the operation between 2 and 3 months of age, a time that corresponds to the nadir of their physiologic anemia. Consequently, blood replacement may be necessary with relatively little blood loss. All blood loss in infants and children should be replaced in one way or another. Accurately measuring blood loss and accurately assessing the acceptable blood loss in the infant are vital to any replacement regimen. The magnitude of blood loss is determined by weighing sponges, using calibrated miniaturized suction bottles, and estimating visually. The concept of allowable red cell loss or allowable blood loss is a preferable guide to blood replacement.[50,51] Normovolemic hemodilution to a predetermined hematocrit can be achieved with crystalloid or colloid solutions.

Frequently, the biggest challenge for anesthesiologists managing infants of this size is maintenance of body temperature. Hypothermia can affect the physical characteristics of inhalation anesthetics as well as the pharmacokinetic and pharmacodynamic effects of intravenous agents. For the inhalation agents, hypothermia not only lowers the minimum alveolar concentration, but also increases the tissue solubility.[52] Thus, for any inspired concentration in a hypothermic patient, an increased amount of anesthetic will be delivered to the tissues to meet a decreased anesthetic requirement. Studies on the effects of hypothermia suggest that hypothermia decreases the requirements for nondepolarizing muscle relaxants[53,54] as well as alters the pharmacokinetics of barbiturates and narcotics.[55–57]

The large surface-to-volume ratio and relative lack of insulating tissue in infants and young children, coupled with the cold operating room, exposure of body cavities to low environmental temperatures, infusions of cold fluid, and ventilation with dry gases, increase the potential for hypothermia during surgery. Therefore, great effort must be made to guard against heat loss both before and during surgery. It is essential that each operating room be equipped with an individual thermistor-control unit so that the room temperature can be adapted to meet the needs of each child. Operating room temperatures of 27–29°C (80–85°F) are frequently needed for infants. Radiant heaters minimize heat loss and are frequently used during the induction of anesthesia until the patient's skin is prepared and draped. Warming mattresses are especially effective in reducing conductive heat loss in infants with a surface area of less than 0.5 m^2.[58] Inspiratory gases should be heated and humidified, and intravenous fluids and blood products should be warmed before administration. Since the head constitutes a large component of the child's body surface area, wrapping the head in plastic after the induction of anesthesia can further limit evaporative and radiational forms of heat loss.

The pharmacology of anesthetic agents in infants and children with hepatic disease has not been fully evaluated. Although the liver is the major site of drug biotransformation, the effects of hepatic dysfunction on drug elimination and disposition are inconsistent. The degree of liver dysfunction and a drug's ability to bind to plasma proteins are important variables in determining drug kinetics in patients with liver disease. For drugs with a high hepatic extraction ratio, hepatic clearance is sensitive to changes in hepatic blood flow, whereas for drugs with a low hepatic extraction ratio, hepatic drug clearance becomes a function of intrinsic hepatic enzyme activity and protein binding. Thus, the reported inconsistent effect of liver disease on drug pharmacology may be a function of the heterogeneous pathophysiology of liver disease with respect to hepatocellular function, protein binding, and hepatic blood flow. For hepatic disease that preserve hepatic blood flow but impair hepatocellular function, the pharmacokinetic profile of a drug with a high hepatic extraction ratio will be relatively unaffected, but for a drug with a low hepatic extraction ratio, similar hepatic pathophysiologic impairment would result in a pronounced change in the drug's disposition and elimination.[59]

In general, liver function is well preserved in the first few months of life in children with biliary atresia. However, as children get older and ductal fibrosis begins, liver dysfunction ensues. Consequently, in children who return for repeated surgical procedures, the pharmacology of intravenous anesthetic agents and adjuncts may be altered. However, little information is available on the pharmacologic properties of anesthetic agents in children with liver disease. In a study of pediatric patients with cholestatic liver disease who were evaluated for liver transplantation, Davis and others noted that the pharmacokinetics of alfentanil in

Table 11-1. A Comparison of the Pharmacokinetics of Alfentanil in Children with Cholestatic Hepatic Disease and Normal Control Children*

	$t_{1/2} \alpha$ (min)	$t_{1/2} \beta_{120}$ (min)	Cl_{120} (mL/kg/min)	Vd_{120} (L/kg)
Children with cholestatic disease	2.7 ± 1.0	45.8 ± 13.3	7.59 ± 3.6	0.46 ± 0.16
Normal control children	3.3 ± 2.5	41.6 ± 16	7.25 ± 4.3	0.40 ± 0.21

*Mean ± SD
$t_{1/2} \alpha$: distribution 1/2 life
$t_{1/2}$? life
Cl_{120} clearance based on a 2 hour collection period
Vd_{120} value division based on a 2 hour collection period

these patients were similar to the kinetics in similar age-matched children with normal hepatic function.[60] This observation is in contrast to the finding that adults with alcoholic liver disease had a slower clearance and longer elimination half-life compared with adult control subjects with normal liver function.[61] It is not clear whether the pharmacokinetic differences between children and adults are a result of differences in the underlying pathophysiology of the respective liver disease, cholestatic versus hepatocellular dysfunction, or differences in the study designs (Table 11-1). Other studies comparing opioid pharmacokinetics in adults with normal and abnormal liver function have shown that liver disease does not affect the disposition and elimination of fentanyl and morphine.[62,63] Similar studies in children have not been carried out.

The pharmacokinetics of muscle relaxants in adults with hepatic dysfunction have been studied. Of the nondepolarizing muscle relaxants, pancuronium, vecuronium, and atracurium are significantly metabolized. Of the three, the pharmacokinetics of only pancuronium and vecuronium are prolonged in patients with hepatic or biliary disease. Atracurium, which is degraded by esterase hydrolysis and Hofmann elimination, is unaffected by liver disease. Recent studies on doxacurium, a potent benzylisoquinolinium, nondepolarizing neuromuscular blocking agent, suggest that in adults, plasma clearance, volume of distribution at steady state, and mean residence times are unaffected by liver disease.[64] Initial pharmacokinetic studies on mivacurium, a new, short-acting, nondepolarizing muscle relaxant whose metabolism appears to occur in the plasma (presumably by plasma esterases and butyrlcholinesterase) suggest that mivacurium clearance and mean residence times are prolonged in patients until liver failure.[65]

Although the experimental evidence in rats suggests that postanesthetic hepatic dysfunction following the use of halothane is similar in cirrhotic and noncirrhotic rats, we tend to prefer isoflurane to halothane as the inhalation anesthetic during liver surgery.[66] Gelman, Fowler, and Smith have shown that hepatic oxygen supply is better maintained with isoflurane than with halothane.[66a] In addition, in hypoxic rat models, the incidence of hepatic centrilobular necrosis was least with isoflurane compared with halothane, nitrous oxide, and fentanyl.[67] Consequently, isoflurane in an oxygen and air mixture is most commonly administered to patients undergoing surgery for biliary atresia.

Recovery from Anesthesia

In infants with biliary atresia undergoing the Kasai procedure or in children having other forms of biliary surgery, if major fluid shifts have not occurred, blood loss has been minimal, and the patient is warm, then all efforts are made to reverse the muscle relaxation and extubate the trachea at the end of the procedure. In children with other organ system failures (i.e., sepsis, cholangitis, pneumonia), and in those who are cold at the end of the procedure (<34°C) or have had more than one blood volume transfusion, extubation is delayed until the patient is warm and hemodynamically stable. In these patients, postoperative recovery and monitoring occurs in an intensive care setting.

Surgical Hepatocellular Diseases

Primary tumors of the liver are relatively uncommon. Pediatric hepatic tumors comprise about 10% of abdominal solid tumors in children. A broad but modified classification of hepatic tumors is presented in Table 11-2.[68,69] Benign hepatic cysts and tumors account for one-third of such cases, whereas malignant hepatic tumors constitute the remaining two-thirds.[70] The predominant malignant tumors are hepatocellular carcinoma and hepatoblastoma. Hemangioma, focal nodular hyperplasia, hemangioen-

Table 11-2. Classification of Liver Tumors

Benign	Malignant
Non-neoplastic tumors	*Epithelial tumors*
Focal nodular	Hepatoblastoma
hyperplasia	Hepatocellular
Epithelial tumors	carcinoma
Hepatic adenoma	*Mesenchymal tumors*
Nonparasitic cyst	Mixed mesenchymoma
Mesenchymal tumors	Rhabdomyosarcoma
Mesenchymal hamartoma	Angiosarcoma
Capillary hemangio-	Teratocarcinoma
endothelioma	*Sarcoma*
Cavernous hemangioma	
Lymphangioma	
Teratoma	

dothelioma, and mesenchymal hamartoma are the most common benign lesions.

Nonmalignant Tumors

Congenital cysts usually can be detected in the physical examination, and the diagnosis can be confirmed by ultrasonography. Surgical excision may require a wedge resection or lobectomy, but for cysts involving both lobes of the liver, internal drainage into a Roux-en-Y is the preferred treatment. A rare entity involving cysts of the liver is seen in patients with polycystic disease of the liver and kidney. With time, liver and kidney function deteriorates, and death occurs at an early age.

Mesenchymal hamartoma has been the term used to describe a large mass composed of multiple cysts of various sizes. The term also refers to cystic mesenchymal hamartoma, lymphangioma, cavernous lymphangiomatoid tumor, and bile cell fibroadenoma. This tumor usually arises in the first year of life. It can be highly vascular, and its large number of arteriovenous shunts may precipitate congestive heart failure. Surgical resection for the predominantly cystic lesions can be performed by a Rouxen-Y technique, or the cyst can be opened into the free peritoneal cavity for drainage and reabsorption.

Hepatic adenoma is a rare hepatic tumor in children and is usually associated with glycogen storage disease, type I glucose phosphate deficiency, and galactosemia.[71,72] Hepatic adenomas are vascular tumors, and symptoms of the tumor are frequently caused by pain from either rupture or infarction of the tumor. Surgical treatment involves a wedge resection or lobectomy.

Focal nodular hyperplasia is a circumscribed lesion in the liver that occurs in both adults and children. The pathogenesis of this lesion in children remains unknown. The childhood onset is between 7 and 10 years of age. In women, oral contraceptives have been implicated in the development of focal nodular hyperplasia and hepatic adenomas. Clinical symptoms and signs of focal nodular hyperplasia may include asymptomatic hepatomegaly, an abdominal mass, and/or mild to moderate epigastric pain. Resection of the circumscribed area is generally curative.

Cavernous hemangioma and hemangioendothelioma are neoplasms of very young children, usually detected during infancy. These tumors are highly vascular, and the large number of arteriovenous shunts may precipitate congestive heart failure. Signs range from asymptomatic hepatomegaly to high-output congestive heart failure, bleeding diathesis, and hemoperitoneum from tumor rupture. Forty percent of children with hemangioendothelioma of the liver have associated cutaneous hemangiomas as well. One or both lobes of the liver can be involved, although most tumors resolve on their own. The signs and symptoms in older children tend to be less severe than in younger infants. Because the natural tendency of these tumors is to enlarge and then to involute spontaneously, differences between symptoms in young and older infants may be related to the stage of the tumor and the tumor's natural history.

The medical treatment of these patients includes digitalis and diuretics in the first few months of life. In infants with high-output congestive heart failure, such medical management is often unsuccessful. In children who have some response to medical management, irradiation, cyclophosphamide, and steroids can be added to the treatment regimen. If congestive heart failure is unresponsive to medical management, hepatic artery ligation or embolization should be performed.[73]

Malignant Tumors

Hepatoblastoma and hepatocellular carcinoma constitute over half of the primary hepatic tumors of childhood.[70] In children, hepatoblastoma usually occurs before 2 years of age and presents as an increasing abdominal mass; anemia, jaundice, and ascites are infrequent findings. Boys predominate at a ratio of 1.5:1. Two to three percent of patients have an associated hemihypertrophy.[74] Findings of liver function tests are frequently normal. Hepatoblastoma has also been associated with isosexual precocity caused by the liver's ectopic gonadotropic production and with the Beckwith-Wiedemann syndrome.[75] The tumor is usually in the right lobe, but in 15–30% of patients, it is bilateral. The prognosis is most favorable when the tumor is confined to the right lobe and thus accessible for total excision. However, it is rare for tumors to be completely removed. Most patients having tumor excision are stage II, III, or IV (i.e., have miscroscopic tumor margins, gross tumor, or metastasis still present after resection). Some patients who undergo excision have treatment with chemotherapeutic agents before surgery. Most recurrences and/or metastases appear 12–18 months after surgery; in these cases death occurs in 2–3 years. The overall survival rate is 35% for patients with hepatoblastoma.

Hepatocellular Carcinoma

Compared with hepatoblastoma, hepatocellular carcinoma has an older age of presentation (10–14 years).[76,77] However, one survey has found two age peaks in children with hepatocellular carcinoma. One peak occurred in children under 4 years of age and the second between 12 and 15 years of age. Typically, patients with hepatocellular carcinoma have systemic symptoms of weight loss, jaundice, fever, and lethargy. Unlike adults with this tumor, only about 5% of the children have an associated cirrhosis.[78] Although hepatocellular carcinomas frequently have a benign histologic appearance, they tend to have a poor prognosis. The prognosis of survival in children with the disease is 5–10%. As with hepatoblastoma, boys predominate with a ratio of 1.3:1. Hepatocellular carcinoma has been associated with von Gierke's disease (type I glycogenosis), cystinosis, extrahepatic biliary atresia, α_1-antitrypsin hypoplasia of the intrahepatic bile ducts, tyrosinemia, Wilson's disease, giant cell hepatitis, and Sotos' syndrome.[79-82] Patients with the chronic form of hereditary tyrosinemia who survive beyond 2 years of age have a 40% chance of developing hepatocellular carcinoma.

Other malignant tumors of the liver, namely, embryonal rhabdomyosarcoma and malignant mesenchymal tumors, are extremely rare. Embryonal rhabdomyosarcoma occurs in the intrahepatic and common bile duct. The symptoms are jaundice, malaise, and fever. Age of onset is between 2 and 4 years. Local resection of the tumor is rarely curative; the average length of survival after the appearance of symptoms is 5–6 months. The malignant mesenchymal tumor occurs between the ages of 6 and 10 years.[82] It is a highly aggressive tumor, and patients have an average survival period of a year after symptoms appear.

Intrahepatic Abscess

Intrahepatic abscesses in children are rare. Two major types occur. One results from infestation due to *Entamoeba histolytica*; the other, pyogenic abscess, from a bacterial infection. Amebic hepatic abscess is seen in populations where intestinal amebiasis is common. Among patients with intestinal amebiasis, the incidence of hepatic involvement ranges from 1% to 25%.[83] The lesion tends to be more common in the right lobe and can be single or multiple. Clinically, children have hepatomegaly, right upper quadrant tenderness, anemia, and increased leukocytosis. Results of liver function tests frequently are normal except for elevated alkaline phosphatase, decreased albumin, and increased serum globulin levels. The major complications of amebic hepatic abscesses include secondary infection and rupture into the peritoneal and/or pleural cavity or lung. At one time, treatment consisted of surgical drainage and administration of amebicidal drugs. Currently, a regimen of metronidazole is the principal form of therapy.

Pyogenic abscesses in children are extremely rare. The causes of hepatic pyogenic infection include portal sepsis, biliary sepsis, systemic sepsis, trauma, infection of contiguous structures, (i.e., appendiceal abscess), and cryptogenic causes. Kaplan and Feigin reported that systemic sepsis accounted for 40% of the hepatic abscesses in patients who did not have chronic granulomatous disease.[84] In neonates less than 6 weeks of age, hepatic abscesses were associated with omphalitis and umbilical vein catheterization. Chronic granulomatous disease is a sex-linked recessive trait in which the polymorphonuclear leukocytes have normal phagocytosis but defective bactericidal function, and patients with this disease are predisposed to hepatic abscess.[85] Clinically, pyogenic liver abscess is her-

alded by chills, fever, hepatomegaly, and right upper quadrant tenderness. There can be one or more lesions, and most involve the right lobe of the liver. Treatment of suppurative hepatic abscesses includes drainage and prolonged antimicrobial therapy. *Staphylococcus aureus,* gram-negative rods, and anaerobic organisms are the most frequent pathogens. Mortality ranges from 25% to 75%.[85]

Anesthetic Management

Anesthetic management for children undergoing hepatic lobe resection or tumor resection involves the same principles that guide the anesthetic care of patients with biliary atresia. Methods of maintaining adequate respiratory ventilation, temperature homeostasis, cardiovascular stability, and fluid management were described earlier. Some patients receive adjunct chemotherapy before surgery. Thus, the chemotherapeutic protocol must be reviewed. Frequently, doxorubicin, an antihracycline, is a major component of the chemotherapy regimen. Doxorubicin may be associated with a dose-dependent, irreversible cardiomyopathy. Although the appearance of a cardiomyopathy is rare with doses less than 200 mg/m^2,[86] cellular lesions can be seen on endomyocardial biopsy.[87] With doxorubicin doses of 200–550 mg/m^2, the appearance of cardiomyopathy is unpredictable, but with doses greater than 550 mg/m^2 the incidence increases. In a study of pediatric patients treated with doxorubicin for childhood leukemia, Lipshitz and others noted in patients who received at least 280 mg/m^2 of doxorubicin that one to 15 years following treatment, 65% of these patients had echocardiographic evidence of increased afterload and/or decreased myocardial contractility.[88] In addition to the total dose of doxorubicin, the investigators also noted that the patient's age at the onset of treatment was an important predictive factor of myocardial dysfunction. Thus the loss of myocytes from doxorubicin in early childhood may cause a loss of left ventricular mass and clinically significant myocardial dysfunction later in life. Therefore, in all patients receiving chemotherapy or patients who have had chemotherapy, a careful physical examination and history should be obtained to evaluate any signs and symptoms of heart failure and to assess cardiac toxicity and cardiac reserve. Because of the potential for massive blood loss in patients undergoing hepatic resection, concerns regarding massive blood replacement are addressed here.

Blood Replacement

In situations in which acute massive blood loss might occur, adequate venous access and invasive monitoring are essential. Two or three large-bore peripheral intravenous catheters are inserted, and a central venous pressure catheter is placed to monitor cardiac filling pressures. Ideally, the intravenous catheters should be placed in the upper extremities. The radial artery, or sometimes the femoral artery, is cannulated, not only to monitor moment-to-moment changes in blood pressure, but also to sample the blood for blood gas, blood chemistry, and blood coagulation profile determinations. Because of the potential for large fluid shifts, a urinary catheter is placed to measure urine output and gauge the adequacy of the perfusion to the kidneys.

Given the difficulty in achieving hemostasis in the resected surfaces of the liver in addition to pre-existing coagulopathies caused by intrinsic liver disease, massive blood volume replacement is a frequent component of the anesthetic resuscitation in children undergoing hepatic resection. Massive blood replacement, defined as the replacement of at least one blood volume, causes a number of physiologic changes that may have anesthetic and surgical consequences. These physiologic alterations include disorders of coagulation, hypothermia, and electrolyte imbalance.

Coagulation defects frequently result in nonsurgical bleeding in patients receiving massive transfusions.[89] Dilutional thrombocytopenia, loss of clotting factors, blood incompatibility, and disseminated intravascular coagulation (DIC) are the major causes. Studies of acute dilutional thrombocytopenia in adults and children suggest that platelet counts of less than 50–100 × 10^9/L correlate with clinical bleeding. The need for platelets perioperatively can be predicted by the preoperative platelet count. Coté and others have shown that the calculated reduction in platelets for a given blood loss is less than the observed platelet count.[90] This is because of platelet mobilization from the bone marrow, lungs, and lymphatic tissue. In addition, Coté and colleagues noted that the starting platelet count was an important factor in determining the need for

platelets during massive blood transfusions (Figure 11-4).[90] The higher the initial platelet count, the more blood volumes could be lost before the administration of platelets was necessary.

When the amount of blood loss approaches one blood volume, levels of labile clotting factors are greatly reduced. Normal clotting requires 20% of factor V and 30% of factor VIII. Most clotting factors are stable in stored blood, but levels of factors V and VIII decrease over time. By 21 days after collection, factors V and VIII decrease to 15% and 50% of their initial activity, respectively.[91] Fresh whole blood may be effective in reversing the coagulopathy associated with massive blood transfusions. Manno and others in a double-blind study involving postoperative pediatric cardiac surgical patients have demonstrated that the transfusion of whole blood less than 48 hours old was associated with significantly less postoperative bleeding than the transfusion of packed red cells, fresh frozen plasma, and platelets.[92] However, most blood banking institutions use component therapy, and fresh whole blood may be difficult to obtain. The composition of the blood components can vary and are listed in Table 11-3.

In the absence of dilutional thrombocytopenia, persistent oozing in a massively transfused patient raises the possibility of blood incompatibility or disseminated intravascular coagulopathy (DIC). General anesthesia frequently masks many of the clinical manifestations of a transfusion reaction. However, tachycardia, hypotension, hemoglobinemia, hemoglobinuria, and non-surgical bleeding require the anesthesiologist to rule out the diagnosis. In patients suspected of a transfusion reaction, it is essential that adequate fluids be administered and that urinary alkalinization and diuresis ensue in order that hemoglobin precipitation in the kidney tubules and acute tubular necrosis are avoided.

DIC is difficult to diagnose and may be hard to distinguish from the underlying coagulopathy associated with liver disease.

Hypothermia

As previously stated, the small child's thermoregulatory mechanisms can be easily overwhelmed, and the transfusion of cold blood products can lead to hypothermia. In the small child, hypothermia can

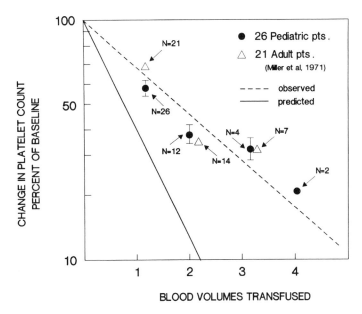

Figure 11-4. Percent of change in platelet count versus blood volumes transfused in adults and children. The broken line represents observed values, whereas the solid line represents calculated values. (Reproduced with permission from Coté, C.J., Liu, L.M.P. and Szyfelbein, S.K. (1985) Changes in serial platelet counts following massive blood transfusions in pediatric patients. *Anesthesiology* 62:197–201.

significantly affect drug pharmacodynamics and pharmacokinetics. Thus, prevention of hypothermia is an essential element of pediatric anesthetic management. A number of warming devices to lessen the effect of cold blood transfusion are available; however, these devices generally do not allow rapid infusion. Heating lamps, room temperature control, devices that heat and humidify inspiratory gases, and warming blankets are standard in all operating rooms that are equipped for children. Efforts to maintain body temperature must continue intraoperatively. If possible, the head should be wrapped in plastic, and if the intestines are exposed, they should be covered and placed in a plastic bag. Both of these measures help reduce heat loss by radiation.

Table 11-3. Differences in Composition of Major Blood Products

	Normal Whole Blood (in vivo)	Citrated Whole Blood (2 weeks old) ACD/CPD	Citrated Packed Red Blood Cells*	Frozen Packed Red Blood Cells	Fresh Frozen Plasma
pH	7.4	6.6–6.9	6.6–6.9	6.6–7.2	6.6–6.9
Pco_2	35–45	180–210	180–210	0–10	180–210
Base deficit (mmol/l)	0	9–15	9–15	?	9–15
Potassium (mmol/l)	3.5–5.0	18–26	18–26	1–2	4–8
Citrate	None	++++	++	None	++++
Factors V and VIII (%)	Normal	20–50	20–50	None	85–100
Fibrinogen	Normal	Normal	Normal	None	Normal
Platelets ×10·ll	240–400	None	None	None	None
2–3 DPG	Normal	3% of normal	3% of normal	Nearly normal	ND
Hematocrit (%)	35–45	35–45	60–70	50–95	ND
Temperature (°C)	37	4–6	4–6	4–6	Cold

Modified from Miller, R. D. (1973) *Refresher Courses in Anesthesiology* 1:101.

*Citrated whole blood and citrated packed red blood cells (PRBCs) have the same chemical composition, but citrated PRBCs have considerably less plasma volume.

ACD/CPD

2–3 DPG: 2,3diphosphoglycerate

ND

Electrolyte Imbalance

In banked blood, potassium gradually leaks from red cells into plasma and after 21–35 days of storage may reach concentrations of 25 mmol/L (see Table 11-3). The potential for hyperkalemia exists in patients who receive massive blood products, especially through central venous catheters; however, hyperkalemia is rarely a problem in whose patients with adequate renal function and in whom the blood is transfused through peripheral venous catheters.

Ionized hypocalcemia secondary to citrate binding of calcium is frequently a complication of blood product administration.[93] The hemodynamic effects of hypocalcemia include hypotension, low cardiac output, and elevated central venous and left atrial filling pressures. These effects generally appear when blood, fresh frozen plasma, and albumin are infused rapidly. Because of the way blood is fractionated into its components, fresh frozen plasma contains the greatest amount of citrate per unit volume of any blood product. Coté showed that infusion of fresh frozen plasma at rates of 1–2.5 mL/kg/min was associated with transient decreases in ionized calcium and with significant decreases in arterial blood pressure.[94] Inhalation anesthetics accentuate the hemodynamic effects of citrate toxicity.[94] In asymptomatic patients, it is unclear whether hypocalcemia needs to be treated.[95,96] In symptomatic patients, equipotent doses of calcium chloride or calcium gluconate are equally efficacious in increasing ionized calcium and in ameliorating the hemodynamic changes.

Portal Hypertension

Extrahepatic, intrahepatic, or suprahepatic obstruction of portal blood flow can result in portal hypertension. Thus, depending on the site of obstruction, liver function may be well preserved or marginal.

Extrahepatic obstruction causes 50–70% of portal hypertension in children and is thought to arise from portal vein thrombosis secondary to umbilical vein catheter insertion, intra-abdominal sepsis, and/or dehydration. In Gaucher's disease, arteriovenous fistulas may develop in the spleen and lead to portal hypertension. Arteriovenous fistulas that occur in the liver and bowel can also lead to portal hypertension.[97] However, in two-thirds of the cases of extrahepatic obstruction, no specific cause can be found. Usually, recanalization occurs and collateral venous channels form, resulting in cavernous transformation of the portal vein. In some children, there is an association of pulmonary hypertension with portal hypertension from cavernous transformation. The associated pulmonary arteriopathy involves medial muscular hypoplasia and hypertrophy. The muscularization extends into the peripheral pulmonary arteries and eventually results in intimal fibroelastosis.[98] Liver function in these patients is well preserved, and bleeding episodes are usually self-limiting and decrease in frequency with age. Medical management generally has been successful, but recently several researchers have demonstrated the feasibility and long-term patency of portasystemic shunts in children 1–16 years of age.[99–102]

Intrahepatic obstruction is associated with intrinsic liver disease. The causes of liver disease associated with cirrhosis are listed in Table 11-4. Many of the known causes of cirrhosis are insidious in onset and often do not progress to portal hypertension until relatively late in childhood. Suprahepatic obstruction (Budd-Chiari syndrome) has been linked to the use of oral contraceptives, and associated with suprahepatic webs, and diaphragms. Hepatic vein occlusions are associated with vasculitis, sickle cell anemia, polycythemia, and leukemia. In patients with suprahepatic obstructions, hepatocellular function deteriorates because of the high-grade outflow blockage.

Shunt Procedures

In the past, effective and reliable portal decompression procedures often were limited by the age of the patient and the size of the vessels to be anastomosed. There has been a high incidence of shunt thrombosis in patients under 10 years of age or if the portavenous anastomosis was less than 10 mm in diameter. However, in 76 children (mean age 7 years) Alvarez and colleagues (1983a, 1983b) demonstrated patency in 92% of shunts placed for portal hypertension,[99,100] and Bismuth, Franco, and Alagille reported a 94% patency rate in children.[102] The type of shunt depends on the patient's underlying disease and anatomy.[103] The hemodynamic and flow characteristics of the shunt vary with the type of shunt and the extent of portal hypertension. The end-to-side portacaval shunt bypasses the liver.

Table 11-4. Causes of Cirrhosis in Infancy and Childhood

Infection	*Obstructive Biliary Disease*
Neonatal viral infection	Extrahepatic atresia
Rubella	Choledochal cyst
Cytomegalovirus	Intrahepatic cholestasis
Coxsackie virus	Congenital hepatic fibrosis
ECHO virus	Infantile polycystic disease
	of liver
Herpes simplex	
Toxoplasmosis	*Vascular Disease*
Acute viral hepatitis	Constrictive pericarditis
Chronic active hepatitis	Pulmonary hypertension
Syphilis	Hepatic vein obstruction
Cholangitis	*Miscellaneous*
Metabolic	Cystic-fibrosis
Galactosemia	Histiocytosis X
Fructosemia	Malnutrition
Glycogen-storage	Drugs, toxins
disease types III, IV	
Niemann-Pick disease	Parenteral nutrition
	(prolonged)
Wolman's disease	Inflammatory bowel
	disease

Cholesterol ester-storage disease
Gaucher's disease
Hurler's disease
Tyrosinemia
Cystinosis
Wilson's disease
α_1-Antitrypsin deficiency
Sickle-cell disease
Thalassemia
Hemochromatosis
Cerebrohepatorenal (Zellweger)
Copper overload

Side-to-side portacaval, splenorenal, and mesocaval shunts direct only a portion of the splanchnic flow into the systemic circulation. With these latter shunts, there is a potential for reversal of flow in the portal vein (Figure 11-5). This may be a factor in late-onset encephalopathy. Clatworthy has noted the feasibility of a central splenorenal shunt and mesocaval shunt in children.[104] Voorhees and colleagues reported that the selective distal splenorenal shunt selectively decompressed the esophageal varices while maintaining portal venous flow.[105] Although the distal splenorenal operation has been successful in children,[106–108] with the success of pediatric patients undergoing liver transplantation, small children with portal hypertension may benefit further by undergoing orthotopic liver transplantation.

Anesthetic Management

Anesthetic considerations for children undergoing shunt procedures are similar to those in the two preceding discussions. Shunt procedures have a tendency to cause quite a bit of blood loss, and, except in patients with prehepatic portal obstruction, end-stage liver disease with minimal hepatic reserve complicates perioperative management. Blood loss can occur as a consequence of the surgical procedure, but it can also occur as a direct complication of the portal hypertension. Hematemesis from esophageal varices, though generally self-limiting, can result in life-threatening exsanguination.

As previously mentioned, the site of obstruction influences the nature of the underlying liver function. Children with intrahepatic and suprahepatic obstruction frequently have underlying cirrhosis. Consequently, the preoperative evaluation of these children must include evaluation for the signs and symptoms of cirrhosis, namely, ascites, splenomegaly, thrombocytopenia, vitamin K deficiency, and neurologic impairment. The patient's respiratory status also must be addressed. Significant alveolar-to-arterial oxygen gradients may exist. Children with end-stage liver disease (cirrhosis) frequently have arterial oxygen partial pressures of 60 or 70. This relative hypoxemia is thought to be due to increased intra-abdominal pressure (ascites), causing relative cephalad displacement of the diaphragm and, in turn, compression and atelectasis of the lung. Other causes of hypoxemia in these patients include pulmonary arteriovenous shunts and parenchymal lung disease. Patients with cirrhosis and portal hypertension frequently have low platelet counts and abnormal coagulation profiles. In patients with prolonged prothrombin times, vitamin K is administered preoperatively. Failure to correct the clotting deficiency may require the administration of fresh frozen plasma or cryoprecipitate. Because of the patient's autoanticoagulated state, premedication is given either orally or intravenously.

Patients with ascites are considered at risk for aspiration. Consequently, a rapid-sequence induction of anesthesia is preferred with cricoid pressure and intravenous thiopental and succinylcholine. After the airway is secured, anesthesia is maintained with oxygen, air, and isoflurane. Nitrous oxide is avoided because it distends the bowel. Atracurium, a nondepolarizing muscle relaxant that does not re-

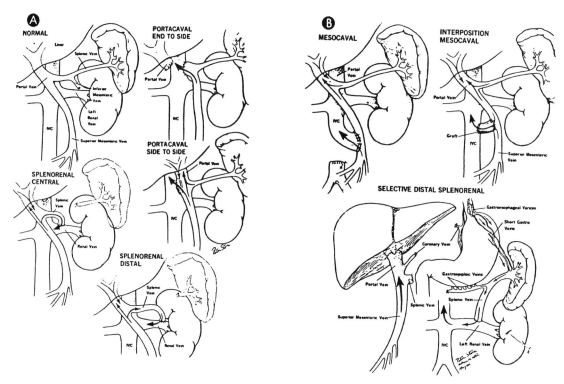

Figure 11-5. Types of portosystemic shunts. (a) In the end-to-side portacaval shunt, all portal flow is diverted to the systemic circulation. In the side-to-side portacaval shunt, the major direction of portal flow is to the systemic circulation, but the capacity for hepatic portal perfusion is retained, depending on the resistance within the liver. Flow dynamics are such that there is a potential for reversal of flow in the portal vein (hepatofugal), shown by broken arrow. In central splenorenal shunt, the principal direction of portal flow is to the systemic circulation. Placing the shunt centrally minimizes angulation of the splenic vein (spleen removed). In distal splenorenal shunt, the major direction of portal flow is to the systemic circulation. Perfusion of the liver with portal blood and potential hepatofugal flow is shown (spleen removed). (b) Mesocaval shunt. The vena cava is transected and the proximal cava is anastomosed to the side of the superior mesenteric vein. The major direction of visceral flow is toward the vena cava. Hepatopetal, as well as potential for hepatofugal, flow is depicted. The interposition mesocaval shunt is hemodynamically similar to the mesocaval shunt. In the selective distal splenorenal shunt, the portal flow is partitioned. Portal inflow to the liver is preserved, while gastroesophageal varices are simultaneously decompressed through short gastric veins and then to the systemic circulation by a distal splenorenal shunt. (Printed with permission from Altman, R.R. (1986) Portal Hypertension. In *Pediatric Surgery* 4th ed. (Welch, K.J., Randolph, J.G., Ravitch, M.M., O'Neill, J.A. and Rowe, M.I. (Eds). pp. 1075–82.)

quire the liver for metabolism, is administered to facilitate muscle relaxation and allow a lower inspired concentration of the potent inhalation agent. Because of the possibility that halothane produces hepatotoxic reductive agents in the presence of tissue hypoxia, isoflurane is frequently used instead as the potent inhalation agent. There is considerable controversy regarding the sensitivity to narcotics of the central nervous system in patients with cirrhosis. Because nitrous oxide is not used, we generally do not administer intraoperative narcotics unless the patient is hemodynamically compromised and is unable to tolerate inhalation anesthesia. However, opioids are administered toward the end of anesthesia and in the postoperative period to alleviate postoperative pain.

Because of the underlying cirrhosis and abnormal coagulation profile, these operative procedures are often lengthy, and blood loss can be excessive. As in patients undergoing liver resection, three large-bore peripheral intravenous catheters are required. Both arterial and central venous pressure catheters are essential for monitoring moment-to-moment changes in the patient's cardiovascular status. The adequacy of ventilation is assessed by blood gas determination, and oxygenation is monitored by pulse oximetry. A urinary catheter is inserted to enable measurement of urine output and renal perfusion. Frequently, patients with hepatic insufficiency require diuretics (furosemide and spironolactone) to correct their sodium and water imbalance. Diuretics should be administered up until operation and may even be needed intraoperatively. Incision through the abdominal cavity in a patient with cirrhosis can lead to significant hemodynamic changes due to release of intra-abdominal pressure, drainage of the ascites, and translocation of fluid from the intravascular compartment. This intravascular fluid depletion can precipitate further liver and renal dysfunction. Spontaneous onset of progressive renal disease frequently occurs in patients with end-stage liver disease. In children undergoing evaluation for possible liver transplantation, Ellis, Avner, and Starzl found a 5% rate of preoperative renal failure, defined as glomerular filtration rate (GFR) ≤ 20 mL/1.75 m². Because renal function in these patients is sensitive to changes in circulating volume, adequate intravascular volume must be maintained. If blood and fluid resuscitation does not restore an adequate urine output (0.5 mL/kg/min), then dopamine is given (5 µg/kg/min).

As with pediatric patients undergoing liver transplantation, hemodynamic instability can be common in children with portal hypertension. Although hypotension is usually related to a decreased circulating blood volume and low ionized calcium level secondary to massive blood volume replacement, other causes should be considered, namely, impaired venous return resulting from compression of the vena cava, acidosis, underlying sepsis, and hypothermia. If volume resuscitation is adequate, the administration of dopamine is begun. Because cardiovascular stability is important in these patients, and because their renal function may be marginal, diligence in replacing blood loss and maintaining an adequate circulating blood volume cannot be overstressed.

Summary

Pediatric anesthesia involves the anesthetic management of patients undergoing rapid change and growth in both the structure and the function of organs. Anesthetic considerations for children undergoing various types of hepatic surgery necessitate not only a knowledge of the underlying disease and its pathophysiologic significance, but also an understanding of the developmental changes that occur with age and maturation. It is meticulous attention to detail, the understanding of age-related changes in physiology and their pharmacological implications, and the realization that infants and children are not miniature adults that have improved the perioperative morbidity and mortality in these patients.

References

1. Shim, W.K.T., Kasai, M. and Spence, M.A. (1974) Racial influence on the incidence of biliary atresia. *Progressive Pediatric Surgery,* 6:53.
2. Lilly, J.R. and Chandra, R.S. (1974) Surgical hazards of co-existing anomalies in biliary atresia. *Surgery, Gynecology and Obstetrics,* 139:49.
3. Nietgen, G.W., Vacanti, J.P. and Perez-Atayde, A.R. (1992). Intrahepatic bile duct loss in biliary atresia despite portoenterostomy: A consequence of ongoing obstruction. *Gastroenterology* 102:2126.
4. Ohi, R., Hanamatsu, M., Mochizuki, I., Chiba, T. and Kusai, M. (1985) Progress in the treatment of biliary atresia. *World Journal of Surgery,* 9:285.
5. Lilly, J.R. (1976) The surgery of biliary hypoplasia. *Journal of Pediatric Surgery* 11:815.
6. Kasai, M., Kimura, S., Asakura, Y. et al. (1968) Surgical treatment of biliary atresia. *Journal of Pediatric Surgery* 3:665.
7. Lilly, J.R. (1986) The jaundiced infant. In: *Pediatric Surgery,* 4th ed. (Welch, K.J., Randolph, J.G., Ravitch, M.M., O'Neill, J.A. and Rowe, M.I. (eds.). pp. 1047–1054.
8. Barkin, R.M. and Lilly, J.R. (1980) Biliary atresia and the Kasai operation: Continuing care. *Journal of Pediatrics* 88:1015.
9. Kasai, M. (1974) Treatment of biliary atresia with special reference to hepatic portoenterostomy and its modifications. *Progressive Pediatric Surgery* 6:5.
10. Odievre, M., Valayer, J., Razemon-Pinta, M. et al. (1976) Hepatic portoenterostomy or cholecystostomy in the treatment of extrahepatic biliary atresia. *Journal of Pediatrics* 88:774.
11. Altman, R.P., Chandra, R., Lilly, J.R. (1975). Ongoing cirrhosis after successful porticoenterostomy in infants with biliary atresia. *Journal of Pediatric Surgery* 10:685.
12. Kasai, M., Watanabe, I. and Ohi, R. (1975). Follow-up studies of long-term survivors after hepatic portoenterostomy for 'noncorrectable' biliary atresia. *Journal of Pediatric Surgery* 10:173.
13. Chiba, T., Ohi, R., Nio, M. and Ibrahim, M. (1992) Late complications in long term survivors of biliary atresia. *European Journal of Pediatric Surgery* 2:22.
14. Laurent, J., Gauthier, F., Bernard, O. et al. (1990) Long-term outcome after surgery for biliary atresia. Study of 40 patients surviving for more than 10 years. *Gastroenterology* 99:1793.

15. Engelskirchen, R., Holschneider, A.M., Gharib, M. and Vente, C. (1991) Biliary atresia—a 25-year survey. *European Journal of Pediatric Surgery* 1:154.

16. Kasai, M., Ohi, R. and Chiba, T. (1986) Long term survivors of biliary atresia. In: *Biliary Atresia Proceedings of the 4th International Symposium on Biliary Atresia.* Sendai, 1986, Professional Postgraduate Services, Tokyo, p. 277.

17. Starzl, T.E., Iwatsuki, S. and Shaw, P.W. (1986) Liver transplantation. In: *Pediatric Surgery,* (Welch, K.J. et al. eds). Chicago, Year Book Medical Publishers, Inc. 1, 373.

18. Falchetti, D., deCarvalho, B., Clapuyt, P., deVille deLeoyet deHeuptinne, B., Claus, D. and Otte, J.B. (1991) Liver transplantation in children with biliary atresia and polysplenic syndrome. *Journal of Pediatric Surgery* 26:528.

19. Lloyd-Still, J.D. (1991) Impact of orthotopic liver transplantation on the mortality from pediatric liver disease. *Journal of Pediatric Gastroenterology and Nutrition* 12:305.

20. O'Neill, J.A. (1986) Choledochal cyst. In: *Pediatric Surgery,* 4th ed., (Welch, K.J., Randolph, J.G., Ravitch, M.M., O'Neill, J.A. and Rowe, M.I. eds). pp. 1056–1059.

21. Kasai, M., Asakura, Y. and Taira, Y. (1970) Surgical treatment of choledochal cyst. *Annals of Surgery* 172:844.

22. Todani, T., Narusue, M., Watanabe, Y. *et al.* (1978) Management of congenital choledochal cyst with intrahepatic involvement. *Annals of Surgery* 187:272.

23. Friesen, R.H., and Lichtor, J.L. (1982) Cardiovascular depression during halothane anesthesia in infants: A study of three induction techniques. *Anesthesia and Analgesia* 61:42.

23a. Friesen, R.H., and Lichtor, J.L. (1983) Cardiovascular effects of inhalation induction with isoflurane in infants. *Anesthesia and Analgesia* 62:411.

24. Rackow, H., Salanitre, E. and Green, L.T. (1961) Frequency of cardiac arrest associated with anesthesia in infants and children. *Pediatrics* 28:697.

25. Salanitre, E. and Rackow, H. (1969) The pulmonary exchange of nitrous oxide and halothane in infants and children. *Anesthesiology* 30:388.

26. Eger, El., Bahlman, S.H. and Munson, E.S. (1971) The effect of age on the rate of increase of alveolar anesthetic concentration. *Anesthesiology* 35:365.

27. Rackow, H. and Salanitre, E. (1974) The pulmonary equilibration of cyclopropane in infants and children. *British Journal of Anesthesia* 46:35.

28. Gibbs, C.P., Munson, E.S. and Tham, M.K. (1975) Anesthetic solubility coefficients for maternal and fetal blood. *Anesthesiology* 43:100.

29. Steward, D.J. and Creighton, R.E. (1978) The uptake and excretion of nitrous oxide in the newborn. *Canadian Anaesthetists Society Journal* 25:215.

30. Brandom, B.W., Brandom, R.B. and Cook, D.R. (1983) Uptake and distribution of halothane in infants: In vivo measurements and computer simulations. *Anesthesia and Analgesia* 62:404.

31. Lerman, J., Gregory, G.A., Willis, M.M. and Eger, El. II. (1984) Age and solubility of volatile anesthetics in blood. *Anesthesiology* 61:139.

32. Cook, D.R., Brandom, B.W., Shiu, G. and Wolfson, B.W. (1981) The inspired median effective dose, brain concentration at anesthesia, and cardiovascular index for halothane in young rats. *Anesthesia and Analgesia* 60:182.

33. Gregory, G.A., Eger, El. II and Munson, E.S. (1969) The relationship between age and halothane requirements in man. *Anesthesiology* 30:488.

34. Nicodemus, H.F., Nassiri-Rahimi, C. and Bachman, L. (1969) Median effective dose (ED_{50}) of halothane in adults and children. *Anesthesiology* 31:344.

35. Gregory, G.A., Wade, J.G., Beihl, D.R., Ong, B.Y. and Sitar, D.S. (1983) Fetal anesthetic requirement (MAC) for halothane. *Anesthesia and Analgesia* 62:9.

36. Lerman, J., Robinson, S., Willis, M.M. and Gregory, G. (1983) Anesthetic requirements for halothane in young children 0–1 month and 1–6 months of age. *Anesthesiology* 59:421.

37. Taylor, R.H. and Lerman, J. (1992) Induction, maintenance, and recovery characteristics of desflurane in infants and children. *Canadian Journal of Anaesthesia* 39:6.

38. Duncan, P., Gregory, G.A. and Wade, J.A. (1981) The effects of nitrous oxide on the baroreceptor response of newborn and adult rabbits. *Canadian Anaesthetists Society Journal* 18:339.

39. Gregory, G.A. (1982) The baroresponses of preterm infants during halothane anesthesia. *Canadian Anaesthetists Society Journal* 29:105.

40. Wear, R., Robinson, S. and Gregory, G.A. (1982) The effect of halothane on the baroresponse of adult and baby rabbits. *Anesthesiology* 56:188.

41. Gootman, P.M., Gootman, N. and Buckley, B. (1983) Maturation of central autonomic control of the circulation. *Federation Proceedings* 42:1648.

42. Shires, T., Williams, J. and Brown, F. (1961) Acute changes in extracellular fluids associated with major surgical procedures. *Annals of Surgery* 154:810.

43. Rowe, M.I. and Arango, A. (1971) The neonatal response to massive fluid infusion. *Journal of Pediatric Surgery* 6:365.

44. Rowe, M.I. and Arango, A. (1975) The choice of intravenous fluid in shock resuscitation. *Pediatric Clinics of North America* 22:269.

45. Rowe, M.I. and Arango, A. (1976) Colloid versus crystalloid resuscitation in experimental bowel obstruction. *Journal of Pediatric Surgery* 11:635.

46. Bennett, E.J. (1975) Fluid balance in the newborn. *Anesthesiology* 43:210.

47. Holliday, M.A. and Segar, W.E. (1957) The maintenance need for water in parenteral fluid therapy. *Pediatrics* 19:823.

48. Roy, R.N. and Sinclair, J.C. (1975) Hydration of the low-birth-weight infant. *Clinical Perinatology* 2:393.

49. Bell, E.F. and Oh, W. (1979) Fluid and electrolyte balance in very low birth weight infants. *Clinical Perinatology* 6:139.

50. Bourke, D.L. and Smith, T.C. (1974) Estimating allowable hemodilution. *Anesthesiology* 41:609.

51. Furman, E.B., Roman, D.G., Lemmer, L.A.S., Hairabet, J., Jasinska, M. and Laver, M.B. (1975) Specific therapy in water, electrolyte and blood-volume replacement during pediatric surgery. *Anesthesiology* 42:187.

52. Eger, E. (1974). *Anesthetic Uptake and Action.* Baltimore, Williams and Wilkins, pp. 1–25.

53. Ham, G.C., Miller, R.D., Benet, L.Z. et al. (1978) The pharmacokinetics and pharmacodynamics of *d*-tubocurarine during hypothermia in the cat. *Anesthesiology* 49:324.

54. Miller, R.D., Agoston, S., Van der Pol, F. et al. (1978) Hypothermia and pharmacokinetics and pharmacodynamics of pancuronium in the cat. *European Journal of Clinical Pharmacology* 32:373.

55. Koren, G., Barker, C., Goresky, G. et al. (1987) The influence of hypothermia on the disposition of fentanyl—human and animal studies. *European Journal of Clinical Pharmacology* 32:373.

56. Kadar, D., Tang, B.K. and Conn, A.W. (1982) The fate of phenobarbitone in children in hypothermia and at normal body temperature. *Canadian Anaesthetists Society Journal* 29:16.

57. Rink, R.A., Gray, I., Rueckert, R.R. and Slocum, H.C. (1956) The effect of hypothermia on morphine metabolism in an isolated perfused liver. *Anesthesiology* 17:377.

58. Goudsouzian, N.G., Morris, R.H. and Ryan, J.F. (1973) The effects of a warming blanket on the maintenance of body temperatures in anesthetized infants and children. *Anesthesiology* 39:351.

59. Williams, R. (1984) Drug administration in hepatic disease. *New England Journal of Medicine* 309:1616.

60. Davis, P.J., Stiller, R.L., Cook, D.R., Brandom, B.W., Davis, P. and Scierka, A.M. (1989) Effects of cholestatic hepatic disease and chronic renal failure on alfentanil pharmacokinetics in children. *Anesthesia and Analgesic* 68:579.

61. Ferrier, C., Marty, J., Bouffard, M.D., Haberer, J.P., Levron, J.C. and Duvaldestin, M.D. (1985) Alfentanil pharmacokinetics in patients with cirrhosis. *Anesthesiology* 62:480.

62. Haberer, J.P., Schoeffler, P., Couderc, E. and Duvaldestin, P. (1982) Fentanyl pharmacokinetics in anaesthetized patients with cirrhosis. *British Journal of Anaesthesia* 54:1267.

63. Patwardhan, R.V., Johnson, R.F., Hoyumpa, A. Jr. et al. (1981) Normal metabolism of morphine in cirrhosis. *Gastroenterology* 81:1006.

64. Cook, D.R., Freeman, J.A., Lai, A.A. et al. (1991) Pharmacokinetics and pharmacodynamics of doxacurium in normal patients and in those with hepatic or renal failure. *Anesthesia and Analgesia* 72:145.

65. Cook, D.R., Freeman, J.A., Lai, A.A. et al. (1992) Pharmacokinetics of mivacurium in normal patients and in those with hepatic or renal failure. *British Journal of Anaesthesia* (In press).

66. Baden, J.M., Kundomal, Y.R., Luttropp, M.E., Maze, M. and Kosek, J.C. (1985) Effects of volatile anesthetics or fentanyl on hepatic function in cirrhotic rats. *Anesthesia and Analgesia* 64:1183.

66a. Gelman, S., Fowler, K.C. and Smith, L.R. (1984) Liver circulation and function during isoflurane and halothane anesthesia. *Anesthesiology* 61:726.

67. Fassoulaki, A., Eger, El., Johnson, B.H. et al. (1984) Nitrous oxide, too, is hepatotoxic in rats. *Anesthesia and Analgesia* 63:1076.

68. Edmondson, H.A. (1956) Differential diagnosis of tumors and tumor-like lesions of liver in infancy and childhood. *American Journal of Diseases of Children* 91:168.

69. deLorimier, A.A. (1977) Hepatic tumors of infancy and childhood. *Surgery Clinics of North America* 57:443.

70. Exelby, P.R., Filler, R.M. and Grosfeld, J.L. (1975) Liver tumors in children in particular reference to hepatoblastoma and hepatocellular carcinoma: American Academy of Pediatrics surgical section survey–1974. *Journal of Pediatric Surgery* 10:329.

71. Howell, R.R., Stevenson, R.E., Ben-Menachem, Y., Phyliky, R.L. and Berry, D.H. (1976) Hepatic adenomata with type 1 glycogen storage disease. *Journal of the American Medical Association* 236:481.

72. Edmonds, A.M., Hennigar, G.R. and Crooks, R. (1952) Galactosemia: Report of a case with autopsy. *Pediatrics* 10:40.

73. deLorimier, A.A., Simpson, E.B., Baum, R.S. and Carlsson E. (1967) Hepatic-artery ligation for hepatic hemangiomatosis. *New England Journal of Medicine* 277:333.

74. Geiser, C.F., Baez, A., Schindler, A.M. and Shik, V.E. (1970) Epithelial hepatoblastoma associated with congenital hemihypertrophy and cystathionuria. *Pediatrics* 46:66.

75. Sotelo-Avila, C., Gooch, W.M., III (1976) Neoplasms associated with the Beckwith-Wiedenmann syndrome. *Perspectives in Pediatric Pathology* 3:255.

76. Exelby, P.R., El-Domeri, A., Huvos, A.G. and Beattie, E.J. Jr. (1971) Primary malignant tumors of the liver in children. *Journal of Pediatric Surgery* 6:272.

77. Fraumeni, J.F., Jr, Rosen, P.J., Hull, E.W., Barth, R.F., Shapiro, S.R. and O'Connor, J.F. (1969) Hepatoblastoma in infant sisters. *Cancer* 24:1086.

78. Jones, E. (1960) Primary carcinoma of the liver with associated cirrhosis in infants and children: Report of a case. *Archives of Pathology* 75:5.

79. Zangeneh, F., Limbeck, G.A., Brown, B.I. et al. (1969) Hepatorenal glycogenosis (type I glycogenosis) and carcinoma of the liver. *Journal of Pediatrics* 74:73.

80. Palmer, P.E. and Wolfe, J.H. (1970) α-antitrypsin deposition in primary hepatic carcinomas. *Archives of Pathology and Laboratory Medicine* 100:232.

81. Weinberg, A.G., Mize, C.E. and Worthen, H.G. (1976) The occurrence of hepatoma in the chronic form of hereditary tyrosinemia. *Journal of Pediatrics* 88:434.

82. Dehner, L.P. (1978) Hepatic tumors in the pediatric age group: A distinctive clinicopathologic spectrum. *Perspectives in Pediatric Pathology* 4:217.

83. DeBakey, M.E. and Jordan, G.L. Jr. (1977) Hepatic abscesses, both intra- and extrahepatic. *Surgery Clinics of North America* 57:325.

84. Kaplan, S.L. and Feigin, R.D. (1976) Pyogenic liver abscess in normal children with fever of unknown origin. *Pediatrics* 58:614.

85. Chusid, M.J. (1978) Pyogenic hepatic abscess in infancy and childhood. *Pediatrics* 62:554.

86. Lenaz, L. and Page, J.A. (1976) Cardiotoxicity of adriamycin and related anthracyclines. *Cancer Treatment Reviews* 3:111.

87. Bristow, M.R., Mason, J.W., Billingham, M.E. and Daniels, J.R. (1978) Doxorubicin cardiomyopathy. Evaluation by phonocardiography, endomyocardial biopsy and cardiac catheterization. *Annals of Intestinal Medicine* 88:168.

88. Lipschitz, S.E., Colan, S.D., Gelber, R.D., Perez-Atayde, A.R., Sallan, S.E. and Sanders, S.P. (1991) Late cardiac effects of doxorubicin therapy for acute lymphoblastic leukemia in childhood. *New England Journal of Medicine* 324:808.

89. Miller, R.D., Robbins, T.O., Targ, M.I. et al. (1974) Coagulation defects associated with massive blood transfusions. *Annals of Surgery* 174:794.

90. Coté, C.J., Liu, L.M.P., Szyfelbein, S.K., Goudsouzian, N.G. and Daniels, A.L. (1985) Changes in serial platelet counts following massive blood transfusion in pediatric patients. *Anesthesiology* 62:197.

91. Kruskall, M. S., Mintz, P.D., Bergin, J.J., et al. (1983) Transfusion therapy in emergency medicine. *Annals of Emergency Medicine* 17:327.

92. Manno, C.S., Hedberg, K.W., Kim, H.C. et al. (1991) Comparison of the hemostatic effects of fresh whole blood, stored whole blood, and components after open heart surgery in children. *Blood* 77:930.

93. Denlinger, J.K., Nahrwold, M. L., Gibbs, P.S. and Lecky, J.H. (1976) Hypocalcemia during rapid blood transfusion in anaesthetized man. *British Journal of Anaesthesia* 48:995.

94. Coté, C.J. (1987) Depth of halothane anesthesia potentiates citrate-induced ionized hypocalcemia and adverse cardiovascular events in dogs. *Anesthesiology* 67:676.

95. Linko, K. (1986) Electrolyte and acide-base disturbances caused by blood transfusions. *Acta Anaesthesiologica Scandinavica* 30:139.

96. Kahn, R.C., Jascott, D., Carlon, G.C. et al. (1979) Massive blood replacement: Correlation of ionized calcium, citrate, and hydrogen ion concentration. *Anesthesia and Analgesia* 58:274.

97. Shulman, R.J., Holmes, R., Ferry, G.D. and Finegold, M. (1986) Splanchnic and vascular malformations and development of portal hypertension. *Journal of Pediatric Surgery* 21:355.

98. Silver, M.M., Bohn, D., Shawn, D., Shuckett, B., Eich, G. and Rabinovitch, M. (1992) Association of pulmonary hypertension with congenital portal hypertension in a child. *Journal of Pediatrics* 120:321.

99. Alvarez, F., Bernhard O., Brunelle, F. et al. (1983) Portal obstruction in children. I. Clinical investigation and hemorrhage risk. *Journal of Pediatrics* 103:696.

100. Alvarez, F., Bernhard, O., Brunelle, F. et al. (1983) Portal obstruction in children. II. Results of surgical portosystemic shunts. *Journal of Pediatrics* 103:703.

101. Bismuth, H., Franco, D. (1976) Portal diversion for portal hypertension in early childhood. *Annals of Surgery* 180:439.

102. Bismuth, H., Franco, D. and Alagille, D. (1980) Portal diversion for portal hypertension in children, the first ninety patients. *Annals of Surgery* 192:18.

103. Altman, R.P. (1986) Portal hypertension. In *Pediatric Surgery* 4th ed. (Welch, K.J., Randolph, J.G., Ravitch, M.M., O'Neill, J.A. and Rowe, M. I. eds). pp. 1075–1082.

104. Clatworthy, W.H. (1991) Big shunts for small patients with portal hypertension: A bit of history. *Journal of Pediatric Surgery* 25:1087.

105. Voorhees, A.B., Chaitman, E., Schneider, S. et al. (1973) Portasytemic encephalopathy in the noncirrhotic patient. *Archives of Surgery* 107:659.

106. Rodgers, B.M. and Talbert, J.L. (1979) Distal splenorenal shunt for portal decompression in children. *Journal of Pediatric Surgery* 14:33.

107. Maksoud, J.G and Mils, S. (1982) Distal splenorenal shunt (DSS) in children. *Annals of Surgery* 195:401.

108. Maksoud, J.G., Goncalves, M.L., Porta, G., Miura, I. and Velhote, C.O. (1981) Endoscopic and surgical management of portal hypertension in children: Analysis of 123 cases. *Journal of Pediatric Surgery* 26:178.

109. Ellis, D., Avner, E.D. and Starzl, T.E. (1986) Renal failure in children with hepatic failure undergoing liver transplantation. *Journal of Pediatrics* 108:393.

Chapter 12
Obstetric Patients with Liver Disease

Raymond D. Seifert and Yoogoo Kang

The management of hepatic impairment is dramatically complicated when the patient is also pregnant. Yet, with an understanding of the pathophysiology of hepatic failure and maternal–fetal medicine, these patients can be successfully treated, with encouraging outcomes for both mother and child. Therefore, clinicians need to be familiar with the physiologic changes that occur during pregnancy and the multiorgan pathophysiologic conditions unique to patients with liver disease. This chapter presents the various liver diseases that complicate pregnancy, the effects of pregnancy on hepatic function, and medical and anesthetic management.

Physiologic Changes during Pregnancy

A comprehensive review of the physiologic changes that occur during pregnancy can be found in several sources and is beyond the scope of this chapter.[1–3] However, major alterations involving each organ system deserve a brief description.

The Cardiovascular System

Changes in the cardiovascular system are summarized in Table 12-1. Cardiac output increases 40% because of an increase in blood volume and a decrease in peripheral vascular resistance. Total blood volume increases approximately 1,500 mL, and plasma volume increases nearly twice as much as the red blood cell volume, producing the "anemia of pregnancy." Vasodilation caused by increased progesterone and prostacyclin levels decreases blood pressure approximately 15% and increases blood flow to the uterus, kidneys, and extremities.[4,5] A grade II/VI flow murmur can result from this hyperdynamic circulatory system, but grade III/VI murmurs, diastolic murmurs, arrhythmia, or cardiomegaly frequently signal a compromised circulatory system.

Significant hypotension can develop from as early as week 20 of gestation if the parturient assumes the supine position, allowing the uterus to compress the abdominal aorta and inferior vena cava.[6] Aortocaval compression decreases venous return and cardiac output and raises uterine venous pressure. This, in turn, results in decreased uterine perfusion pressure because autoregulation does not exist in the uterus. The consequences can range from mild changes in the fetal heart rate to sustained fetal bradycardia and fetal acidosis: systolic blood pressure < 70 mmHg is associated with sustained fetal bradycardia.[7,8] The effects of the aortocaval compression improve when the woman returns to the lateral position.[9] Therefore, the supine position should be avoided at all costs by using a left uterine displacement device (e.g., commercial devices, pillows, blankets). A net increase in oxygen transport

Table 12-1. Changes in the Cardiovascular System during Pregnancy

Blood volume	+35%
Plasma volume	+45%
Red blood cell volume	+20%
Cardiac output	+40%
Stroke volume	+30%
Heart rate	+15%
Total peripheral resistance	+15%
Mean arterial pressure	−15%
Central venous pressure	0
Femoral venous pressure	+15 mmHg

Modified from Gutsche, B.B. (1979) Maternal physiologic alterations during pregnancy. In *Anesthesia for Obstetrics*, (Shnider, S.M. and Levinson, G., eds.) Baltimore: Williams and Wilkins, p. 6.

to the tissues is seen during pregnancy because increased cardiac output, decreased blood viscosity, lower systemic vascular resistance, hyperventilation, and shift of P_{50} to the right offset the effects of the anemia of pregnancy (16–19.5 mL/dL).[10,11]

The Respiratory System

An increased progesterone level augments minute ventilation approximately 50% by raising the respiratory rate and tidal volume (Table 12-2). Total lung capacity is only slightly reduced, if at all.[12] However, functional residual capacity, expiratory reserve vol-

Table 12-2. Changes in the Respiratory System during Pregnancy

Minute ventilation	+50%
Alveolar ventilation	+70%
Tidal volume	+40%
Respiratory rate	+15%
Dead space	0
Airway resistance	−36%
Total lung capacity	−0–5%
Inspiratory lung capacity	+5%
Functional residual capacity	−20%
Expiratory reserve volume	−20%
Residual volume	−20%
Vital capacity	0
Closing volume	0
Total compliance	−30%
Lung compliance	0
Chest wall compliance	−45%

Modified from Gutsche, B.B. (1979) Maternal physiologic alterations during pregnancy. In *Anesthesia for Obstetrics*, (Shnider, S.M. and Levinson, G., eds.) Baltimore: Williams and Wilkins, p. 4.

ume, and residual volume are reduced approximately 20% by the upward pressure of the abdominal contents, particularly in the supine position. Decreased functional residual capacity, increased oxygen consumption, and early airway closure predispose the pregnant patient to hypoxemia.

The Central Nervous System

Mean alveolar concentration levels of anesthetics are decreased by 20–40% during pregnancy,[13] possibly owing to the increased levels of progesterone and beta-endorphins.[14] Pregnant patients require a lower total volume of local anesthetics to produce adequate levels of epidural anesthesia because of increased pressure in the epidural space from venous engorgement, increased cerebrospinal fluid pressure from uterine contractions,[15] and possibly increased sensitivity to local anesthetics.[16] Although plasma cholinesterase activity is reduced approximately 25% during pregnancy,[17] prolonged neuromuscular blockade after the administration of usual doses of succinylcholine is relatively uncommon.

The Digestive System

Esophageal reflux and decreased gastric outflow are likely to develop in pregnancy owing to the positional changes in the digestive system, higher levels of progesterone, and lower levels of motilin.[18–20] Secretion of gastrin by the placenta causes increased gastric acid secretion. Therefore, the risk for aspiration pneumonitis is greater during pregnancy.[21] A higher incidence (as much as 66%) of esophageal varices is seen in late pregnancy from increased venous flow through the azygos system.[22–24]

The Hepatic System

Hepatic function and hepatic blood flow are essentially unchanged during a normal pregnancy. However, the proportion of the cardiac output directed to the liver decreases from 35% to 29%.[25] "Sluggish gallbladder of pregnancy" and increased lithogenecity of the bile salts predispose the patient to cholecystitis.[23,26]

Table 12-3. Changes in Laboratory Values during Pregnancy

Laboratory Test	Percent Change
Hemoglobin	−20
Hematocrit	−20
Blood urea nitrogen (BUN)	−40
Creatinine	−40
Glucose (fasting)	−10 to 0
Glucose (postprandial)	0
Prothrombin time	0
Partial thromboplastin time	0
Platelet count	−20
Aspartate aminotransferase (AST)	0
Alanine aminotransferase (ALT)	0
Lactate dehydrogenase (LDH)	0
Albumin	30
Alkaline phosphatase	+200
Bilirubin	−6 to 2
Cholesterol	+50
Triglycerides	+300

Laboratory values reflecting hepatic function show a variety of changes during pregnancy (Table 12-3). The transaminases, aspartate aminotransferase (AST) and alanine aminotransferase (ALT), remain at normal levels during pregnancy but may increase slightly as term approaches.[27] Lactate dehydrogenase remains essentially unchanged during pregnancy. The alkaline phosphatase level increases throughout pregnancy and reaches nearly twice the normal value at full term, owing to placental secretion of alkaline phosphatase and fetal bone maturation.[28] Total serum bilirubin may increase slightly but rarely is greater than 2 mg/dL.[29] One in five pregnancies is accompanied by an increased direct fraction of bilirubin despite a normal total bilirubin level, possibly from reduced maximal bilirubin excretory capacity.[30] Triglycerides increase by as much as 300%, and cholesterol increases by 50–100%.[31] Alpha-fetoprotein can be detected in pregnant women, and increased levels of alpha-fetoprotein have been associated with fetal neural tube defects, anencephaly, and maternal hepatocellular carcinoma.

The Renal System

Serum blood urea nitrogen (BUN) and serum creatinine levels fall to about 40% of normal values owing to increased glomerular filtration rate and renal plasma flow. Renal dysfunction should be suspected if a pregnant woman has "normal" nonpregnancy values for either BUN or creatinine.

Glucose Metabolism

Although blood glucose levels frequently remain within the normal range, pregnancy results in a diabetogenic condition. Human placental lactogen promotes lipolysis, inhibits gluconeogenesis, increases insulin release, and induces a resistance to insulin. Also, estrogen and progesterone cause beta-cell hyperplasia and greater insulin production.[32]

The Hematopoietic and Coagulation Systems

The hemoglobin concentration falls during pregnancy, but it should not be less than 1.7 mmol/L (11 g/dL). When anemia occurs, it is most commonly caused by iron deficiency. During the third trimester, the increased levels of circulating estrogens and cortisol raise the leukocyte count.[33] Pregnancy induces a hypercoagulable state. Levels of factors I (fibrinogen), VII, VIII, and X increase dramatically, and the platelet count decreases approximately 20% because of the increased plasma volume. However, prothrombin time, bleeding time, platelet function, and fibrinolytic activity are unaltered by pregnancy.

Pathophysiologic Changes Seen in Liver Disease

The pathophysiologic changes in patients with liver disease deserve a brief description because they mimic or potentiate the physiologic changes of pregnancy.

A hyperdynamic circulatory system is a well-known feature in patients with severe liver disease and includes high cardiac output, tachycardia, low peripheral vascular resistance, low arterial blood pressure, and arteriovenous shunting. Because patients in this state have little remaining cardiac reserve, they may not be able to cope with the added demand or stress of pregnancy or of labor.

Hypoxemia and respiratory alkalosis are common and are associated with "true shunts" in the lung, ventilation/perfusion mismatch from pleural effusions and ascites, and impaired hypoxic pulmonary vasoconstriction.[34] Therefore, pregnant patients with hepatic dysfunction are prone to becoming severely hypoxemic. Hepatic encephalopathy should be differentiated from neurologic changes associated with pregnancy, because preeclampsia or eclampsia presents a grave prognosis. The hepatorenal syndrome is common and may be caused by increased aldosterone levels, reduced plasma volume, and increased renal tubular reabsorption of sodium. Other types of organ dysfunction in patients with liver disease include displacement of the diaphragm by ascites, malabsorption, reduced gastrointestinal tract motility, glucose intolerance, insulin resistance, anemia, pancytopenia, and coagulopathy.

Hepatic Dysfunction during Pregnancy

The incidence of pregnancy complicated by liver disease is relatively low, although a broad spectrum of liver diseases can develop: from mild, reversible, and nonicteric hepatic dysfunction at one end to fulminant hepatic failure at the other. The incidence of jaundice during pregnancy varies from 1:1,500 to 1:5,000 normal pregnancies.[35,36] Viral hepatitis caused by hepatitis A, B, or non-A, non-B and by herpes simplex virus remains the most common cause of icteric hepatic dysfunction, accounting for 40% of cases.[35,37] The incidence of non-icteric hepatic dysfunction is unknown. Cholestasis is responsible for approximately 20% of patients with non-icteric hepatic dysfunction.

Liver Disease Occurring after but Unrelated to Pregnancy

Viral Hepatitis

Viral hepatitis, the most common cause of jaundice during pregnancy, occurs more frequently in pregnant women than in either men or nonpregnant women.[38] Pregnant women are prone to a fulminant and often fatal process.[39,40] Premature birth, in one study, was two to three times more common in patients with hepatitis.[41]

Patients with acute viral hepatitis A develop generalized malaise, fever, nausea and vomiting, right upper quadrant tenderness, and jaundice. A marked increase in the results of liver function tests enables the distinction between acute hepatitis A and cholestasis or acute fatty liver (AFL) of pregnancy. The last two entities cause only a modest increase in liver enzymes. Management consists of supportive therapy, and symptoms should abate in 2–3 weeks. Chronic hepatic dysfunction is uncommon, and fetal wasting has not been shown to be greater in patients with acute hepatitis A except in severe cases. Transmission of the virus to the fetus does not lead to chronic liver disease in the neonate.

The signs and symptoms of acute hepatitis B are essentially the same as for hepatitis A. Detection of the surface antigen (HB_sAg) in the maternal serum confirms the diagnosis, and patients usually recover completely. Mortality of pregnant patients with a clinical picture of viral hepatitis is greater when serologic markers are not found,[38,42] suggesting that hepatic diseases other than hepatitis B may account for the high mortality in pregnancy.

The hepatitis B virus does not readily cross the placenta, although it may occur when the mother is a chronic carrier (persistent HB_sAg) or when active hepatitis B virus is present during the third trimester. Infants usually acquire the virus by exposure to maternal blood during delivery. About 40–50% of all infants born to mothers with hepatitis B are positive for HB_sAg.[43] Low titers of HB_sAg have been detected in the breast milk of mothers who are antigen positive. However, breast-feeding probably is an unusual means of transmission of the disease. The natural history for infants of mothers with hepatitis B is unknown. Approximately 50% of infants born to mothers with non-A, non-B hepatitis have increased liver enzymes at birth. These infants apparently do not develop chronic liver disease,[44] although some develop chronic liver disease and hepatoma. It has been recommended that infants born to mothers who are HB_sAg positive receive hepatitis immune globulin at birth.

Acute fulminant hepatitis, though rarely seen in pregnancy, is life-threatening in this situation. Therefore, a correct diagnosis, by liver biopsy, is of paramount importance. Management of patients with acute fulminant hepatitis is controversial. There have been case reports of successful delivery as well as reports of maternal and fetal demise with either immediate or delayed delivery.

Drug-Induced Hepatitis

Given the reluctance of expectant mothers to ingest medication and of obstetricians to prescribe it for them, there is little information available regarding drug-induced hepatic injury. Furthermore, there is no evidence of an increased incidence of drug-induced hepatotoxicity during pregnancy. The clinical course of tetracycline-induced fatty infiltration of the liver is similar to that of AFL of pregnancy[45] and carries a maternal mortality approaching 80%. Hepatotoxicity has been reported with the use of erythromycin estolate,[46] halothane,[47] and methoxyflurane.[48]

Biliary Tract Diseases

Biliary colic, frequently caused by decreased gallbladder motility, is not uncommon during pregnancy, but obstructive jaundice is rare.[49] Acute cholecystitis usually responds to conservative therapy. However, cholecystectomy can be performed without an increase in maternal or fetal morbidity.[23] Pregnant women can also have pancreatitis, which usually is associated with cholelithiasis,[50,51] AFL of pregnancy, or preeclampsia.[52]

Systemic Infection

Profound hepatic derangement can follow septicemia, particularly with severe pyelonephritis.

Alcoholic Liver Disease

Maternal alcoholism is associated with an increased risk of first trimester fetal wasting and a higher incidence of congenital anomalies in infants of mothers who are heavy drinkers (39%) compared with nondrinkers (9%).[53] Fetal alcohol syndrome consists of craniofacial dysplasia, intrauterine growth retardation, cardiac anomalies, and mental retardation. Babies born to alcoholic mothers may have hypoglycemia, tremors, and difficulties with temperature regulation. Management of alcoholic pregnant women is supportive and may include sedation. Maternal counseling is highly recommended to prevent difficulties with future pregnancies.

Hepatic Tumors

Although rare during pregnancy, primary hepatoma carries a very high maternal mortality (up to 100%).[54] Cavernous hemangioma is the most common benign tumor encountered during pregnancy. The tumor can increase in size during pregnancy

and cause abdominal discomfort. Hepatic adenoma has been associated with the use of oral contraceptives. Because these adenomas can grow and rupture, they are considered a contraindication to pregnancy until the tumor has resolved or has been surgically removed.

Budd-Chiari Syndrome

Hepatic venous thrombosis is uncommon during pregnancy. It usually is associated with the use of oral contraceptives[55] or occurs during the early postpartum period.[56,57] The prognosis is grave without expeditious lifesaving intervention, that is, liver transplantation. Isolated cases of hepatic arterial thrombosis have been reported;[58] some patients have completely recovered.

Hepatic Dysfunction as a Result of Pregnancy

Hyperemesis Gravidarum

Severe cases of intractable nausea and vomiting can result in mild hepatic dysfunction, and supportive therapy with hospitalization is necessary. Serum bilirubin is usually less than 2.5 mg/dL but can rise above 4.0 mg/dL.[59] Generally, the histologic findings of liver biopsy are normal. The jaundice is of no prognostic significance, and there are no associations of this syndrome with chronic liver disease.

Intrahepatic Cholestasis of Pregnancy

Intrahepatic cholestasis of pregnancy (ICP) is the second most common cause of jaundice, and it may be caused by increased levels of female hormones. An autosomal-dominant pattern of inheritance has been found and there may be an association with the A31,B8 haplotype. Certain ethnic groups, namely Scandinavians, Chilean Indians, and Poles, are more susceptible to ICP. A high incidence of fetal prematurity (30%) and perinatal mortality (10%) has been reported.[60] The recurrence of ICP during future pregnancies has been reported to be as high as 30–70%.[61]

This disease presents a wide spectrum of symptoms and signs, from pruritus (pruritus gravidarum) to intense itching and clinical jaundice (obstetric hepatosis). Pruritus may be accompanied by nausea, vomiting, malaise, and right upper quadrant pain after the 30th week of pregnancy. Bilirubin levels are often increased but are usually less than 5 mg/dL.[62] Alkaline phosphatase levels tend to increase, and determination of isoenzyme levels confirms the hepatic, rather than the placental, origin. Although serum AST and ALT levels are increased, they usually remain below five times their normal values. Therefore, tests of serum AST and ALT may be useful in distinguishing ICP from viral hepatitis. Liver biopsy may show a normal or a nonspecific cholestatic pattern.[63]

Treatment of ICP is supportive. Antihistamines are ineffective in the treatment of pruritus, but it can be reduced with cholestyramine, 12–24 g/day in three divided doses.[30] Because cholestyramine binds iron and fat-soluble vitamins, it should be supplemented with an iron preparation and vitamin K. Phenobarbital may be effective by enzyme induction or a choleretic effect.[64] S-adenosyl-L-methionine reversed cholestasis in laboratory animals and in women with ICP in one study, possibly by the inactivation of estrogen metabolites, increasing the rate of bile secretion, or by hepatocyte protection against cholestasis.[65]

Preeclampsia and Eclampsia

Preeclampsia is defined as the triad of hypertension, generalized edema, and proteinuria in the gravid patient after the 24th week of gestation. A generalized vasoconstriction secondary to an imbalance between the vasodilating prostacyclin and the vasoconstricting thromboxane is believed to cause this condition. This vasoconstricted state decreases the blood flow to the uterus, liver, and kidneys, while increasing blood viscosity and platelet adhesiveness. Fibrin deposits are seen within the hepatic sinusoid.[66] Liver dysfunction is caused by edema and ischemia from reduced hepatic blood flow. In severe cases, periportal hemorrhage and spontaneous rupture of the liver can occur. This life-threatening condition requires rapid diagnosis and aggressive therapy. Peritoneal lavage has the highest and quickest diagnostic yield, and abdominal computerized tomography and ultrasound provide accurate information. Once the diagnosis is made, immediate delivery of the fetus and surgical repair of the liver are indicated.[67]

A peculiar subset of patients with the HELLP syndrome (hemolysis, elevated liver enzymes, and low platelet count) has been described.[68] This syndrome is seen in as many as 12% of preeclamptic patients,[69] and it may constitute a subgroup of preeclampsia. The HELLP syndrome also occurs in patients suffering from AFL of pregnancy.

Acute Fatty Liver of Pregnancy

AFL is a rare disease (1:1,000,000 pregnancies), and the etiology of this devastating condition remains obscure.[70,71] Symptoms and signs usually are not seen until the 32nd to 38th week of gestation, and they may completely mimic those of preeclampsia: mild hypertension, generalized edema, and proteinuria. However, the clinical course is that of a fulminant disease, with rapid deterioration including severe hepatic failure, encephalopathy, hypoglycemia, thrombocytopenia, coagulopathy, and pancreatitis. An increased leukocyte count ($>15 \times 10^9$) may be the only laboratory finding suggestive of AFL. The definitive diagnosis is made by liver biopsy, although coagulopathy may prohibit the procedure. Microvascular fatty infiltration of hepatocytes is characteristic, but pathologic findings can range from those typifying acute viral hepatitis to ballooned vacuolated cells.[71] The pathologic findings seen in Reye's syndrome have been seen in patients with AFL; the relation between the two diseases is unknown.[72]

Management is strictly supportive and similar to that of patients suffering from fulminant hepatic failure. Care is taken to avoid hypoglycemia, provide adequate nutrition, correct coagulopathy, and support renal function with monitored volume expansion, mannitol, furosemide, or dopamine. An extremely high mortality has been reported in pregnant women (70%) and fetuses (80%),[73] although some investigators offer a less ominous prediction.[74] Obstetric management is controversial. Early cesarean section has been recommended,[49,75] but it carries an increased risk in the presence of hepatic failure and coagulopathy. Successful full-term pregnancy following an episode of AFL has been reported,[76] and future pregnancy is not contraindicated. The hepatic histologic findings in infants who do not survive may be similar to those in the mother.

Primary Hepatic Pregnancy

The fetus usually implants on the inferior surface of the right lobe of the liver in this very unusual complication. Patients usually have abdominal pain and often have frank blood in the abdominal cavity. Immediate surgical delivery of the fetus and repair of the liver is mandatory.

Pregnancy Occurring in Patients with Preexisting Liver Disease

Cirrhosis and Portal Hypertension

Patients with cirrhosis and portal hypertension often were unable to conceive because of inhibited ovulation. However, with improved medical therapy, more women with hepatic dysfunction now are able to conceive. Pregnancy alone does not hasten the natural progression of the underlying liver disease, unless hepatic function worsens early in the pregnancy. The presence of esophageal varices before conception, however, increases the risk of maternal variceal hemorrhage and possibly death. Therefore, the risk of pregnancy should be carefully evaluated, and contraception may be recommended in patients with severe liver disease.

Massive variceal bleeding can occur without warning in 25–45% of pregnant cirrhotic women,[77] and a high perinatal mortality (18%) has been reported in this situation.[78] Many factors can contribute to this increased risk of variceal hemorrhage: increased blood volume, inferior vena caval compression by the gravid uterus, increased venous pressure during uterine contractions, and Valsalva maneuvers during fetal expulsion. Therefore, Valsalva maneuvers are to be avoided in the second stage of labor, and the use of outlet forceps is recommended under pudendal or regional anesthesia. The indications for cesarean section are the same as those for noncirrhotic patients. If variceal hemorrhage occurs, treatment should be instituted immediately: balloon tamponade, sclerotherapy if indicated, and rapid blood replacement via large-bore intravenous catheters.

Chronic Active Hepatitis

The results of liver function studies are abnormal in 30% of pregnant women with chronic active hepatitis.[30] The incidence of perinatal mortality is similar to that of cirrhotic mothers (18%), but long-term survival is unaffected by the disease state.[79] However, poor maternal and fetal outcome

has been found when the mother had persistent HB_s Ag.[80] Patients with chronic active hepatitis are at increased risk for developing pregnancy-induced hypertension. Azathioprine has not been reported to be teratogenic in the immunosuppressant doses used in patients with chronic active hepatitis.[23]

Chronic Persistent Hepatitis

Patients with this condition have a relatively uneventful pregnancy. In addition, pregnancy does not worsen this disease process, and no increase in neonatal morbidity or mortality has been reported.[81]

Primary Biliary Cirrhosis

Successful pregnancy has been reported for women with primary biliary cirrhosis. Although cholestasis may worsen during pregnancy, it abates after delivery.[82]

Wilson's Disease

Patients with Wilson's disease have had successful pregnancies if their disease is controlled by penicillamine or if they are in the early, asymptomatic stages of the disease.[83] Symptoms appear to diminish during pregnancy because of fetal requirement of copper and an increased serum ceruloplasmin level during pregnancy.[84]

Amebic Abscess of the Liver

Caused by *Entamoeba histolytica*, amebic abscess of the liver is seen in endemic areas. Fever and malaise are usual symptoms. The results of liver function studies may be normal, with an occasional mild increase in the serum bilirubin level. Stool cultures may be negative, and ultrasound of the liver indicates the presence of intrahepatic cysts. The abscess is treated with metronidazole.

Other Diseases

Patients with familial hyperbilirubinemia have had successful deliveries, and patients with Gilbert's syndrome (unconjugated hyperbilirubinemia) are at no increased risk for maternal and fetal morbidity or mortality.[85] The Dubin-Johnson syndrome (conjugated hyperbilirubinemia) is aggravated by pregnancy but resumes its prepregnancy state after delivery.[86] The increase in serum bilirubin levels results from the decrease in the maximum bilirubin secretory capacity that occurs during pregnancy.[87] Familial intrahepatic cholestasis, Alagille's syndrome (arteriohepatic dysplasia), and Bylers' syndrome (congenital absence of the bile ducts) are worsened by pregnancy.[88]

Pregnancy after Orthotopic Liver Transplantation

The experience with women who became pregnant after liver transplantation at the University of Pittsburgh was recently reviewed.[89] Seventeen patients delivered 20 children after successful orthotopic liver transplantation. One patient delivered twins, and two patients had two subsequent pregnancies. All patients were receiving standard immunosuppression that included prednisone, cyclosporine, and azathioprine. Liver function did not change in 12 pregnancies and eight were complicated by abnormal liver function tests of varying degrees. One patient had biopsy verified rejection. Thirteen deliveries were by cesarean section and seven were spontaneous vaginal deliveries at term. Indications for cesarean section were premature rupture of the membrane and pregnancy-induced hypertension. Eleven of 12 children older than one year had normal developmental patterns, and one child had a slow speech developmental pattern. All eight children younger than one year of age had reached appropriate developmental milestones for their age. Therefore, women can successfully conceive and deliver after orthotopic liver transplantation, but there appears to be an increased risk of prematurity, hypertension, and mild to moderate hepatic dysfunction.

Anesthetic Considerations for Pregnant Patients with Liver Disease

Concerns about anesthesia in patients with liver disease are described in previous chapters and other comprehensive reviews.[70] This section is limited to the salient issues involving the pregnant patient with significant hepatic dysfunction.

As with any patient, the goals of the anesthetist are to provide the mother with adequate amnesia, analgesia, and muscle relaxation during surgery while maintaining the physiologic state of both mother and fetus. Patients with mildly abnormal liver function can be treated as healthy pregnant women, providing blood coagulability is within normal limits. However, all pregnant patients with liver disease should be considered at a high risk for aspiration pneumonitis, and 30 mL of a nonparticulate antacid should be administered at least 20 minutes before the administration of any anesthetic. If time permits, 150 mg of ranitidine hydrochloride and 10 mg of metoclopramide hydrochloride are given orally the night before surgery and intravenously on the morning of surgery.

When fetal well-being is not of concern during a surgical procedure, as with therapeutic abortions, anesthetic management is similar to that for other patients with liver disease. When fetal well-being must be considered, such as during a cerclage procedure for imminent abortion, the fetal heart tone should be monitored to detect and prevent any significant fetal distress.

Vaginal Delivery

During labor and delivery, repeated Valsalva maneuvers should be avoided to reduce the risk of life-threatening variceal hemorrhage. Therefore, controlled second stage of labor is recommended, and the delivery is performed with outlet forceps or vacuum extraction. Vaginal delivery can be facilitated by the use of local anesthesia for episiotomy, pudendal nerve block, spinal anesthesia, epidural anesthesia, or inhalation analgesia. A pudendal nerve block should be used only when its benefit outweighs the risk of hematoma. Spinal and epidural anesthesia can be used when coagulation is relatively normal: prothrombin time and activated partial thromboplastin time < 1.5 times control and platelet count > $100 \times 10^7/L$.

Inhalation analgesia is preferable to regional anesthesia in patients with coagulation abnormalities. Inhalation analgesia is induced with 30–50% nitrous oxide in oxygen with or without other potent inhalation anesthetics, such as enflurane (0.1–0.5%) or isoflurane (0.1–0.5%). The anesthetist must maintain communication with the patient at all times, because overdose of anesthetics can occur easily and aspiration of gastric contents is an ever-present danger. The uptake of both insoluble and soluble anesthetics is facilitated because of decreased functional residual capacity and increased minute ventilation. Animal studies showed a 20–40% decrease in minimum alveolar concentration (MAC) during pregnancy,[13] and 50% below MAC values appears to be sufficient in pregnant women. If the patient should lose consciousness, 100% oxygen should be administered and the volatile agent stopped. The obstetrician should be alerted to pause momentarily, if possible, until the patient regains consciousness.

Cesarean Section

For cesarean section in the patient with liver disease, anesthesia can be administered in the same fashion as in the healthy parturient if hepatic function is stable and coagulation is normal. However, patients with moderate to severe liver disease should be prepared adequately before surgical delivery. The ability to administer large volumes of blood products rapidly is mandatory because of the risk of intraoperative massive hemorrhage and bleeding from esophageal varices. The use of at least two large-bore intravenous catheters (>16 gauge) before the induction of anesthesia and invasive monitoring of arterial, central venous, and pulmonary arterial pressure may be necessary in severe cases. Adequate supplies of blood products should be available: 10 units each of packed red blood cells and fresh frozen plasma. Platelets should be prepared when the platelet count is less than 75×10^9/L. Left-sided uterine displacement should be performed in all patients to avoid aorto-caval compression.

Regional anesthesia is generally preferred to general anesthesia in the healthy parturient, and this rule also applies to the parturient with hepatic dysfunction. However, the choice of anesthetic is determined by factors such as the urgency of delivery or the presence of coagulopathy. In the absence of coagulopathy, regional anesthesia can be used in the standard fashion. Both the amide and ester types of local anesthetics may have a more prolonged and pronounced effect because of decreased hepatic degradation and the low cholinesterase activity. Also, drugs that inhibit the cytochrome P-450 system (cimetidine and probably ranitidine) may decrease the clearance of certain drugs with a high hepatic extraction ratio, such as lidocaine.[90] Theoretically, local anesthetic toxicity can develop if repeated doses of local anesthetics are administered within the epidural space, although no data are available. Details on choosing a local anesthetic and the merits of each type of regional anesthesia can be found elsewhere.[91,92] Prehydration with 1,000 mL of balanced salt solution is recommended before the induction of regional anesthesia. However, volume overloading may be a problem in patients with an uncertain intravascular volume state, and regional anesthesia is best avoided in those patients. After regional anesthesia is induced, supplemental oxygen should be administered.

When general anesthesia is to be used, a rapid sequence induction with cricoid pressure or awake intubation is used to secure the airway. Thiopental (3–4 mg/kg) is frequently chosen as an induction agent. Ketamine hydrochloride is an alternative agent for the hypotensive or hypovolemic patient, but the dose should be limited to 1 mg/kg because of the high incidence of neonatal depression with its use.[93] A nondepolarizing muscle relaxant, given frequently to prevent fasciculation, is unnecessary in patients receiving magnesium therapy for preeclampsia or preterm labor.[94] Succinylcholine (1.5 mg/kg) provides adequate relaxation for intubation of the trachea. After the airway is secured, the surgeon can begin the operation, during which anesthesia is maintained with 50% nitrous oxide in oxygen. A potent inhalation agent may be added until the umbilical cord is clamped, but the concentration of the agent should be limited, enflurane to 0.75% and isoflurane to 0.5%, to minimize neonatal depression.[95] Halothane should be avoided because it reduces hepatic blood flow[96,97] and is associated with unexplained halothane hepatitis. When muscle relaxation is required, atracurium besylate is a logical choice because its action is not influenced by liver disease. Succinylcholine also can be used, but paralysis may occasionally be prolonged.[98]

Maternal hyperventilation should be avoided because hypocapnia reduces both uterine[99] and hepatic blood flow. Use of a higher inspired oxygen concentration should be considered, and oxygen saturation should be monitored by pulse oximetry or arterial blood gas tension. Great caution is advised when a nasogastric tube is needed to empty the stomach; most of these patients have esophageal varices, and epistaxis can occur from swollen nasal mucosa.

After the umbilical cord is clamped, general anesthesia can be deepened if necessary. Excessive use of narcotics or sedatives should be avoided to expedite postoperative neurologic assessment of the patient. The trachea should not be extubated until the patient is fully conscious and the airway reflex is intact at the end of surgery or in the recovery room.

In conclusion, the pregnant patient with liver disease presents many challenges to the clinician. Proper management promotes successful conception and delivery and has enabled more women with hepatic dysfunction to become pregnant. This challenge can be met only by the teamwork of specialists sincerely interested in caring for these patients and by good communication between physicians and patients. Can we offer any greater gift than the joy known only to those who have children?

References

1. Hytten, F. and Chamberlain, G. (1980) *Clinical Physiology in Obstetrics*. Oxford: Blackwell Scientific Publications.
2. Gibbs, C. (1981) Maternal physiology. *Clin Obstet Gynecol* 24:525–43.
3. Cheek, T.D. and Gutsche, B.B. (1987) Maternal physiologic alterations during pregnancy. In *Anesthesia for Obstetrics*, 2nd ed., (Shnider, S.M. and Levinson, G. eds). Baltimore: Williams and Wilkins, pp. 3–13.
4. Clark, K.E., Austin, J.E. and Seeds, A.E. (1982) Effects of bisenoic prostaglandins and arachidonic acid on the uterine vasculature. *Am J Obstet Gynecol* 142:261–68.
5. Ylikorkala, O., Jouppila, P., Kirkinen, P. and Viinikka, L. (1983) Maternal prostacyclin, thromboxane, and placental blood flow. *Am J Obstet Gynecol* 145:730–32.
6. Eckstein, K.L. and Marx, G.F. (1974) Aortocaval compression and uterine displacement. *Anesthesiology* 40:92–96.
7. Hon, E.H., Reid, B.L. and Hehre, F.W. (1960) The electronic evaluation of the fetal heart rate. II. Changes with maternal hypotension. *Am J Obstet Gynecol* 79:209–15.
8. Zilianti, M., Salazar, J.R., Aller, J. and Aguero, O. (1970) Fetal heart rate and pH of fetal capillary blood during epidural analgesia in labor. *Obstet Gynecol* 36:881–86.
9. Scott, B.D. (1973) Inferior vena caval occlusion in late pregnancy. In *Parturition and Perinatology*, Marx, G.F. (ed). Philadelphia: F.A. Davis Co, p. 42.
10. Bonica, J.J. (1981) Maternal physiologic and psychologic alterations. In *Obstetric Anesthesia and Perinatology*, (Cosmi, E.V. ed). New York: Appleton-Century-Crofts, pp. 28–29.
11. Kambam, J.R., Handte, R.E., Brown, W. and Smith, B.E. (1983) Effect of pregnancy on oxygen dissociation. *Anesthesiology* 59:A395.
12. Leontic, E.A. (1977) Respiratory disease in pregnancy. *Med Clin North Am* 61:111–28.
13. Palahniuk, R.J., Shnider, S.M. and Eger, E.I. II (1974) Pregnancy decreased the requirements for inhaled anesthetic agents. *Anesthesiology* 41:82–83.
14. Steinbrook, R.A., Carr, D.B., Datta, S., et al. (1982) Dissociation of plasma and cerebrospinal fluid beta-endorphins immunoreactivity levels during pregnancy and parturition. *Anesth Analg* 61:893–97.
15. Marx, G.F., Oka, Y. and Orkin, L.R. (1967) Cerebrospinal fluid pressures during labor. *Am J Obstet Gynecol* 84:213–19.
16. Datta, S., Lambert, D.H., Gregus, J., Gissen, A.J. and Covino, B.G. (1983) Differential sensitivities of mammalian nerve fibers during pregnancy. *Anesth Analg* 62:1070–72.
17. Shnider, S.M. (1965) Serum cholinesterase activity during pregnancy, labor and puerperium. *Anesthesiology* 26:335–39.
18. Marx, G.F. (1975) Physiology of pregnancy. In *ASA Refresher Course in Anesthesiology*, Hershey, S.C. (ed). Philadelphia: J.B. Lippincott, pp. 117–28.
19. Csapo, A. (1956) Progesterone block. *Am J Anat* 98:273–91.
20. Christofides, N.D., Ghatei, M.A., Bloom, S.R., Barbog, C. and Gillmer, M.D.G. (1982) Decreased plasma motilin concentrations in pregnancy. *Br Med J* 285:1453–54.
21. Roberts, R.B. and Shirley, M.A. (1976) The obstetrician's role in reducing the risk of aspiration pneumonitis with particular reference to the use of oral antacids. *Am J Obstet Gynecol* 124:611–17.
22. Kerr, M.G., Scott, D.B. and Samule, E. (1964) Studies of the inferior vena cava in late pregnancy. *Br Med J* 1:532–35.
23. Riely, C.A. (1987) The liver in pregnancy. In *Diseases of the Liver*, 6th ed, (Schiff, L. and Schiff, E.R. ed,). Philadelphia: J.B. Lippincott, pp. 1059–73.
24. Britton, R.C. (1982) Pregnancy and esophageal varices. *Am J Surg* 143:421–25.
25. Laakso, L., Ruotsalainen, P., Punnonen, R. and Maatel, A. (1971) Hepatic blood flow during late pregnancy. *Acta Obstet Gynecol Scand* 50:175–78.
26. Ylostalo, P., Kirkinen, P., Heikkinen, J., et al. (1982) Gallbladder volume and serum bile acids in cholestasis of pregnancy. *Br J Obstet Gynaecol* 89:59–61.
27. Noller, L.K. (1981) Liver disease in pregnancy. In *Principles and Practice of Obstetrics and Perinatology*, vol. 2, (Iffy, L. and Kaminetzky, H.A. eds). New York: Wiley Medical Publishers, pp. 1327–59.
28. Sussman, H.H., Bowman, M. and Lewis, J.L. (1968) Placental alkaline phosphatase in maternal serum during normal and abnormal pregnancy. *Nature* 218:359–60.
29. McNair, R.D. and Jaynes, R.V. (1960) Alterations in liver function during normal pregnancy. *Am J Obstet Gynecol* 80:500–05.
30. Gitlin, N. (1985) Liver disease in pregnancy. In *Liver and Biliary Disease*, (Wright, R. ed). Philadelphia: W.B. Saunders, pp. 1121–34.
31. Svanborg, A. and Vikrot, O. (1965) Plasma lipid fractions, including individual phospholipids at various stages of pregnancy. *Acta Med Scand* 178:615–30.
32. Kalkhoff, R.K., Kissebah, A.H. and Kim, H.J. (1979) Carbohydrate and lipid metabolism during normal pregnancy: Relationship to gestational hormone action. In

The Diabetic Pregnancy. A Perinatal Perspective. (Merkatz, I.R. and Adams, P.A.J. eds). New York: Grune and Stratton, pp. 3–21.

33. Pitkins, R.M. and Witte, D.L. (1979) Platelet and leukocyte counts in pregnancy. *JAMA* 242:2696–98.

34. Brown, B.R. Jr. (1988) *Anesthesia in Hepatic and Biliary Tract Disease.* Philadelphia: F.A. Davis Co, pp. 151–60.

35. Haemmerli, U.P. (1966) Jaundice during pregnancy with special emphasis on recurrent jaundice during pregnancy and its differential diagnosis. *Acta Med Scand* 179(suppl. 444):1–111.

36. Richard, R.L., Willocks, J. and Dow, T.G. (1976) Jaundice in pregnancy. *Scot Med J* 15:52–57.

37. Goyert, G.L., Bottoms, S.F. and Sokol, R.J. (1985) Anicteric presentation of fatal herpetic hepatitis in pregnancy. *Obstet Gynecol* 65:585.

38. Khurro, M.S., Telli, M.R., Skidmore, Sofi, M.A. and Khuroo, M.I. (1981) Incidence and severity of viral hepatitis in pregnancy. *Am J Med* 70:252–55.

39. Borhanmanesh, F., Haghighi, P., Hekmat, K., Rezaizadeh, K. and Ghavami, A.G. (1973) Viral hepatitis during pregnancy: Severity and effect on gestation. *Gastroenterology* 64:304–12.

40. Gelpi, A.P. (1979) Viral hepatitis complicating pregnancy: Mortality trends in Saudi Arabia. *Int J Gynaecol Obstet* 17:73–77.

41. Mallia, C.P. and Narncekivell, A.F. (1982) Fulminant virus hepatitis in late pregnancy. *Ann Trop Med Parasitol* 76:143–46.

42. Hieber, J.P., Dalton, D., Shorey, J. and Combes, B. (1977) Hepatitis and pregnancy. *J Pediatr* 91:545–70.

43. Derso, A., Boxall, E.H., Tarlow, M.J. and Flewett, T.H. (1978) Transmission of HBsAg from mother to infant in four ethnic groups. *Br Med J* 1:949–52.

44. Tong, M.J., Thursby, M., Rakela, J. et al. (1981) Studies on the maternal-infant transmission of the viruses which cause acute hepatitis. *Gastroenterology* 80:999–1004.

45. Combes, B., Whalley, P.J. and Adams, R.H. (1972) Tetracycline and the liver. *Prog Liver Dis* 4:589–96.

46. McCormack, W.M., George, H., Donner, A., et al. (1977) Hepatotoxicity of erythromycin estolate during pregnancy. *Antimicrob Agents Chemother* 12:630–35.

47. Holden, T.E. and Sherline, D.M. (1972) Hepatitis and hepatic failure in pregnancy. *Obstet Gynecol* 40:586–93.

48. Rubinger, D., Davidson, J.D. and Melmed, R.N. (1975) Hepatitis following the use of methoxyflurane in obstetric analgesia. *Anesthesiology* 43:593–95.

49. Miller, J.P. (1977) Diseases of the liver and alimentary tract. *Clin Obstet Gynecol* 4:297–317.

50. Jouppila, P., Mokka, R. and Larmi, T.K.I. (1974) Acute pancreatitis in pregnancy. *Surg Gynecol Obstet* 139:879–82.

51. McKay, A.J., O'Neill, J. and Imrie, C.W. (1980) Pancreatitis, pregnancy, and gallstones. *Br J Gynaecol* 87:47–50.

52. Wilkinson, E.J. (1973) Acute pancreatitis in pregnancy: A review of 98 cases and a report of 8 new cases. *Obstet Gynecol Surv* 28:281–303.

53. Ouellette, E.M., Rosett, H.L., Rosman, P. and Wiener, L. (1977) Adverse effects on offspring of maternal alcohol abuse during pregnancy. *N Engl J Med* 297:528–30.

54. Egwuatu, V.E. (1980) Primary hepatocarcinoma in pregnancy. *Roy Soc Trop Med Hyg* 74:793–94.

55. Tsung, S.H., Han, D., Loh, W. and Lin, J.I. (1980) Budd-Chiari syndrome in women taking oral contraceptives. *Ann Clin Lab Sci* 10:518–21.

56. Rosenthal, T., Shani, M., Deutsch, V. and Samra, H. (1972) The Budd-Chiari syndrome after pregnancy: Report of two cases and a review of the literature. *Am J Obstet Gynecol* 113:789–92.

57. Gatell-Artigas, J.M., Sala-Estabanez, J. and Aused-Faure, M.R. (1982) Pregnancy and the Budd-Chiari syndrome. *Dig Dis Sci* 27:89–90.

58. Dammann, H.G., Hagemann, J., Runge, M. and Klippel, G. (1982) In vivo diagnosis of massive hepatic infarction by computed tomography. *Dig Dis Sci* 27:73–79.

59. Adams, R.H., Gordon, J. and Combes, B. (1968) Hyperemesis gravidarum: I. Evidence of hepatic dysfunction. *Obstetrics and Gynecology* 31:659–64.

60. Reid, R., Ivey, K.J., Rencoret, R.H. and Storey, B. (1976) Fetal complications of obstetric cholestasis. *Br Med J* 1:870–72.

61. Geall, M.G. and Webb, M.J. (1974) Liver disease in pregnancy. *Med Clin North Am* 58:817–22.

62. Haemmerli, U.P. and Wyss, H.I. (1967) Recurrent intrahepatic cholestasis of pregnancy. Report of 6 cases and review of the literature. *Medicine* 46:299–321.

63. Adlercreutz, H., Svanborg, A. and Anberg, A. (1967) Recurrent jaundice in pregnancy: I. A clinical and ultrastructural study. *Am J Med* 42:335–40.

64. Espinoza, J., Barnafi, L. and Schnaidt, E. (1974) The effect of phenobarbital on intrahepatic cholestasis of pregnancy. *Am J Obstet Gynecol* 119:234–38.

65. Frezza, M., Pozzato, G., Chiesa, L., Stramentinoli, G. and di Padova, C. (1984) Reversal of intrahepatic cholestasis of pregnancy in women after high dose S-adenosyl-L-methionine administration. *Hepatology* 4:274–78.

66. Arias, F. and Mancilla-Jimenez, R. (1976) Hepatic fibrinogen deposits in pre-eclampsia: Immunofluorescent evidence. *N Engl J Med* 295: 578–82.

67. Henny, C.P., Lim, A.E., Brummelkamp, W.H., Buller, H.R. and Ten Cate, J.W. (1983) Review of the importance of acute multidisciplinary treatment following spontaneous rupture of the liver capsule during pregnancy. *Surg Gynecol Obstet* 156:593–98.

68. Weinstein, L. (1982) Syndrome of hemolysis, elevated liver enzymes and low platelet count: A severe consequence of hypertension in pregnancy. *Am J Obstet Gynecol* 142:159–67.

69. MacKenna, J., Dover, N.L. and Brame, R.G. (1983) Preeclampsia associated with hemolysis, elevated liver enzymes, and low platelets: An obstetric emergency? *Obstet Gynecol* 62:751–54.

70. Brown, B.R. Jr. (1988) *Anesthesia in Hepatic and Biliary Tract Disease.* Philadelphia: F.A. Davis Co.

71. Standers, H.J. and Cadden, J.F. (1934) Acute yellow atrophy of the liver in pregnancy. *Am J Gynecol* 28:61–69.
72. Sherlock, S. (1983) Acute fatty liver of pregnancy and the microvesicular fat disease. *Gut* 24:265–69.
73. Varner, M. and Rinderknecht, N.K. (1980) Acute fatty metamorphosis of pregnancy. A maternal mortality and literature review. *J Reprod Med* 24:177–80.
74. Housh, M., Levine, S., Ahola, S. et al. (1984) Acute fatty liver of pregnancy: Survival with early Caesarean section. *Dig Dis Sci* 29:449–52.
75. Iber, F.L. (1965) Jaundice in pregnancy: A review. *Am J Obstet Gynecol* 91:721–53.
76. MacKenna, J., Pupkin, M., Crenshaw, C., McLeod, M. and Parker, R.T. (1977) Acute fatty metamorphosis of the liver: A report of two patients who survived. *Am J Obstet Gynecol* 127:400–04.
77. Varma, R.R., Michelsohn, N.H., Borkowf, H.I. and Lewis, J.D. (1977) Pregnancy in cirrhotic and noncirrhotic portal hypertension. *Obstet Gynecol* 50:217–22.
78. Cheng, Y.S. (1977) Pregnancy in liver cirrhosis and portal hypertension. *Am J Obstet Gynecol* 128:812–22.
79. Steven, M.M., Buckley, J.D. and MacKay, I.R. (1979) Pregnancy in chronic active hepatitis. *Quarterly Journal of Medicine* 48:519–33.
80. Schweitzer, I.L. and Peters, R.L. (1976) Pregnancy in hepatitis B antigen positive cirrhosis. *Obstet Gynecol* 48:53–56.
81. Infeld, D.S. and Borkowf, H.T. (1979) Chronic persistent hepatitis and pregnancy. *Gastroenterology* 77:524–27.
82. Whelton, M.J. and Sherlock, S. (1968) Pregnancy in patients with hepatic cirrhosis: Management and outcome. *Lancet* ii:995–98.
83. Walshe, J.M. (1977) Pregnancy in Wilson's disease. *Quarterly Journal of Medicine* 46:73–83.
84. Burrows, S. and Pekala, B. (1971) Serum copper and ceruloplasmin in pregnancy. *Am J Obstet Gynecol* 109:907–09.
85. Friedlaender, P. and Osler, M. (1967) Icterus and pregnancy. *Am J Obstet Gynecol* 97:894–900.
86. Cohen, L., Lewis, C. and Arias, I.M. (1972) Pregnancy, oral contraceptives, and chronic familial jaundice with predominantly conjugated hyperbilirubinemia. *Gastroenterology* 62:1182–90.
87. DiZoglio, J.D. and Cardillo, E. (1973) The Dubin Johnson syndrome and pregnancy. *Obstet Gynec* 42:560–63.

88. Romero, R., Reese, E.A., Riely, C. and Hobbins, J.C. (1983) Arteriohepatic dysplasia in pregnancy. *Am J Obstet Gynecol* 147:108–09.
89. Scantlebury, V., Gordon, R., Tzakis, A., et al., (1990) Childbearing after liver transplantation. *Transplantation* 49:317–21.
90. Brown, B.R. Jr. (1988c) *Anesthesia in Hepatic and Biliary Tract Disease*. Philadelphia: F.A. Davis Co, pp. 67–91.
91. Bromage, P.R. (1987) Choice of local anesthetic in obstetrics: General considerations. In *Anesthesia for Obstetrics*, 2nd ed, (Shnider, S.M. and Levinson, G. eds). Baltimore: Williams and Wilkins, pp. 59–68.
92. Shnider, S.M. (1987) Regional anesthesia for labor and delivery. In *Anesthesia for Obstetrics*, 2nd ed, (Shnider, S.M. and Levinson, G. ed). Baltimore: Williams and Wilkins, pp. 109–22.
93. Shnider, S.M. (1987) Anesthesia for Cesarean section. In *Anesthesia for Obstetrics*, 2nd ed, (Shnider, S.M. and Levinson, G. eds). Baltimore: Williams and Wilkins, pp. 59–178.
94. DeVore, J.S. and Asrani, R. (1980) Magnesium sulfate prevents succinylcholine-induced fasciculations in toxemic parturients. *Anesthesiology* 52:76–77.
95. Abboud, T.K., Kim, S.H., Henriksen, E.H. et al. (1985) Comparative maternal and neonatal effects of halothane and enflurane for cesarean section. *Acta Anaesth Scand* 29:663–68.
96. Hughes, R.L., Mathie, R.T., Campbell, D. and Fitch, W. (1980) Effects of enflurane and halothane on liver blood flow and oxygen consumption in the greyhound. *Br J Anaesth* 52:1079–86.
97. Thompson, I.D., Fitch, W., Hughes, R.L. and Campbell, D. (1983) Effect of increased concentrations of carbon dioxide during halothane anesthesia on liver flow and hepatic oxygen consumption. *Br J Anaesth* 55:1231–37.
98. Blitt, C.D., Petty, W.C., Alberternst, E.E. and Wright, B.J. (1977) Correlations of plasma cholinesterase activity and duration of action of succinylcholine during pregnancy. *Anesth Analg* 56:78–81.
99. Levinson, G., Shnider, S.M., deLorimier, A.A. and Steffenson, J.L. (1974) Effects of maternal hyperventilation on uterine blood flow and fetal oxygenation and acid-base status. *Anesthesiology* 40:340–47.

FOUR

Intensive Care

Chapter 13
Acute Liver Failure

Graeme Alexander

There are few conditions in which the onset is so dramatic and progression to multiorgan failure so rapid as in acute liver failure, yet the survival of a patient with acute liver failure is professionally satisfying because these patients can make a complete clinical recovery with a return to normal health and activity. The principles of the care of such patients are first, to recognize the prognosis, which includes recognition of the etiology; second, to determine whether a liver transplant is indicated; and finally, whether or not a liver transplant is indicated, to maintain the patient in the best possible state in the hope, or expectation (depending on etiology), that liver regeneration will occur or that a graft will become available. Liver transplantation for patients with acute liver failure has dramatically altered the outlook, and it is important to recognize that small therapeutic manipulations, which may only gain the patient 6 or 12 hours, may have a profound effect on outcome if this is sufficient to allow the patient to go to surgery in a stable condition for transplantation to proceed.

Definitions

For many years, the diagnosis of fulminant hepatic failure has been based on the definition of Trey and Davidson, that is, the onset of encephalopathy within 8 weeks of the onset of symptoms.[1] More recently, Gimson and colleagues described a group of patients with a poor prognosis in whom the onset of encephalopathy occurred between 8 weeks and 6

months from the onset of symptoms, which was defined as late-onset hepatic failure.[2] During this time, French workers with great experience in the field of liver failure had developed a different terminology that included the delay between the onset of jaundice (rather than symptoms) and encephalopathy, as well as factor V estimation. At a recent meeting of European experts, a consensus for the definition of liver failure was reached;[3] in this definition, the time from the onset of jaundice (which is easier to define than the onset of symptoms in many cases) to the time of the onset of encephalopathy (which is generally easy to recognize) is essential (Table 13-1).

The importance of this new definition is illustrated (see later) by the fact that the best models for determining prognosis in acute liver failure place great emphasis on the speed with which the disease progresses—paradoxically, patients with the fastest onset do rather better than those with slower onset.

Etiology

In the U.K., more than 50% of patients presenting with acute liver failure are due to paracetamol poisoning. For reasons that are unclear, paracetamol poisoning is less common in almost every other part of the world. More than one-third of the remaining cases are due to a *presumed* viral hepatitis which, in the majority of cases, is not hepatitis A, B or C.[4] There are no clues to the etiology in the majority of these patients, although a small proportion do have infection with herpes simplex virus type I or II,

Table 13-1. Time from Onset of Jaundice to Onset of Encephalopathy

Hyperacute liver failure	Fewer than 7 days
Acute liver failure	7 days to less than 1 month
Subacute liver failure	1–6 months

cytomegalovirus, Epstein-Barr virus, or herpes zoster virus (Table 13-2). It is also essential to recognize that a proportion of cases are due to drug reactions (Chapter 18).

Hepatitis B is a rare cause of acute liver failure in the U.K., but is the most common cause of viral hepatitis leading to liver failure in France.[5] It is important to recognize that at the time of presentation with acute liver failure due to hepatitis B, viral replication has ceased in the majority or will cease within a short time after admission.[6] There are, however, recent reports of acute liver failure due to a mutant hepatitis B virus in which viral replication is ongoing in the liver and the precise proportion of cases due to this mutation is not yet known.[7]

It is essential that patient care is not compromised in any way by the fact that the patient may have a virus transmittable to staff (who should be vaccinated).

By and large, the etiology of acute liver failure is important only in the effect it has on prognosis, but one or two points merit consideration. If a patient with hepatitis-B virus–related liver failure undergoes a liver transplant at an early stage, there is a risk of infection of the liver graft. Perioperative immune globulin and probably immune globulin for

Table 13-2. Causes of Acute Liver Failure

Paracetamol Poisoning	Amanita Phalloides *Poisoning*
Viral Hepatitis	*Idiosyncratic Drug Reactions*
Non-A/non-B hepatitis	Halothane
Hepatitis A	Isoniazid
Hepatitis B	Rifampicin
Hepatitis B + D	Nonsteroidal anti-
Hepatitis E	inflammatory drugs
Herpes simplex virus I	*Uncommon Causes*
Herpes simplex virus II	Wilson's disease
Herpes zoster virus	Hyperthermia
Cytomegalovirus	Massive malignant
Epstein-Barr virus	infiltration of liver
	Amyloid
Acute Fatty Liver of	
Pregnancy	

the ensuing 12 months at least is recommended currently.[8] Patients with underlying malignant disease or amyloid infiltration of the liver can be difficult to distinguish from patients with other causes of acute liver failure; however, it is clear that such patients are not good candidates for liver transplantation. If these diagnoses are a distinct clinical possibility, then measures should be taken to make a more confident diagnosis before transplantation. This may include transjugular liver biopsy or even an exploratory laparotomy immediately before continuing with a liver transplantation. Diagnosis of acute fatty liver of pregnancy is usually easy to make, and it is essential in this setting that the pregnancy is terminated as quickly as possible. The dramatic improvement in mortality over the last 10 years in this group is undoubtedly attributable not just to better intensive care but to early termination of pregnancy.

Prognosis

Liver transplantation should be regarded as an adjunct to medical therapy for acute liver failure; early recognition of patients who should be transplanted because their prognosis is awful and recognition that patients have moved from a *good* prognosis group to a *bad* prognosis group is essential. A number of studies have been performed looking at prognostic determinants in patients with acute liver failure, but it is important to recognize that these reflect the experience of a particular center and should not be adopted uncritically in their entirety. Instead, these data must be viewed in the light of the local experience in the medical management of acute liver failure and, in addition, in the light of local results for liver transplantation for patients with acute liver failure. The balance may change from one center to another. The largest such analysis to date was based on 588 patients with grade III or IV encephalopathy admitted between 1973 and 1985 to the Liver Failure Unit at King's College Hospital, London, and retrospectively validated on a further 175 admissions between the years 1986 and 1987.[9]

As can be seen from Table 13-3, etiology has a critical bearing on outcome. First, the prognostic indicators were different for those with paracetamol-induced liver damage and those with other etiologies, perhaps reflecting that paracetamol poisoning

Table 13-3. Indications for Transplantation in Acute Liver Failure

Paracetamol	Nonparacetamol
Arterial pH <7.30	Prothrombin time >100 s
or (in the absence of above)	*or any* three of the following:
All three of the following:	Unfavorable etiology
Prothrombin time >100 s	(i.e., not hepatitis A or B
Creatinine >300 μmol/L	virus infection)
Grade III encephalopathy	Jaundice >7 days before
	encephalopathy
	Age <10 or >40 years
	Prothrombin time >50 s
	Serum bilirubin >300
	μmol/L

represents a single insult to the liver followed, in uncomplicated cases, by liver regeneration, whereas with other etiologies there is a more persistent insult. In addition, for those with non-paracetamol poisoning, patients with hepatitis A or B did much better than patients with other etiologies. The recommended indications for transplantation in acute liver failure, based on that analysis, are shown in Table 13-3.

Using these criteria for patients with acute liver failure *not* due to paracetamol, 95.5% of fatal cases were identified, while in those who did not meet the criteria the survival was 81.8%. For those with paracetamol-induced liver failure, the criteria identified 77% of fatal cases with a survival rate of 88.6% in those who did not meet the criteria. It is noteworthy that some patients who would now be considered for transplantation would have survived their episode of acute liver failure, but they represent a minority. Similarly, a small proportion of patients who would not currently be considered liver transplantation candidates would have died. The merits of this particular analysis are that the clinical information and the laboratory investigations required to determine high-risk patients are readily available at any hospital in the U.K. Although the French system of identification of patients with a poor prognosis, based on a factor V estimation, undoubtedly provides a prognostic guide equivalent to that identified by O'Grady and coworkers,[9] the lack of availability of factor V assay as an on-call procedure for hospitals in the U.K. makes it unlikely this system will be adopted or that the factor V will be added to assessment in the U.K. in the immediate future.

The Role for Liver Transplantation in Acute Liver Failure

The criteria for liver grafting used on the liver unit at King's College Hospital are shown in Table 13-3, but it is important to recognize that there are medical contraindications to transplantation. These include uncontrolled sepsis, refractory hypotension, and brain stem dysfunction. Refractory hypotension is defined as a systolic blood pressure of less than 90 mmHg, despite adequate intravascular resuscitation and appropriate inotropic support. Sepsis is common in this group of patients, and transplantation of patients with active sepsis is associated with recurrent sepsis in the immediate postoperative period following induction of immunosuppression. There are very few ways to estimate brain stem function in the comatose, ventilated, and paralyzed patient with hepatic encephalopathy. It may be clear, if intracranial pressure monitoring is available, that a patient has become brain dead. However, in many circumstances this will not be available, and in most centers it is current policy not to proceed further if the pupils are fixed, dilated, and unresponsive to treatment.

In general, the results of liver transplantation for acute liver failure are less satisfactory than the first reports would have suggested, with current practice giving 5-year actuarial survival rates of 55–70% in the majority of centers worldwide.[10,11] However, it is likely that the criteria for transplantation have broadened over this time, and this does not actually represent an underachievement. The main causes of death in the postoperative period are acute graft failure, sepsis, and multiorgan failure.

Liver transplantation for acute liver failure due to paracetamol poisoning is much more contentious, but given that many of these patients are young and do not intend suicide, the fact that these patients have taken an overdose should not necessarily eliminate them from consideration. Many patients recovering from paracetamol overdose regret the overdose and have a normal psychological and social outcome; the same is proving true of patients undergoing liver transplantation for paracetamol poisoning.[12] However, in a patient who has taken a paracetamol overdose with a potentially poor outcome, evidence of serious psychiatric disorder should be sought at an early stage if at all possible. Often the patient will be admitted before significant encephalopathy develops when a full history should be taken. At this stage also, discussion with the general practitioner and family is essential to determine the psychological prognosis.

Management of the Complications of Acute Liver Failure

Hepatic Encephalopathy

In a patient with a fluctuating mental state, it is essential to exclude hypoglycemia, which is best done by hourly estimation of the blood sugar. It is also important to recognize that narcotic and sedative drugs are frequently used before the onset of encephalopathy and may exacerbate the situation. A recent observation indicated that 95% of a series of 36 patients who survived liver failure and 75% of 49 patients who died with liver failure had received narcotic or sedative drugs before the onset of encephalopathy.[12a]

Current thinking suggests that hepatic encephalopathy may be precipitated or exacerbated by increased activity of the inhibitory gamma-amino butyric acid (GABA)-ergic neurotransmitter system. In animals, visually evoked response patterns in acute liver failure resemble those induced by benzodiazepines (BZD), which exert their sedative effect by interacting with the central GABA-BZD receptor complex,[13] leading to the hypothesis that hepatic encephalopathy might be associated with increased tone of the GABA-ergic system.[14] The GABA-BZD receptor is a supramolecular complex comprising distinct binding sites for GABA, BZD, and barbiturates. Binding of GABA to its receptor induces conformational change after which the chloride ionophore is opened with an influx of chloride ions into the postsynaptic neuron. Benzodiazepines augment the chloride flux in the presence of GABA. In experimental models of acute liver failure, administration of GABA or BZD antagonists (flumazenil and others) have been shown to transiently ameliorate hepatic encephalopathy.[15,16] Clinical improvement was associated with improvement in EEG and visual evoked responses.[15–17] In clinical trials, flumazenil has been associated with improvement in a proportion of patients with acute liver failure to cirrhosis.[18] The results of two controlled clinical trials to date are contradictory regarding the clinical usefulness of flumazenil. Although in an ideal setting it would be advantageous to ameliorate hepatic encephalopathy, manipulation by the use of agonists or antagonists to the GABA-BZD receptor does not ameliorate the underlying condition and is best regarded as peripheral to the care of the patient.

Intracranial Hypertension

Evidence of raised intracranial pressure is present in 86% of patients progressing to grade III or IV encephalopathy, and this complication is the major cause of morbidity and mortality at this stage of the illness.[19,20] Successful treatment is dependent on early recognition of the complication to permit therapeutic intervention before irreversible brain injury has occurred.

In the initial phase, the early signs of raised intracranial pressure include extensor posturing, teeth grinding, opisthotonus, papillary abnormalities, and systolic hypertension.[21] However, the care of such patients almost invariably involves paralysis and ventilation, which means that the only sign of raised intracranial hypertension is systolic arterial hypertension. It is important to realize that this is a reflex, the function of which is to allow continued perfusion of the brain and is not, in itself, a clinical indication to lower the blood pressure. As the disease progresses, this reflex may be lost following which pupillary abnormalities may be the only sign of raised intracranial pressure—and this is a late sign, by which stage treatment may be ineffective.

To overcome the limitations of the clinical diagnosis of intracranial hypertension, a variety of monitoring techniques have been used. The most reliable has proved to be extradural intracranial pressure monitoring in conjunction with arterial pressure monitoring. Local hemorrhage, despite severe coagulopathy, is rare and may be associated with poor surgical technique; thrombocytopenia is a contraindication to insertion of an intracranial pressure monitor and an arbitrary "safe limit" of 50×10^9/L for platelets has been recommended. The advantage of intracranial pressure monitoring is that it allows ready determination of cerebral perfusion pressure. In a recent study, the use of intracranial pressure monitoring resulted in the recognition of more episodes of intracranial hypertension with a subsequent increase in prescribed treatment.[22] The use of monitors, however, does not improve survival but, in this particular study, improved the duration of survival from a median of 10 hours to a median of

60 hours. It also gave important prognostic information because patients with higher peak intracranial pressures are more likely to die.

A further advantage of the use of intracranial pressure monitoring is in those patients being put forward for liver transplantation. Most centers that have experience of liver transplantation for acute liver failure have also had experience of patients who have failed to regain consciousness postoperatively, despite excellent graft function. In some of these cases, decerebration subsequent to intracranial hypertension in the intraoperative or early postoperative period was thought to be the mode of death. In a small series of patients who had intracranial pressure monitors inserted before liver transplantation for acute liver failure, there was a rise in intracranial pressure from the induction of anesthesia to the preclamp phase with a relative decrease in the intracranial pressure during the anhepatic phase.[23] Importantly, although the levels increased during the reperfusion phase, there were three significant episodes in six patients of intracranial hypertension in the first 10 hours postoperatively. The precise mechanism underlying intracranial hypertension has not been determined, but one possibility is reduced cerebral blood flow with reduced cerebral perfusion pressure leading to hypoxic damage. In a recent study, cerebral blood flow was determined using intravenous [133]xenon with simultaneous estimation of arterial and jugular bulb blood samples.[22] Mean cerebral blood flow was substantially reduced compared with a group of healthy adult controls. Cerebral blood flow correlated strongly with the arteriovenous pCO_2 difference, mean arterial pressure, and arteriovenous glucose difference. Cerebral metabolic rate for oxygen was substantially reduced and correlated with the cerebral blood flow. The implications of these findings are that protection from brain injury should be directed at attempts to increase cerebral blood flow, cerebral oxygenation, and cerebral perfusion pressures.

The patient should probably be nursed flat. The previous recommendation that patients should be nursed at 45° was aimed at reducing cerebral blood flow when early studies had suggested that cerebral blood flow was elevated in most patients with intracranial hypertension. This may be true in a small proportion of patients but, for the majority, it is more appropriate to have them lying flat to increase perfusion pressure. For those with experience of intracranial pressure monitoring, it is clear that stimulation of the patient by tracheal suction, examination of the pupils, or even extraneous stimuli cause increase in intracranial pressure. Tracheal suction should be performed only when essential and can be performed with local anesthesia.

It is important to maintain adequate oxygenation. During episodes of intracranial hypertension, it has been the practice in the past to hyperventilate patients, but it is probably more appropriate to increase inspired oxygen concentrations. First-line interventional therapy is mannitol which was shown, in a controlled clinical trial in 1982, to be an effective therapy for intracranial hypertension.[24] This study also showed that dexamethasone was not advantageous in this particular group of patients. For patients failing to respond to conventional therapy, an infusion of thiopentone has been shown, in a limited uncontrolled study, to reduce intracranial pressure.[25] When given as a dose between 200 mg and 500 mg over a 15-minute period, there was no significant impairment of cerebral perfusion pressure. The mechanism of action is unknown but could be due to a combination of anesthetic activity[26] or cerebral vasoconstriction.[27] One important point that should not be overlooked is that some of these patients undoubtedly have subclinical grand mal seizures, and in some cases, barbiturates may help by a direct effect on seizure activity. In patients with intracranial hypertension that is difficult to control, an EEG may be a worthwhile investigation to determine whether seizure activity is ongoing.

An important source of error in the management of patients with intracranial hypertension has been to concentrate on the intracranial pressure without paying due attention to cerebral perfusion pressure. This should always be maintained above 60 mmHg where possible. It certainly should not be allowed to drop below 40 mmHg. It may be more critical during an episode of intracranial hypertension to increase arterial pressure by the use of, for example, noradrenaline than to treat the intracranial hypertension per se. A recent study suggesting that acetylcysteine has a direct effect on cerebral blood flow merits further consideration.[28]

Renal Failure

Renal failure occurs in 40% to 80% of patients with acute liver failure according to etiology and undoubtedly worsens the prognosis.[29,30] The onset is often rapid, and it must be remembered that the serum urea is a poor guide to renal dysfunction because urea formation is reduced in such patients; failure to recognize renal impairment because of reliance on plasma urea estimation is a common source of error. The pathology appears to be identical to that complicating cirrhosis (i.e., the hepato-renal syndrome characteristically, with a low urinary sodium (<10 mmol/L) and a urine plasma osmolality ratio greater than 1.1 with normal renal histology).[31] However, the diagnosis of hepatorenal failure cannot be considered, on the basis of a low urinary sodium, until hypovolemia has been excluded.

Renal blood flow is reduced in such patients[31–33] and current thinking suggests the basis for this is renal vasoconstriction. This could be due to a number of different factors, many of which could be relevant, including splanchnic pooling, peripheral arterial vasodilation, hormonal imbalance, and the presence of a circulating factor that is directly responsible for hepatorenal failure. One recent line of investigation has been that circulating endotoxin, leading to an inflammatory cascade, has a direct effect on renal perfusion. One consequence of circulating endotoxin is the formation of eicosanoids which comprise the prostaglandins, thromboxane A_2, and the cysteinyl-leukotrienes LTC_4, LTD_4, and LTE_4. PGE_2 and prostacyclin are renal vasodilators, while in contrast, thromboxane A_2, LTC_4, and LTD_4 are renal vasoconstrictors. Recent studies have indicated that there is increased production of thromboxane A_2 in patients with hepatorenal failure, which in that particular study may simply have been a reflection of impaired hepatic function since patients with comparable liver dysfunction, but without renal failure, had similar levels.[34] Two subsequent studies have demonstrated increased cysteinyl-leukotriene production in hepatorenal failure.[35,36] In one of these studies, cysteinyl-leukotriene production was higher in subjects with liver disease and hepatorenal failure[36] when matched with patients with liver disease without renal failure in contrast to the studies of Thromboxane A_2.[34] Undoubtedly, vasodilatory prostaglandins are important in patients with liver disease since it is well documented that administration of nonsteroidal anti-inflammatory drugs to such patients causes a reduction in glomerular filtration rates. There is some evidence that there is decreased renal production of PGE_2 in hepatorenal failure.[37]

Severe acidosis is rarely a consequence of renal impairment and is usually due to lactic acidosis in association with tissue hypoxia, particularly following paracetamol overdose. Hyponatremia is common. It is important to maintain renal blood flow by maintenance of the mean arterial pressure at at least 75 mmHg, with volume replacement and inotropic support (see later). Low-dose dopamine infusions are routinely used, but the evidence for their use in patients with hepatorenal failure, or liver disease at risk of hepatorenal failure, is lacking. If there is no effect, the drug should be stopped.

The risks of conventional hemodialysis in patients with acute liver failure are hypotension, which may exacerbate cerebral edema; direct precipitation of cerebral edema by unknown mechanisms; and an increased risk of hemorrhage with platelet consumption. In a recent study of patients with acute renal failure consequent to acute liver failure, eight of 11 patients undergoing a first hemodialysis developed hypotension with at least a 15 mmHg drop.[38] This was associated with a reduction in cardiac output and was attributed to decreased peripheral venous return. Such a compromise in a patient with already borderline perfusion of the brain would undoubtedly exacerbate intracranial hypertension. Three of four subjects studied with an intracranial pressure monitor in situ had an episode of increased intracranial pressure during hemodialysis that had been observed clinically on many occasions previously.[38] For these reasons, most patients who develop acute renal failure complicating acute liver failure should be dialyzed using continuous arteriovenous or veno-venous high-volume hemofiltration, which has a less pronounced effect on blood pressure and intracranial pressure.[38]

Hepatorenal failure undoubtedly worsens the prognosis but should not be regarded as a contraindication to transplantation. It is a frequent observation that renal function recovers rapidly following transplantation, if the liver graft functions.

Hemodynamics

Acute liver failure is characterized by severe circulatory disturbance, including reduced systemic vascular resistance and an increased cardiac output, which are identical to the changes seen in patients with sepsis and other critical illness. These patients are known to demonstrate pathologic supply dependency for oxygen, even though baseline levels of oxygen uptake in these patients are frequently within the normal range or even below.[39] An increase in oxygen delivery in these patients results in increased oxygen consumption, indicating that the underlying tissue is hypoxic with a tissue oxygen debt. The precise basis for this hypoxia is unknown, but the most relevant factor is likely to be arteriovenous shunting with bypass of respiring tissue. In acute liver failure, blood lactate levels have a significant negative correlation with systemic vascular resistance and oxygen extraction. It is likely that lactic acidosis is a consequence of tissue hypoxia as a direct result of blood being shunted away from actively respiring cells in which anaerobic metabolism becomes essential but is associated with the buildup of lactate.[39] Lactate levels are higher in nonsurvivors than survivors and, in addition, hemodynamic characteristics can also predict survival since patients who died have significantly lower systemic vascular resistance, oxygen consumption, and oxygen extraction ratio. Infusion of prostacyclin to patients who subsequently died resulted in a greater increase in oxygen consumption than in those who survived, suggesting a greater degree of tissue hypoxia.[39,40]

Hypotension is common in these patients and inotropes are frequently required. Adrenaline and noradrenaline have been studied in such patients and are equally effective in increasing mean arterial pressure and systemic vascular resistance index. The use of both agents, however, results in a decrease in oxygen consumption secondary to a decrease in oxygen extraction ratios, indicating that improved arterial pressure was at the expense of increased tissue hypoxia.[41] Because of the previous experience with prostacyclin, which has been shown to increase oxygen delivery and oxygen consumption,[39,40] the combination of adrenaline and prostacyclin or noradrenaline and prostacyclin was also studied. Both these combinations have been shown to result in increased mean arterial pressure without reduction in oxygen consumption, indicating that the combination is probably the best available for patients with acute liver failure who are hypotensive with reduced systemic vascular resistance.[41]

Hemodynamic disturbance is so common in such patients that aggressive hemodynamic monitoring is indicated, and the insertion of a pulmonary artery flow catheter with constant measurement of pulmonary capillary wedge pressure and cardiac output with calculation of oxygen delivery and consumption should be regarded as the norm (Table 13-4). This is particularly important because recent studies have shown that in patients with a

Table 13-4. Targets for Hemodynamic Monitoring

Cardiac index >4.5 L/min/m^2
Oxygen delivery >700 mL/min/m^2
Oxygen consumption >170 mL/min/m^2
Systemic vascular resistance index >700 dyne/sec/cm^5/m^2

pathologic oxygen supply dependency, improved survival can be achieved by monitoring and manipulation of these variables.[42,43]

Acetylcysteine has conventionally been given in the early phase following an overdose of paracetamol.[44] However, two recent studies, one a retrospective analysis[45] and one a prospective analysis,[46] have indicated that acetylcysteine has a substantial effect on mortality when prescribed at a much later stage and almost certainly beyond the stage when an influence on the metabolism of paracetamol could be relevant. Because of this late effect in which it was shown that hypotension, cerebral edema, or renal failure was less likely,[46] the hemodynamic effects of acetylcysteine were investigated. In 12 patients with paracetamol-induced liver failure and eight patients with liver failure of other causes, acetylcysteine was shown to result in an increase in mean oxygen delivery due to an increase in the cardiac index and also was associated with an increase in mean arterial pressure, despite a decrease in systemic vascular resistance.[47] Furthermore, there was an increase in oxygen consumption associated with a substantial increase in oxygen extraction ratio. It is important to note that in this particular study, the hemodynamic effects were independent of etiology and were just as prominent in those who had not ingested paracetamol. When acetylcysteine was infused concurrently with prostacyclin, there was a further increase in the cardiac index with a further increase in the oxygen delivery but no further improvement in oxygen consumption.[47]

Infection

One of the first studies that could differentiate between patients with a poor prognosis and those who were likely to survive was measurement of Kupffer cell function as assessed by clearance of [125]iodine labeled microaggregated albumin.[48] There was massive impairment of Kupffer cell function in those with acute liver failure, particularly in those who died; Kupffer cell function improved in those who survived.[48] Impaired Kupffer cell function may exacerbate the immune deficit well documented in such patients and allow endotoxemia by failure to clear endotoxin from the portal circulation. A consequence of this would be cytokine release and, in addition, a direct effect on hemodynamic indices.[49]

A study in 1982 showed a 22% incidence of bacteremia in fulminant hepatic failure.[50] A recent comprehensive prospective study documented an incidence of bacterial and fungal infection that was so high, patients with acute liver failure should be considered immune deficient in perhaps the same way as patients with leukemia undergoing chemotherapy.[51,52] Fifty consecutive patients were assessed by prospective protocol culture of all possible sites and, in addition, when patients became unwell. In 80% of patients, bacterial infection was proven by culture and a bacterial infection was considered likely in a further 10%, even though cultures were negative; 14% of the patients had more than one proven bacterial infection. The main site of infection was the respiratory tract, which accounted for 47% of infections, with a further 23% in the urinary tract; 25% of infections were associated with bacteremia. Seventy percent of infections were due to gram-positive organisms, over half of which were *Staphylococcus aureus*. Twenty-four of the 30 patients who died during this study had evidence of bacterial infection in the 24 hours preceding death. One further important message from this study was that the usual parameters of active bacterial infection (i.e., a fever or elevation of the white cell count) were absent in more than 30% of patients indicating that for the diagnosis of infection, protocol cultures should be performed in this immunocompromised group.

Thirty-two percent of the same series had definite evidence of fungal infection, which was predominantly candida. Fungal infection was considered a major contributor to death in half of those cases, and all untreated patients died. All those with fungal infection had evidence of active or previous bacterial infection and there was a clearly recognized syndrome associated with fungal infections: deterioration of coma grade after an initial improvement, pyrexia unresponsive to antibiotics, established renal failure, and an elevated white cell count.

The median time of onset for bacterial infection proved to be 4 days and for fungal infection 8 days after starting antibiotics. With such a high rate of infection, which occurred early after admission to a tertiary unit, there is a strong argument for prophylaxis. A prospective controlled trial of selective parenteral and enteral antimicrobial therapy is under way and an early analysis was presented recently that indicates a substantial reduction in the incidence of bacterial and fungal infection in the treated population.[53]

There is considerable interest in cytokines in patients with multiorgan failure, and there are plenty of reasons to assume that cytokines might be relevant in patients with acute liver failure because of the circulating endotoxemia, the Kupffer cell dysfunction, and the high incidence of bacterial infection with both gram-positive and gram-negative organisms. Tumor necrosis factor (TNF) and interleukin-1 (IL-1) production are both elevated in patients with acute liver failure.[54,55] Plasma interleukin-6 (IL-6) and TNF levels are also elevated in acute liver failure and are associated with death and multiorgan failure. It appears from multivariate analysis that IL-6 levels are more closely associated with a poor prognosis.[56] Cytokines or antibodies to cytokines may play a role in the future management of acute liver failure, but there is no role for these at present.

Respiratory Function

The problems with the chest are similar to those experienced in patients with multiorgan failure except that acute respiratory distress syndrome appears to be relatively rare in patients with acute liver failure. Bacterial infection is the most common cause of dysfunction, but such patients are also at risk of intraalveolar hemorrhage and noncardiogenic pulmonary edema. The onset of progressive respiratory difficulty with increasing ventilation pressure and increased shadow on a chest x-ray in a patient with an unknown etiology should raise the possibility of Paraquat poisoning. The presence of hypoxia in association with a normal chest x-ray and no difficulty in ventilation is likely to be due to intrapulmonary vascular shunting—the so-called hepatopulmonary syndrome.[57]

Coagulopathy

The marked elevation of prothrombin time seen in these patients provokes a great deal of anxiety. In practical terms, hemorrhage is not a major clinical problem. The elevation of prothrombin time is *not* a contraindication to the insertion of lines; in an experienced unit, intra-arterial monitor, pulmonary artery catheter, and, where indicated, intracranial pressure monitor as well as a peripheral venous line are part of the normal management of such patients. There is a temptation to correct the abnormal indices by the use of fresh frozen plasma, but this was not shown to be beneficial in a controlled clinical trial[58] and has one major disadvantage—it prevents assessment of progress and prognosis since the prothrombin time forms an important part of patient assessment.

Although the prothrombin time is the most widely used indicator of the severity of liver damage, factor V has the shortest half-life and is therefore a more sensitive yardstick for the assessment of liver function and the synthesis of coagulation factors. This is not available routinely in the U.K., although it is used routinely in France. Circulating levels of antithrombin III are also reduced, the result being that the half-life of administered heparin is dramatically shortened. Heparin requirements are therefore increased in patients with liver disease when they require extracorporeal circuits (e.g., for dialysis) and *not* decreased as is usually thought.

In addition to the decreased synthesis of clotting factors, there is an increase in peripheral consumption, and a low-grade disseminated intravascular coagulation is present in most patients.[59] By and large, however, disseminated intravascular coagulation is not a clinical problem.

There are quantitative and qualitative defects in platelet function and thrombocytopenia can be particularly severe following paracetamol overdose. Thrombocytopenia itself is a much better predictor of hemorrhage, and in the presence of thrombocytopenia an intracranial pressure monitor is contraindicated because of the risk of hemorrhage. Platelet infusions are indicated as in normal clinical practice.

Gastrointestinal Tract

Pancreatitis is a frequent but ill recognized complication of acute liver failure. There are no specific maneuvers that can be used to prevent the condition and treatment is simply supportive.[60] Gastrointestinal hemorrhage was one of the major causes of morbidity and mortality in the early days of treatment of acute liver failure. Controlled clinical trials showing that H$_2$-receptor antagonists reduce the risk of hemorrhage and improve mortality were completed in 1978.[61] There is a theoretical risk of increasing chest infections by the use of drugs that reduce the gastric pH and, for this reason, current prophylaxis against gastrointestinal hemorrhage is with sucralfate. Some patients with acute liver failure or subacute liver failure develop varices and there is a risk of variceal hemorrhage, particularly in patients with subacute liver failure. These should be treated in a conventional manner with vasopressin and nitrates or somatostatin, with endoscopic sclerotherapy where appropriate.

Nutrition is an importance aspect of the care of patients with acute liver failure (Chapter 17). It is conventional to give Parentrovite on admission; this is essential for patients in whom alcohol may be an important etiologic factor. The use of folate and vitamin K is also recommended in such patients. Many of these patients are extremely catabolic and certainly should receive some form of intravenous nutrition. No studies have yet been performed to indicate what the best form of nutrition is, but there appears to be no detrimental effect from the infusion of amino acids and dextrose. The role of lipids in such patients is not established, but uncontrolled observations have indicated that lipids can be cleared quite rapidly in such patients despite severe liver dysfunction.

Liver Regeneration

If there is going to be a breakthrough in the management of acute liver failure in the next few years, it will surely be within the field of liver regeneration. Hepatocyte growth factor (HGF), which masqueraded under a series of names, is a strong mitogen for hepatocytes and for other cell lines.[62,63] It is a heterodimer with two polypeptides derived from proteolytic cleavage of a single chain precursor, and the larger chain has sequence homology with plasminogen. The light chain is a pseudoprotease without a catalytic site. A receptor has also been recently identified.[64] HGF has been detected in the exocrine portion of the pancreas, neurons, thyroid, Brunner's glands, duodenum, endothelial cells, and macrophages, and message has been found, in addition, in the kidneys. Its precise role in acute liver failure has not yet been established. Serum levels are high, but the protein has not yet been identified in regenerating liver cells.[65,66] HGF is detectable in plasma very shortly after any liver injury, and the concentrations that are reached are known to be mitogenic for cultured hepatocytes. The elevation of HGF clearly precedes the initiation of DNA synthesis in vitro. Epidermal growth factor (EGF) and transforming growth factor α (TGFα) are also mitogens for hepatocytes; TGFα is a more potent mitogen.[67] Transforming growth factor β (TGFβ) is an inhibitor of mitosis in hepatocytes.[68] A very important observation is that other inhibitors of mitosis in hepatocytes include interleukin-1 and interleukin-6.[69] There are, in addition, a number of important comitogens (i.e., substances that are mitogenic for hepatocytes only in the presence of other factors including HGF, EGF and TGFα). These include: insulin, glucagon, norepinephrine, vasopressin, angiotensin II, angiotensin III and estrogens.[70]

References

1. Trey, C. and Davidson, C. (1970) *The Management of Fulminant Hepatic Failure.* New York: Grune and Stratton, pp. 282–98.

2. Gimson, A.E., O'Grady, J., Ede, R.J. *et al.* (1986) Late onset hepatic failure: clinical, serological and histological features. *Hepatology* 6:288–94.

3. O'Grady, J.G., Schalm, S.W., Williams R. (1993) Acute liver failure: Redefining the syndromes. Lancet 342:273–75.

4. Sallie, R., Tibbs, C., Silva, A.E. *et al.* (1991) Detection of hepatitis E but not C in sera of patients with fulminant NANB hepatitis. *Hepatology* 14:68A (abstract).

5. Bernuau, J., Rueff, B. and Benhamou, J.P. (1986) Fulminant and subfulminant liver failure: definitions and causes. *Semin Liver Dis* 6:97–107.

6. Gimson, A.E., Tedder, R.S., White, Y.S. *et al.* (1983) Serological markers in fulminant hepatitis B. *Gut* 24:615–17.

7. Liang, T.J., Hasegawa, K., Rimon, N., Wands, J.R. and Ben-Porath, E. (1990) A hepatitis B virus mutant associated with an epidemic of fulminant hepatitis. *N Engl J Med* 324, 24:1705–09.

8. Samuel, D., Bismuth, A., Mathieu, D., et al. (1991). Passive immunoprophylaxis after liver transplantation in HBsAg-positive patients. *Lancet*, i:813–15.

9. O'Grady, J.G., Alexander, G.J.M., Hayllar, K. and Williams R. (1989). Early indicators of prognosis in fulminant hepatic failure. *Gastroenterology* 97:439–45.

10. O'Grady, J.G., Alexander, G.J.M., Thick, M. et al. (1988a). Outcome of orthotopic liver transplantation in

the aetiological and clinical variants of acute liver failure. *Quarterly Journal of Medicine*, 69:817–24.

11. Bismuth, H., Samuel, D., Gugenheim, J., et al. (1987) Emergency liver transplantation for fulminant hepatitis. *Ann Intern Med* 107:337–41.

12. O'Grady, J.G., Wendon, J., Tan, K.C., et al. (1991) Liver transplantation after paracetamol overdose. *British Medical Journal* 303:221–23.

12a. Bernau, personal observation.

13. Schafer, D.F., Pappas, S.C., Brody, L.E., et al. (1984) Visual evoked potentials in a rabbit model of hepatic encephalopathy. I. Sequential changes and comparisons with drug induced comas. *Gastroenterology* 91:540–45.

14. Schafer, D.F. and Jones, E.A. (1982) Hepatic encephalopathy and the gamma-aminobutyric-acid neurotransmitter system. *Lancet* i:18–19.

15. Bassett, M.L., Mullen, K.D., Skolnick, P. and Jones, E.A. (1987) Amelioration of hepatic encephalopathy by pharmacologic antagonism of the GABA/benzodiazepine receptor complex in a rabbit model of fulminant hepatic failure. *Gastroenterology* 93:1069–88.

16. Baraldi, M. Zenaroli, M.L., Ventura, E. et al. (1984) Supersensitivity of benzodiazepine receptors in hepatic encephalopathy due to fulminant hepatic failure in the rat: reversal by a benzodiazepine antagonist. *Clinical Science* 67:167–75.

17. Bosman, D.K., Maas, M.A.W., van den Buijs, C.A. et al. (1989) The effects of benzodiazepine receptor (BZR) antagonists and BZR inverse agonists on hepatic encephalopathy (HE) in the rat. *J Hepatol* Suppl 1:S10.

18. Ferenci, P. (1991) The GABA$_A$-benzodiazepine neurotransmitter system in hepatic encephalopathy. *Acute Liver Failure; Improved Understanding and Better Therapy*, pp. 32–36.

19. Ede, R.J., Gimson, A.E.S., Bihari, D. and Williams, R. (1986) Controlled hyperventilation in the prevention of cerebral oedema in fulminant hepatic failure. *J Hepatol* 2:43–51.

20. Ware, A.J., D'Agostino, A.N. and Combes B (1971). Cerebral oedema: A major complication of massive hepatic necrosis. *Gastroenterology* 61:877–84.

21. Ede, R.J., and Williams, R. (1986) Hepatic encephalopathy and cerebral oedema. *Semin Liver Dis* 6:107–18.

22. Keays, R., Alexander, G.J.M. and Williams, R. (1991) Intracranial pressure monitoring and cerebral blood flow measurements in fulminant hepatic failure. *Acute Liver Failure; Improved Understanding and Better Therapy*, pp. 45–47.

23. Keays, R., Potter, D., O'Grady, J., et al. (1991) Intracranial and cerebral perfusion pressure changes before, during and immediately after orthotopic liver transplantation for fulminant hepatic failure. *Quarterly Journal of Medicine*, 79:425–33.

24. Canalese, J., Gimson, A.E.S., David, C. et al. (1982) Controlled trial of dexamethasone and mannitol for

the cerebral oedema of fulminant hepatic failure. *Gut* 23:625–29.

25. Forbes, A., Alexander, G.J.M., O'Grady, J.G., et al. (1989) Thiopental infusion in the treatment of intracranial hypertension complicating fulminant hepatic failure. *Hepatology* 10:306–10.

26. Steen, P.A. and Michenfelder, J.D. (1978) Cerebral protection with barbiturates: relation to anesthetic effect. *Stroke* 9:140–42.

27. Shapiro, H.M., Galindo, A., Wyte, S.R. et al. (1973) Rapid intraoperative reduction of intracranial pressure with thiopentone. *Br J Anaesth* 45:1057–62.

28. Harrison, P.M., Wendon, J.A., Keays, R. et al. (1991) Modulation by N-Acetylcysteine of cerebral blood flow in fulminant hepatic failure (abst). *J Hepatology* 13(supply 2):74.

29. Wilkinson, S.P., Blendis, I.K., and Williams, R. (1974) Frequency and type of renal and electrolyte disorders in fulminant hepatic failure. *Br Med J* i:186–89.

30. O'Grady, J., Gimson, A.E.S., O'Brien, C.J. et al. (1988) Controlled trials of charcoal haemoperfusion in fulminant hepatic failure. *Gastroenterology* 94:1186–92.

31. Ring-Larsen, H. and Palazzo, U. (1981) Renal failure in fulminant hepatic failure and terminal cirrhosis: A comparison between incidence, types, and prognosis. *Gut* 22:585–91.

32. Guarner, F., Gimson, A.E.S., Hughes, R.D. and Williams, R. (1987) Renal function in fulminant hepatic failure: haemodynamics and renal prostaglandins. *Gut* 28:1643–47.

33. Wilkinson, S.P., Arroyo, V.A., Moodie H. et al. (1976) Abnormalities of sodium excretion and other disorders of renal function in fulminant hepatic failure. *Gut* 17:501–05.

34. Moore, K.P, Ward, P., Taylor, G. and Williams, R. (1991) Systemic and renal production of thromboxane A_2 and prostacyclin in decompensated liver disease and hepatorenal syndrome. *Gastroenterology* 100:1069–77.

35. Huber, M., Kastner, S. Scholmerich, J. et al. (1989) Analysis of cysteinyl leukotrienes in human urine: Enhanced excretion in patients with liver cirrhosis and hepatorenal syndrome. *Europ J Clin Invest* 19:53–60.

36. Moore, K.P., Taylor, G.W., Maltby, N., et al. (1990) Increased cysteinyl-leukotriene production in hepatorenal syndrome. *J Hepatol* 11:263–71 (*sic*).

37. Govindarajan, S., Nast, C.C., Smith, W.L. et al. (1987) Immunohistochemical distribution of renal prostaglandin endoperoxide synthase and prostaglandin synthase: Diminished endoperoxide synthase in the hepatorenal syndrome. *Hepatology* 7:654–59.

38. Moore, K., Taylor, G., Ward, P. and Williams, R. (1991) Aetiology and management of renal failure in acute liver failure. *Acute Liver Failure; Improved Understanding and Better Therapy*, pp. 47–53.

39. Bihari, D.J., Gimson, A.E. and Williams, R. (1986) Cardiovascular, pulmonary and renal complications of fulminant hepatic failure. *Semin Liver Dis* 6:119–28.

40. Bihari, D.J. and Tinker, J. (1988) The therapeutic value of vaso-dilator prostaglandins in multiple organ failure associated with sepsis. *Intensive Care Medicine* 15:2–7.

41. Wendon, J.A., Harrison, P.M., Keays, R., et al. (1992) Effects of vasopressor agents and epoprostenol on systemic hemodynamics and oxygen transport in fulminant hepatic failure. *Hepatology* 15:1067–71.

42. Edwards, J.D., Brown, G.C., Nightingale, P. et al. (1989) Use of survivor's cardiorespiratory values as therapeutic goals in septic shock. *Crit Care Med* 17:1098–1103.

43. Shoemaker, W.C., Kram, H.B. and Appel, P.L. (1990) Therapy of shock based on pathophysiology, monitoring, and outcome prediction. *Crit Care Med* 18:519–25.

44. Prescott, L.F., Illingworth, R.N., Critchley, J.A.J.H., et al. (1979) Intravenous N-acetylcysteine: the treatment of choice for paracetamol poisoning. *British Medical Journal* 2:1097–1100.

45. Keays, R., Harrison, P.M., Wendon, J.A., et al. (1991) Intravenous acetylcysteine in paracetamol induced fulminant hepatic failure: a prospective controlled trial. *British Medical Journal* 303:1026–29.

46. Harrison, P.M., Keays, R., Bray, G.P. et al. (1990) Improved outcome of paracetamol-induced fulminant hepatic failure by late administration of acetylcysteine. *Lancet* i:1572–73.

47. Harrison, P.M., Wendon, J.A., Gimson, A.E.S. et al. (1991) Improvement by acetylcysteine of hemodynamics and oxygen transport in fulminant hepatic failure. *N Eng J Med* 324:1852–57.

48. Canalese, J., Gove, C., Gimson, A.E.S. et al. (1982) Reticuloendothelial system and hepatocyte function in fulminant hepatic failure. *Gut* 23:265–69.

49. Suffredeni, A.F., Fromm, R.E., Parker, M.M. et al. (1989) The cardiovascular response of normal humans to the administration of endotoxin. *N Eng J Med* 321:280–87.

50. Wyke, R.J., Canalese, J.C., Gimson, A.E.S. et al. (1982) Bacteraemia in patients with fulminant hepatic failure. *Liver* 2:45–52.

51. Rolando, N., Harvey, F., Brahm, J. et al. (1990) Prospective study of bacterial infection in acute liver failure: an analysis of fifty patients. *Hepatology* 11:49–53.

52. Rolando, N., Harvey, F., Brahm, J. et al. (1991) Fungal infection: A common, unrecognised complication of acute liver failure. *J Hepatol* 12:1–9.

53. Rolando, N., Gimson, A.E.S., Kalayci, C. et al. (1990) Prospective study of selective parenteral and enteral antimicrobial regime (SPEAR) in fulminant hepatic failure (abstract). *Hepatology* 12:1012.

54. De la Mata, M., Meager, A., Rolando, N. et al. (1990) Tumour necrosis factor production in fulminant hepatic failure: Relation to aetiology and superimposed infection. *Clini Exp Immunol* 82:479–84.

55. Muto, Y., Nouri-Aria, K.T., Meager, A. et al. (1988) Enhanced tumour necrosis factor and interleukin-1 in fulminant hepatic failure. *Lancet* ii:72–74.

56. Sheron, N., Goka, J., Wendon, J. et al. (1990) Highly elevated plasma cytokines in fulminant hepatic failure: Correlations with multi-organ failure and death (abstract). *Hepatology* 12:939.

57. Bihari, D.J., Gimson, A.E. and Williams, R. (1986) Cardiovascular, pulmonary and renal complications of fulminant hepatic failure. *Semin Liver Dis* 6:119–28.

58. Gazzard, B., Henderson, J. and Williams, R. (1975) Early changes in coagulation following paracetamol overdose and a controlled trial of fresh frozen plasma therapy. *Gut* 16:617–20.

59. O'Grady, J.G., Langley, P.G., Isola, L.M. et al. (1986) Coagulopathy of fulminant hepatic failure. *Semin Liver Dis* 6:159–63.

60. Ede, R.J., Moore, K.P., Marshall, W.J. and Williams, R. (1988) Frequency of pancreatitis in fulminant hepatic failure using isoenzyme markers. *Gut* 29:778–81.

61. Macdougall, B. and Williams, R. (1978) H_2-receptor antagonist in the prevention of acute upper gastrointestinal haemorrhage in fulminant hepatic failure. *Gastroenterology* 74:464–65.

62. Michalopoulos, G., Houck, K., Dolan, M. and Novicki, D.L. (1983) Control of proliferation of hepatocytes by two serum hepatopoietins. *Fed Proc* 42:1023.

63. Nakamura, T., Nawa, K. and Ichihara, A. (1984) Partial purification and characterisation of hepatocyte growth factor from serum of hepatectomised rats. *Biochem Biophys Commun* 122:1450–59.

64. Zarnegar, R. and Michalopoulos, G.K. (1990) Identification and partial characterisation of binding sites for hepatopoietin A (hepatocyte growth factor). (In press).

65. Lindroos, P., Zarnegar, R. and Michalopoulos, G.K. (1990) Hepatocyte growth factor (hepatopoietin A) rapidly increases in plasma prior to DNA synthesis and liver regeneration stimulated by partial hepatectomy and CC14 administration. (In press).

66. Tsubouchi, H., Niitani, Y., Hirono, S. et al. (1991) Levels of the human hepatocyte growth factor in serum of patients with various liver diseases determined by an enzyme-linked immunosorbent assay. *Hepatology* 13:1–5.

67. Brenner, D.A., Koch, K.S. and Leffert, H.L. (1989) Transforming growth factor-alpha stimulates proto-oncogene c-jun expression and a mitogenic program in primary cultures of adult rat hepatocytes. *DNA* 8:279–85.

68. Carr, B.I., Hayashi, I., Branum, E.L. and Moses, H.L. (1986) Inhibition of DNA synthesis in rat hepatocytes by platelet-derived type transforming growth factor. *Cancer Res* 46:2330–34.

69. Nakamura, T., Arakaki, R. and Ichihara, A. (1988) Interleukin-1 is a potent growth inhibitor of adult rat hepatocytes in primary culture. *Exp Cell Res* 179:488 –97.

70. Michalopoulos, G.K. (1991) Overview of liver regeneration. *Acute Liver Failure; Improved Understanding and Better Therapy*, pp. 85–89.

Chapter 14

Intensive Care of Patients after Liver Surgery

Gilbert R. Park and K.E.J. Gunning

After prolonged or difficult hepatic surgery a patient's stay in the intensive care unit may be divided into two phases. The initial phase covering the first hours after the procedure is a time of stabilization, effectively a continuation of the intraoperative management, with close cardiorespiratory and biochemical monitoring. The second phase is a period of recovery. It is dominated by the need for pain relief and resumption of respiratory function. The latter stage may be characterized by important metabolic changes associated with a change in liver function, in a patient who may previously have been in end-stage liver failure. This change may be an improvement, for example, after the relief of biliary obstruction. Alternatively, there may be deterioration in a patient with end-stage liver disease who is unable to withstand the stress of surgery and anesthesia. All are factors that can influence the function of the liver, kidneys, and other organs. The main aim of management is to maintain hepatic blood flow and oxygenation.

Ventilatory Support

During transfer from the operating room to the intensive care unit, cardiovascular monitoring should be continued and ventilatory support maintained. A volume-controlled fluid-logic ventilator that allows air entrainment can be used. This avoids the use of 100% oxygen with its attendant high risk of absorption atelectasis.[1,2] During transfer the inspired gases can be humidified using a heat and moisture exchanger. Because microbiological contamination of the ventilator and the subsequent transfer of these organisms represents a risk to these patients, a heat and moisture exchanger combined with a microbiological filter should be used.[3]

On arrival in the intensive care unit, the patient will usually need ventilatory support with a volume-controlled ventilator. Later, synchronized intermittent mandatory ventilation (SIMV) is used to allow patient triggering at an early stage.

A positive end expiratory pressure (PEEP) of 5 cm H_2O is usually used. The use of PEEP helps maintain arterial oxygenation with a low F_1O_2 by preventing the development of areas of atelectasis. The decrease in hepatic blood flow seen when PEEP is used is directly related to the decrease in cardiac output.[4] This can be overcome by increasing the intravascular volume to maintain cardiac output.[5] The small decrease in renal function that occurs with PEEP of this level does not appear to be clinically significant.[6]

The ventilator is adjusted to maintain normocarbia, since both hyperventilation and hypoventilation have deleterious effects on hepatic oxygen consumption and splanchnic blood flow.[7-9] A heat and moisture exchanging filter, identical to the one used on a transport ventilator, can be used to provide humidification.

In the uncomplicated patient, weaning from artificial ventilation is usually done easily within the first 8–12 hours. If there is poor gas exchange or renal function or a major complication such as abdominal bleeding or pyrexia then weaning should be delayed. Effective analgesia is vital during weaning and is discussed below and in chapter 5.

If the patient develops respiratory insufficiency after tracheal extubation, reintubation of the trachea and the reinstitution of ventilatory support should not be delayed. Patients do not tolerate a period of inadequate, spontaneous ventilation well, and eventually ventilatory support will be needed as an emergency procedure. The liver, already stressed by the operation, may be unnecessarily damaged by hypoxia.

Lung water increases after major surgery and this may result in pulmonary edema. It may occur in both adults and children. Riegle and colleagues reported the development of radiographically proven pulmonary edema in 44% of their pediatric patients after liver transplantation.[10] The Birmingham group has also commented on the sensitivity of patients with chronic liver disease to fluid loads.[11]

The factors responsible for this include a large intraoperative blood transfusion, fluid shifts, and hormonal changes in response to stress. Surgical trauma results in tissue edema that accumulates for several hours after the end of the operation and is later absorbed into the circulation. Antidiuretic hormone is increased because of the raised mean intrathoracic pressure owing to artificial ventilation and the application of PEEP. In addition, opioids, administered for analgesia, will also lead to water retention,[12] further exacerbating the increase in lung water.

The clinical diagnosis of fluid overload and consequent pulmonary edema is difficult in patients receiving controlled ventilation; fine crackles are heard only when extreme pulmonary edema exists. Right atrial pressure and pulmonary capillary wedge pressure may be artificially elevated during mechanical artificial ventilation, unless the patient is temporarily disconnected from the ventilator during measurement. These measurements are, anyway, of dubious value in the diagnosis of noncardiogenic pulmonary edema. Although radiology may help, it can be difficult to diagnose the presence of early pulmonary edema on a portable, supine chest x-ray in a patient receiving artificial ventilation.

It was hoped that the lung water computer might provide a solution to the diagnosis of excessive lung water. This technique uses changes in diffusible or nondiffusible indicators to calculate extravascular lung water. In the diffusible indicator technique, alterations in thermal conductivity are used and 3% saline, chromium tagged red cells, albumin, or indocyanine green are used as nondiffusible indicators.[13] However, it carries with it the need for both pulmonary and femoral artery catheterization and has proved unreliable.

Because of the difficulties in diagnosing pulmonary edema, we give a small intravenous dose of frusemide (5 mg in the adult, 1–2 mg in the child) before weaning from artificial ventilation. It is usually followed by a prompt and large diuresis in those patients who are water and probably salt overloaded. Indeed, Tew and Park have shown that large doses of diuretics may be unnecessary in many critically ill patients, urine output increasing by 133% for each 0.1 mg/kg of frusemide given.[14] The use of small doses of frusemide, repeated as necessary, may avoid the adverse effects of an unnecessarily large diuresis[15] caused by larger doses. Furthermore, Johnston and colleagues have shown that the nondiuretic hemodynamic effects of frusemide (venodilation) are small with doses as low as 5 or 10 mg.[16] Therefore, small doses of frusemide may cause less hemodynamic disturbance than larger ones.

After tracheal extubation, opacification of the right lower zone on the chest x-ray is common. The factors contributing to this include:

Pleural effusion. During surgery, trauma to the right hemidiaphragm results in a sympathetic effusion. Additionally, ascitic fluid, often present preoperatively as part of severe liver disease, recurs after surgery and drains through peritoneal-pleural channels in the right hemidiaphragm into the pleural space. Their presence was shown in a patient admitted to the intensive care unit before liver transplantation in whom 6 L of ascitic fluid was drained when a right internal jugular line was inadvertently placed into his pleural cavity. Vargus-Tank and colleagues have also demonstrated the existence of peritoneal-pleural connections using air in cadavers, and a radiotracer method in patients.[17] In seven of 65 autopsies and two of eight patients, air or radiotracer passed rapidly into the chest showing the presence of these channels.

Surgical retraction of the diaphragm. This causes atelectasis by direct pulmonary trauma.

Paralysis of the right phrenic nerve. During liver transplantation and other surgical procedures when the suprahepatic inferior vena cava is cross clamped, the clamp may trap the right phrenic nerve paralyzing the right hemidiaphragm in approximately 10% of patients. Recovery is usually seen over 2–4 weeks. If there is profuse abdominal bleeding after operation this increases intra-abdominal pressure leading to ischemia of the diaphragm. This has led to bilateral diaphragmatic palsies that can take a long time to recover.[18]

Liver size. This is important only during liver transplantation. Although the donor organ is, wherever possible, matched for recipient size, the difficulties of donor availability may not always make a perfect match possible. When a large donor liver is transplanted into a small recipient, then the diaphragm will be elevated, interfering with ventilation at the right base. Bronchial breathing may be heard on auscultation of the chest in such circumstances and is an indicator of compression of the lung rather than collapse or infection.

Intra-Abdominal collections. Perihepatic collections of blood or pus will also elevate the hemidiaphragm, leading to collapse of the right base of the lung.

Pain. If adequate analgesia is not provided then patient will not cough, expectorate, or adequately expand the lower parts of the lung. This will result in pulmonary atelectasis and segmental collapse.

The problem of basal pulmonary opacification has almost completely disappeared from our practice. This follows from a more aggressive approach to analgesia and the institution of intermittent positive pressure breathing (IPPB) and physiotherapy four times a day. Although IPPB was shown to be of little benefit in the prophylaxis and treatment of atelectasis in patients after routine surgery, this study was performed in patients after widely differing operations as opposed to our more homogenous group of patients after liver surgery.[19]

Sedation and Analgesia

After liver surgery adequate sedation and analgesia is essential. Analgesia is required because of pain from the large incision and intra-abdominal dissection. Respiratory depression and an antitussive effect are required immediately after operation to enable the patient to tolerate artificial ventilation and the tracheal tube. In a noisy and often brightly lit environment there is a further requirement for anxiolysis and the need for sleep. If complications such as bleeding or infection occur then sedation and analgesia may be necessary to facilitate a more prolonged period of ventilation.

Many analgesics, hypnotics, sedatives, tranquilizers, neuroleptics, and muscle relaxants have been used for analgesia and sedation suggesting that the ideal treatment regimen does not yet exist. In this chapter only the commoner and more useful techniques will be discussed. Other chapters describe these drugs in more detail. For a more comprehensive review the reader is referred to other sources.[20,21]

Over the last few years there has been a change in the depth of sedation thought to be necessary for critically ill patients. Ten years ago most ICUs thought patients should be deeply sedated.[22] More recently Bion and Ledingham have shown that the current aim is to have the patient asleep but easily rousable.[23] Amnesia for unpleasant events and procedures may also be beneficial, and nocturnal sleep is a further need.

Undersedation and inadequate analgesia in critically ill patients have adverse pathophysiologic effects. These include autonomic disturbances, such as hypertension and tachycardia resulting in damage to an ischemic myocardium. The patient who is inadequately sedated may disconnect or dislodge some of the equipment essential to his care, and failure to synchronize with the ventilator may result in hypoxia and hypercarbia. Without adequate analgesia patients, particularly children, breathing spontaneously, may fail to cough and expectorate their sputum effectively. This, combined with underventilation, results in atelectasis, lobar collapse, and an increase in pulmonary shunting of blood that may progress to respiratory failure.

Nurses (who usually decide when and how much sedation a patient receives) prefer over-rather than undersedation. Although undersedation is more obviously dangerous, oversedation is not without hazard. Respiratory depression may occur in the immediate period after operation when any sedative and analgesic drug is given. Hemodynamic effects may also be seen after opiates. Morphine is thought to be worse than the newer synthetic opiates such as fentanyl or alfentanil.

An ileus occurs immediately after liver surgery secondary to the surgical trauma. Opiates may aggravate this by inhibiting gastric emptying, delaying gastrointestinal transit, and constricting smooth muscle.[24] Unnecessarily prolonging an ileus increases the duration of time that parenteral nutrition may be necessary, with its attendant risks. Many authors have shown significant hemodynamic changes in the gastrointestinal tract after giving midazolam, morphine, and fentanyl.[25–27] The clinical significance of changes in gastrointestinal blood flow in patients after liver surgery is difficult to determine but may be important in changing oxygen delivery to the liver.

Cerebral function is depressed with analgesic and sedative drugs. If the duration of action of the drugs is prolonged and unrecognized then cerebral function may be misdiagnosed as cerebral damage. This can result in inappropriate major management decisions.

Infection remains a major cause of mortality and morbidity in the critically ill, and the contribution of sedation to this was described and recognized over 30 years ago.[28,29] Morphine, diazepam, local anaesthetic agents (except bupivacaine), and intravenous induction agents have also been shown to have adverse effects on the immune system.[30,31] Codeine can be manufactured within the body from morphine and is present in papaveretum and has been implicated in the cause of renal failure.[32] Immobility caused by unnecessary prolonged sedation results in increased muscle wasting and nitrogen loss.[33]

Drugs that are Principally Sedative

Benzodiazepines

Many different benzodiazepines are available. The most commonly used ones in critically ill patients are lorazepam,[34] diazepam, and midazolam. In critically ill patients the metabolism and elimination of diazepam may be markedly reduced and its active metabolite, desmethyldiazepam, has an even longer half-life.[35] Midazolam is a water-soluble benzodiazepine with a rapid onset and short duration of action in normal subjects.[36] Its main metabolite, 10H-hydroxymidazolam, is pharmacologically active but has a shorter elimination half-life than midazolam[37] and is probably the most predictable of this group. Flumazenil is a specific benzodiazepine antagonist that acts on the GABA receptors[38,39] and can be used to reverse prolonged sedation, caused by benzodiazepines.[40,41]

Propofol

Di-isopropylphenol in soya bean emulsion is a short-acting anesthetic agent. Its use for providing sedation has been investigated.[42–44] It appears to be safe and predictable but is expensive.

Chlormethiazole

This agent is structurally similar to thiamin (vitamin B_1). It has been widely used in preeclampsia, status epilepticus, and during regional analgesia. It is available only as a 0.8% solution and large volumes may be needed to sedate patients. Because of this, it has not found widespread acceptance in the management of the critically ill. New methods of renal support may overcome this difficulty.[45] Of particular importance is the observation by Modig that this agent may be protective against endotoxemia.[46]

Isoflurane

Kong, Willats, and Prys-Roberts have evaluated isoflurane for sedation of critically ill patients.[47] It is particularly attractive in patients with liver disease because of its low biotransformation and excretion by the pulmonary system. In hepatic and renal failure, concentrations of fluoride may increase to potentially toxic values.[48]

Drugs that are Principally Analgesic

All patients show an immense variation in requirements for opiates, particularly morphine.[49]

Morphine

Morphine is commonly used either alone or as papaveretum to provide analgesia. It is often given by continuous intravenous infusion, although the rationale for this is not clear. It has a highly active metabolite, morphine 6 glucuronide, that accumulates in renal failure.[50]

Pethidine

Although pethidine is used to provide analgesia in the critically ill,[51] its pharmacology in critically ill patients has not been fully evaluated. The clearance of pethidine is decreased in patients with impaired liver function, although the volume of distribution and degree of protein binding are unchanged. This pattern has been seen in patients with cirrhosis and those with viral hepatitis,[52] when a collateral circulation does not develop. Because of this, the prolonged half-life of pethidine in these patients has been attributed to an impaired metabolic function of the liver. In patients with impaired renal function receiving repeated doses of pethidine, accumulation of the major metabolite of pethidine, norpethidine, will occur.[53] This metabolite has a central excitatory action that can lead to fits and other CNS excitatory phenomena.[54]

Phenoperidine

Phenoperidine was thought to be more predictable than other opiates,[55] although others have shown this not to be so.[56] It has a half-life of approximately 60 minutes, and its main metabolites are pethidine and norpethidine. In patients with liver disease phenoperidine has a prolonged elimination half-life and a reduced clearance.[57] This appears to be a result of reduced hepatic metabolism, since the proportion of the dose excreted as pethidine and norpethidine is decreased, while that excreted as phenoperidine is increased. The pharmocokinetics of phenoperidine in renal failure are not known and accumulation of norpethidine might occur.

Fentanyl

This is a synthetic opiate that has been used to provide analgesia for critically ill patients and is usually administered by continuous intravenous infusion. In the critically ill, fentanyl appears to have a prolonged terminal half-life with an enlarged volume of distribution; the clearance and degree of protein binding remain the same.[58,59]

Alfentanil

This short-acting opiate is now being promoted as an analgesic for use by infusion in patients needing ventilatory support.[60] Pharmacokinetic studies in critically ill patients have shown decreased clearances, comparable to those seen in anaesthetized surgical patients.[51,61] A normal clearance in renal failure has been shown,[62] suggesting that alfentanil is a suitable opioid for use in this situation.

Naloxone

Naloxone is a specific opiate antagonist acting at the μ receptors. Its use in sedation and analgesia is limited to assessment of patients who may have prolonged sedation. If used to reverse respiratory depression, it can produce arrhythmias and sudden hypertension because analgesia is also reversed, with respiratory depression, unless an additional method of pain relief is provided.

Regional Anesthesia

When a patient is breathing spontaneously and the trachea has been extubated there is no longer any need for sedation, but there is a continuing need for analgesia. Indeed, this need may be even greater after tracheal extubation. Hypoventilation, because of pain, particularly if combined with a failure to expectorate, will result in areas of collapse, an increase in pulmonary shunting, and the risk of infection and respiratory failure. Opiates can be used but their antitussive and respiratory depressant effects limit their use in this situation. Regional analgesia is superior.[63] Suitable techniques to provide analgesia for patients after liver surgery include epidural analgesia, paravertebral blocks, subarachnoid analgesia, intrapleural catheters, wound perfusion, and intercostal nerve blockade. Spinal analgesia using local anesthetic agents has too short a duration of action to be useful. Intrathecal opioids are unpredictable, although the use of midazolam by this route may warrant investigation in the future.[64,65] Paravertebral nerve blockade and epidural analgesia can both be used with a catheter to provide continuous analgesia. However, they require the use of large needles to insert the catheters, and in patients with liver disease the coexisting coagulopathy makes this hazardous.

Fluid Balance

Maintenance of fluid balance is important particularly in the early period after operation. In the intensive care unit, as during the preceding surgery, the numerical values of fluid input and output can be misleading and they are best assessed from the measurement of cardiovascular parameters and urine output.

On return from the operating room the patient will need fluid in addition to the measured losses. This is partly accounted for by vasodilation, as re-warming occurs, expanding the intravascular volume. There may be a period of continued ooze of blood from dissected surfaces that may not drain externally, but needs blood transfusion.

An often underestimated loss is the exudate from the area of dissection left after skeletonization of the liver. This occurs even in the absence of bleeding and can be an appreciable volume. The patients who appear to lose the largest volumes of exudate are those who have had previous surgery and after operation have a large raw area from extensive dissection.

A further group in whom exudative losses are seen are those patients with polycystic disease of the liver who have had a liver transplant. In this group of patients the discrepancy in size between the large diseased liver and the small donor liver results in little tamponade effect on bleeding or the oozing surface.

Fluid replacement is guided by right atrial pressure or capillary wedge pressure, the hematocrit, and the plasma oncotic pressure. If a patient is hypovolemic and the hematocrit is low then blood is transfused. If however the hematocrit is high then a colloid is transfused.

When a vascular anastomosis has been performed as part of the surgery the hematocrit is maintained in the region of 0.3–0.35 to lessen the risk of thrombosis. Although this has been suggested as the optimal figure for oxygen carriage and tissue delivery,[66] normovolemic hemodilution should only be used in this situation. In those patients without such an anastomosis a normal hemoglobin concentration is maintained. This will improve oxygen delivery to the tissues.

Albumin Replacement

The drainage fluid from the abdominal drains, although blood stained, usually has a low hemoglobin content and consists principally of an exudate. The hematocrit is between 2 and 10% and blood replacement usually is not needed. However, if the hematocrit is greater than 10%, then this is usually an indicator of postoperative bleeding and blood transfusion is appropriate. The exudate has a high concentration of albumin. A liver recently subjected to prolonged surgery can be expected to have a diminished synthetic capability for many substances, including albumin. Because of the high protein content of any exudate loss and diminished synthetic ability of the liver, some intensive care units routinely give albumin rather than wait for the inevitable decrease in the plasma concentration of albumin. Whether this reduces morbidity or mortality in this group is unknown. In the population found in a general intensive care unit the use of albumin, as opposed to other colloids, makes no difference to pulmonary edema, renal failure, length of stay, or mortality.[67]

Renal Dysfunction and Its Prevention after Liver Surgery

Mortality after major liver surgery is closely related to the development of renal failure.[68] The most important causes of renal dysfunction include major blood loss occurring in the perioperative period and the hepatorenal syndrome.

In all patients hemorrhage results in sympathetic vasoconstriction, which mainly affects the afferent glomerular arterioles, with a decrease in renal blood flow and consequent renal ischemia. Sepsis and the use of potentially nephrotoxic drugs, such as the cephalosporin or aminoglycoside groups of antibiotics (especially in combination with loop diuretics) and the immunosuppressant cyclosporin A,[69] may also be causally implicated in some patients.

Many theories exist about the causes of renal dysfunction in patients with liver disease, probably reflecting the many causes of this problem. There are no significant morphologic changes demonstrable in the kidneys of patients with the hepatorenal syndrome. The deterioration in fluid and electrolyte state is purely functional with the kidneys responding appropriately to various neurohumoral mechanisms. Tubular function is normal and indeed the urine produced by these patients is usually concentrated. Koppel and colleagues transplanted kidneys from patients with the hepatorenal syndrome into patients without hepatic dysfunction, but with renal failure, and found that the transplanted kidneys recovered normal function.[70]

There are a variety of endocrinological changes in the hepatorenal syndrome. The first involves increases in aldosterone levels. Adrenal secretion of this hormone increases and since its destruction is dependent on liver function, particularly liver blood flow, its breakdown is reduced in severe liver disease. Increases in the concentration of aldosterone result in sodium retention. The second feature is a decrease in effective plasma volume caused by the redistribution of fluids from the intravascular space to the interstitial fluid compartment, including ascitic fluid. Hypovolemia stimulates volume receptors, found in atria and elsewhere, leading to an increase in secretion of renin and the production of angiotensin I. This enzyme is then changed by converting enzyme, found predominantly in the lung, to angiotensin II. Production of these substances leads to atrial vasoconstriction and an increased resorption of sodium and water in the distal tubules. Plasma concentrations of antidiuretic hormones are also increased in hepatic disease, and this combined with the decreased filtrate delivered to the distal convoluted tubules and collecting system leads to further water retention. Thus total body sodium increases and free water clearance decreases. Other hormonal changes in patients with hepatic failure that influence renal function include an increase in plasma noradrenaline and aldosterone levels to two to five times normal. These concentrations will increase further if patients develop renal failure. In addition, in liver disease there are changes in endogenous renal prostaglandins and vasoactive intestinal polypeptides that further alter intrarenal mechanisms of salt and water excretion.

Assessment of Renal Function

Routine tests of renal function before and after liver surgery include the estimation of plasma urea, creatinine, and creatinine clearance. In most patients these tests will provide an adequate guide to renal function. Interpretation of these results in some patients requires caution.

Plasma urea may be falsely low in patients with severe liver failure. In this situation the liver may no longer be able to break down protein and produce urea. However, if the liver failure is less acute, then plasma urea may be artificially increased because of recent gastrointestinal bleeding resulting in breakdown of blood to urea by bacteria.

In cachectic patients plasma creatinine may be falsely low, even in the presence of severe renal dysfunction and prolonged liver disease. These patients have a reduced muscle bulk and fail to produce creatine for the liver to break down to creatinine. Creatinine clearance is reduced according to the degree of renal dysfunction but continues to provide an adequate guide to renal function.

Deeply jaundiced patients (plasma bilirubin > 300 μmol/L) may provide further difficulties. In these patients the estimation of creatinine itself is unreliable, rendering creatinine clearance estimations valueless. In this situation glomerular filtration rate should be measured using another technique, such as EDTA clearance. Even the use of radiolabeled measurements, which are technically easier to do, may be inaccurate as a result of fluid shifts in the immediate period after operation.[71]

Renal Protection

Dawson showed that giving mannitol to jaundiced patients during surgery reduced the incidence of renal failure by promoting an osmotic diuresis.[72]

Other agents, especially catecholamines, have also been investigated as protective agents. The kidneys are richly innervated with dopaminergic receptors. These are found both in blood vessels[73] and the tubules.[74] It was hoped that stimulation of these receptors with low-dose dopamine[75] and dopexamine[60] might reduce the incidence of renal failure after liver transplantation. In a prospective trial Swygert and colleagues failed to show any benefit from dopamine.[76] Whether dopexamine is effective is unknown. Theoretically, it has advantages since it does not have significant α receptor effects, even at high plasma concentrations. High plasma concentrations are likely with all catecholamines, even when given at low doses, in patients with liver disease.[77]

Although the effects of dopaminergic stimulation on renal function are well described, effects on other organs may also occur. These may include a general increase in splanchnic blood flow that may decrease the incidence of stress ulceration and improve anastomotic healing.

Dopamine has been shown to increase estimated hepatic blood flow (EHBF) under many conditions. These include peritonitis and hemorrhagic shock,[78–80] possibly by increasing the portal venous supply rather than hepatic artery flow.[81] The increased EHBF is usually associated with an increased cardiac output. However, the percentage increase in EHBF is greater than the percentage increase in cardiac output, implying some selective dilatation of the hepatic vasculature.[82] Dopaminergic stimulation increases portal vein blood flow. The hepatic artery also has β_2 receptors that when stimulated result in an increase in flow, although the precise location of the receptors is unclear.[81] One patient has been reported in whom the use of dopexamine (that also has potent β agonist properties) resulted in an increase in hepatic blood flow. This in turn led to an increase in oxygen consumption without an increase in oxygen delivery.[83]

Electrolyte and Acid–Base Balance

The plasma concentrations of potassium is usually low on return from the operating room. Although banked blood has a high potassium content, and might be expected to result in hyperkalemia, it is rapidly absorbed by the transplanted liver after revascularization. Indeed, if hyperkalemia is seen after operation then there is almost certainly major hepatic or renal dysfunction.

After operation plasma glucose continues to be increased, a consequence of stress, the metabolism of citrate, and giving glucose and (if the patient needs immunosuppression) exogenous steroids. The plasma glucose should be measured frequently (every one or two hours initially) at the bedside, using a reflectance meter. Hyperglycemia should be treated with a sliding scale infusion of insulin or a reduction in the amount of dextrose being given.

Ionized calcium is maintained intraoperatively by giving calcium chloride to replace that lost by chelation with citrate transfused in the blood. High ionized calcium levels have been reported after operation as the citrate is metabolized by the transplanted liver.[84] However, these rapidly return to normal.

Autologous blood transfusion may be used during the operation. Most automated systems collect blood from the operative field and heparinize it, after which it separates the red blood cells by centrifugation, washes, and resuspends them in saline. The final hematocrit of the suspension is 60%.[85,86] The infusion of large amounts of washed red cells suspended in 0.9% saline may theoretically lead to biochemical abnormalities such as hypernatremia

and hypokalemia. These have not been shown in patients after liver transplantation.[87]

Gastrointestinal Bleeding

Stress ulceration is a serious complication after liver surgery. The exact cause is unclear but certain risk factors have been identified. These include artificial ventilation, sepsis, hypotension, inotropic support, liver failure, and parenteral nutrition.[88] In addition, after liver surgery patients are at further risk of gastrointestinal bleeding for a number of reasons.

The coagulopathy, often a part of liver disease, increases the risk of bleeding from any source and correction of this reduces the risk of bleeding. Many patients will have portal hypertension and as a consequence esophageal varices. Although the surgical procedure may have returned portal blood pressure to normal the esophagus remains friable. Trauma to esophageal varices can be reduced by the use of a small diameter (12 FG) silicone-coated nasogastric tube. This is the least traumatic size that still allows aspiration of gastric contents. Further down the gastrointestinal tract, additional factors predisposing to this complication include the presence of bile acids in the stomach, the administration of high-dose steroids for immunosuppression after liver transplantation, and the lack of food in the stomach.

In patients with fulminant liver failure antacids are less effective in preventing stress ulceration than the H_2 receptor antagonists.[89] Prophylaxis against this complication can be provided with intravenous ranitidine or cimetidine.[85,90] The former agent is preferred because it is thought to have fewer side effects than cimetidine, notably cytochrome P450 enzyme inhibition.[91] Although ranitidine is both metabolized in the liver and excreted unchanged by the kidneys, delayed metabolism and excretion have been shown in renal disease.[92] Should this complication arise then the normal dose should be halved.

More recently it has been shown that prophylaxis against stress ulceration is better provided with sucralfate. This agent, a nonabsorbable aluminum salt of sucrose octa sulphate, works by increasing the synthesis of mucosal prostaglandins, stimulating mucus and bicarbonate production and increasing mucosal cell renewal; it does not change gastric pH. Both sucralfate and H_2 antagonists are equally effective at preventing stress ulceration.[93]

However, H_2 antagonists increase the gastric pH and this allows bacterial overgrowth to occur. When this happens retrograde pharyngeal colonization with gram-negative and anaerobic organisms may result. Subsequently, these may be aspirated past a cuffed tracheal tube, resulting in a nosocomial pneumonia. Since sucralfate does not increase gastric pH the incidence of bacterial colonization of the stomach and nosocomial pneumonia is lower than in those patients treated with ranitidine.[94,95] Furthermore, sucralfate is easier to give, does not require regular pH monitoring of the nasogastric aspirate, and is cheaper. Because of these features current opinion favors sucralfate rather than H_2 antagonists.[96] Sucralfate prophylaxis has one disadvantage, because gastric pH is not increased if pulmonary aspiration of stomach contents does occur after tracheal extubation then Mendelson's syndrome may develop. Ranitidine can be given, intravenously, one hour before tracheal extubation to prevent this complication.

Pinkleton and Hadzima have shown that enteral alimentation is protective against gastrointestinal bleeding, and is superior to both antacids and H_2 receptor antagonists.[97] Enteral nutrition may act by inducing a dilutional alkalinization of stomach contents or by maintaining nutrition better than parenteral feeding or by increasing gut blood flow. In normal circumstances once patients are established onto either full nasogastric feeding or an adequate diet, prophylaxis against stress ulceration can often be stopped.

Coagulation

After operation when liver function recovers and abdominal bleeding stops, coagulation often returns to the values found before operation. However, if liver function deteriorates then all the coagulation changes associated with acute liver failure will develop (increased prothrombin and kaolin partial thromboplastin time and a decreased fibrinogen concentration and platelet count). The increase in prothrombin time may be used as a measure of liver function. If there is bleeding after operation, needing continued blood transfusion, the dilutional coagulopathy seen intraoperatively continues.

Treatment of both forms of coagulopathy is similar. Thrombocytopenia ($< 50,000 \times 10^9L$) is treated with platelet transfusion. If the plasma urea is increased, because of renal failure, then dDAVP should be given to improve platelet function. Clotting factors are replaced with fresh frozen plasma; if fibrinogen is low then cryoprecipitate may also be given. Vitamin K (10 mg) may also be given to replace any deficiency. Some centers give it routinely after operation for two to three days, in case the patient is deficient. Activation of the coagulation cascade resulting in a consumptive coagulopathy is increasingly recognized.

Thrombosis of the liver and other organs may also be a problem after transplantation. Low levels of antithrombin III activity have been found in some pediatric patients after liver transplantation and may be a contributory factor in hepatic artery thrombosis. Furthermore, low levels of antithrombin III activity may also be a factor in the cause of renal failure, owing to thrombosis in the kidney.[98] When a liver is transplanted for the Budd-Chiari syndrome, thrombosis of the donor liver is a significant risk. When postoperative bleeding stops subcutaneous heparin should be started, followed at 24–48 hours by systemic heparinization and eventually oral anticoagulation.

Postoperative Intra-Abdominal Bleeding

Chronic liver disease frequently results in portal hypertension with large, abnormal blood vessels in both the skin and peritoneum. These are divided during liver surgery and despite meticulous attention to hemostasis, torrential bleeding may occur that can be impossible to stop intraoperatively. On rare occasions the liver, a large vascular organ, may also be inadvertently lacerated resulting in bleeding. If the bleeding cannot be controlled, the abdomen is closed and the patient taken to the intensive care unit for 6–36 hours. During this time the abdomen is allowed to tamponade, which controls the bleeding. The patient is then taken back to the operating room electively for removal of the packs and clot. Abdominal tamponade may be hastened by abdominal binding[99] or by use of pneumatic antishock garments.[100] However, abdominal tamponade is not without hazard. Studies in dogs have reported the changes seen with increasing intra-abdominal pressure;[101-103] cardiac output decreased and systemic vascular resistance increased with increasing intra-abdominal pressure. This effect was most marked in dogs rendered hypovolemic. The reduction in cardiac output was thought to reflect not only an increased systemic vascular resistance but also myocardial depression and a decrease in venous return. Alterations in pleural pressure were insignificant and thought not to contribute to the hemodynamic changes. If oliguria occurs the intra-abdominal pressure should be reduced.[104]

Should adequate replacement of coagulation factors, hemostatic laparotomy, and abdominal tamponade prove unsuccessful at stopping the hemorrhage then vasopressin may be useful in its management. Vasopressin has long been known to reduce portal pressure,[105] and this has led to its use in the control of bleeding, particularly from esophageal varices. We have studied its use for uncontrollable abdominal bleeding in six patients after liver transplantation and four others (two with liver disease) who had continuing intra-abdominal hemorrhage.[106]

Vasopressin controlled intra-abdominal bleeding in two patients after liver transplantation and also in two other patients. In a further two patients vasopressin significantly reduced the rate of bleeding. The physiologic effects of vasopressin varied between patients. There was a general improvement in hemodynamic parameters and six patients (three after liver transplantation and three after other surgery) had a diuresis after its use. Although in some patients vasopressin appears to be useful in the management of massive and uncontrolled intra-abdominal bleeding, because of the risk of ischemic damage to other organs, vasopressin should be used only when conventional medical and surgical therapy has failed.

Infection

This remains one of the major causes of morbidity and mortality after liver surgery. To reduce the incidence, prophylactic antibiotic therapy is usually started before operation and continued for 48 hours afterwards. Regular microbiological screening should be performed on drainage fluids, sputum, and urine. In addition, the tips of all intravenous monitoring lines, drains, and tracheal tubes, etc. should be sent for culture when they are removed from the patient.

The immunosuppressed patient is especially at risk of infection. In an early review, infection was noted to occur in over 70% of patients after liver transplantation.[107]

The diagnosis of infection in a patient after liver transplantation is particularly difficult. Rejection, infection, and infarction will all result in both a pyrexia and an increase in white cell count. Infarction and rejection may be characterized by a deterioration in liver function and an increase in serum transaminase concentrations. Although infection is associated with liver dysfunction,[108] it tends to be predominantly cholestatic in nature. Further diagnostic difficulties may be encountered when deterioration in liver function is seen without a fever. This may also be caused by an infection, rejection, or liver failure. Similarly an increase in white cell count does not always occur with infection.[109] If T-tube drainage of the biliary tract has been placed by the surgeon then both the quantity and quality of bile drained after operation may be indicators of hepatic well-being. Usually copious quantities of dark green or brown bile are seen. If the amount decreases and particularly if the color turns to orange then liver dysfunction may be occurring. If there is uncertainty about the cause of deterioration, urgent liver biopsy should be performed.

The investigation of a pyrexia after liver surgery should include an abdominal ultrasound scan and computerized tomography (CT) to diagnose infected fluid collections. These techniques may be used to guide percutaneous drainage of fluid collections. The defect in the liver after hepatic resection is another potential source for infection. It may become filled with a hematoma which acts as a focus for infection. The presence of a biliary fistula may be demonstrated by transhepatic percutaneous cholangiography.

Infections may be bacterial, fungal, or viral. The high incidence reported by Schroter and colleagues after liver transplantation, during the early part of Starzl's series, reflects difficulties with the biliary drainage and immunosuppression.[107] Cuervas-Mons reviewed the main causes of death in 48 patients and found infection to be the major cause in 21 of them.[110] Of the group in whom infection was the primary cause nine had bacterial, seven fungal, and one a viral infection. Ho reviewed the microbiological course of a further 62 patients after liver transplantation.[111] Twenty-six patients developed 30 episodes of severe fungal infections (superficial infections were excluded). Twenty-two of these were caused by candida, six by aspergillus, one a cryptofungus, and a further one a mucor fungus. Aspergillus infection is particularly serious in the immunocompromised patient.[112] In Ho's series all the patients with this infection died. Aspergillus spores are ubiquitous and may enter the systemic circulation via the portal system. The Kupffer cells may be compromised in the patient after operation both by the severity of illness and the resulting liver injury.[113] After transplantation the need for immunosuppression may further impair immune responses.

Viral infections also occur commonly after transplantation including herpes simplex and cytomegalovirus infection. They may represent reactivation or primary infection from a source such as donated organ or blood products. Ho feels that primary infection is more serious than one resulting from reactivation.[111] Weekly storage of a sample of the patient's serum allows the increase in viral and fungal titers seen with some infections to be measured.

All patients with liver disease should be screened for the hepatitis B antigen. The presence of the surface antigen (HBsAg) indicates potential infectivity. Those patients with the e antigen or no e markers in the presence of HBsAg are potentially highly infectious; special precautions should be taken to prevent infection of the attending personnel and other patients (see chapter 16). Patients with HBsAg who are anti HBe positive can be regarded as low risk. The absence of HBsAg, anti-HBs and/or anti HBc is associated with immunity and loss of infectivity.

Nutrition

Many patients who need liver surgery are malnourished before operation. The catabolic response to surgery worsens this. If the patient needs intensive care for a long time then, unless properly managed, malnutrition may contribute to morbidity and the risk of death. Therefore, periods without nutritional support should be as short as possible.

If it is likely that the patient is not going to start eating quickly parenteral nutrition should be started when hemodynamic stability is achieved, usually within the first 24 hours after operation. This usually consists of a mixture of carbohydrates (dextrose or glucose) and conventional amino acid solutions. They should be started at a low concentration that is increased over the first 24–48 hours to provide 2000 calories as carbohydrate and 14 g nitrogen per day. The patient's energy expenditure[114] and nitrogen requirements[115] can be estimated if required. Hyperglycemia is treated by an insulin sliding scale. If excessive amounts of insulin are needed (> 8 units/hr) to control the blood sugar, the amount of glucose should be decreased.

In the past we have avoided fat emulsions as a routine energy source in these patients because of concerns that they may precipitate cholestatic jaundice. This may have been unfounded, however; see chapter 5 for the risks of the fat overload syndrome.

A study by Benjamin in infants and children[116] and one by Wolfe and colleagues[117] have both shown parenteral nutrition, including lipids, to have no demonstrable effect on hepatic histology. Any changes that were noted were attributed to the prolonged fasting or underlying disease process. Furthermore, Kuse and colleagues have shown that increasing amounts of fat emulsions (50g twice a week, 0.7 g/kg/day and 1.5 g/kg/day) does not lead to significant deterioration in hepatic function or to a fatty liver.[118] Unfortunately this study did not include a control group receiving carbohydrate solutions alone.

The Newcastle group has also shown the beneficial effects of daily administration of a fat emulsion on hepatic drug oxidation.[119] They compared the metabolism of antipyrine in four groups of patients after elective gastrointestinal surgery. The first group received no parenteral nutrition, the second received 2000 Kcal (all as dextrose), a further group received only 1600 Kcal (all as dextrose), and a final group received 2000 Kcal but with 25% of the calories provided by a fat emulsion. In both groups receiving energy only as dextrose, antipyrine clearance decreased by 34% compared with the control group. This was not seen in the group who received the fat emulsion. Because hepatic function needs to be as good as possible in patients after liver surgery, we now routinely add fat to the total parenteral nutrition regimen of these patients.

Enteral feeding should be started when bowel function returns. Bowel sounds and the passage of flatus are indicators of returning gastrointestinal function. However, in patients with a complicated course after operation who need prolonged artificial ventilation, bowel sounds are an unreliable guide of bowel motility.[120] In such patients when a decrease in nasogastric aspirate to levels below 20 mL every four hours is seen, nasogastric feeding is started. Water is first instilled and if this is tolerated without nausea, large volumes of nasogastric aspirate, or abdominal distension, enteral nutrition is commenced with a propriety feed. This is increased in volume and concentration until the patient is receiving adequate nutrition or until a normal diet is resumed.

Cardiovascular System

Bradycardias are sometimes a feature in the more severely ill patients after liver surgery. They may be the result of accumulation of bile salts, bilirubin, and toxic substances that accumulate in liver failure.[121] Alternatively, since they are particularly common during tracheal suction they may represent an increase in sensitivity of the vagus. The bradycardia responds rapidly to atropine or glycopyrrolate. Repeated doses of atropine in patients with renal failure may allow the accumulation of its breakdown product, tropic acid, that is centrally active. Fits have been observed on at least one occasion in a patient when multiple doses of atropine were used for recurrent bradycardias.

Postoperative hypertension, particularly in children, may occur in up to 81% of patients after liver transplantation.[10] The cause is not known, but it responds to treatment with intravenous labetalol or sublingual nifedipine.

Hepatic Dysfunction

There is some evidence that hepatic dysfunction after liver surgery may be improved by infusions of prostaglandins or N-acetylcysteine. Prostaglandin E_2 has been used in acute liver failure and after liver transplantation.[122] It is thought to act by improving hepatic microcirculation and altering cytokine release.

N-Acetylcysteine was first used in the treatment of paracetamol overdose where it acts as a glutathione donor. Harrison and colleagues showed that it improved global oxygen delivery and consumption in patients with fulminant liver failure. They proposed that it acted by stimulating the activity of derived endothelial releasing factor by replenishing tissue sulphydryl groups or increasing cysteine levels.[123]

References

1. Park, G.R. and Johnson, S. (1982). A ventilator for use during mobile intensive care and total intravenous anaesthesia. *Anaesthesia* 37:1204–08.
2. Park, G.R., Manara, A. Bodenham, A. and Moss, C. (1989) An assessment of the Pneupac ventilator. *Anaesthesia* 44:419–24.
3. Shelly, M.P., Park, G.R., Warren, R.E. and Whetstone, R.J. (1986) Portable lung ventilation: The potential risk from bacterial colonisation. *Intensive Care Medicine* 12:328–31.
4. Winso, O., Biber, B., Gustavsson, B. et al. (1986) Portal blood flow in man during graded positive end-expiratory pressure ventilation. *Intensive Care Medicine* 12:80–85.
5. Matuschak, G.M., Pinsky, M.R. and Rogers, R.M. (1987) Effects of positive end-expiratory pressure on hepatic blood flow and performance. *Journal of Applied Physiology* 62:1377–83.
6. Berry, A.J. (1981) Respiratory support and renal function. *Anesthesiology* 55:655–67.
7. Epstein, R.M., Wheeler, H.O., Frumin, M.J. et al. (1961) The effect of hypercapnia on estimated hepatic blood flow, circulating splanchnic blood volume and hepatic sulfobromopthalein clearance during general anaesthesia in man. *Journal of Clinical Investigation* 40:592.
8. Hughes, R.L., Mathie, R.T., Fitch, W. and Campbell, D. (1979) Liver blood flow and oxygen consumption during hypocapnia and IPPV in the greyhound. *Journal of Applied Physiology* 47:290–95.
9. Cooperman, L. H., Warden, J. C. and Price, H. L. (1968) Splanchnic circulation during nitrous oxide anesthesia and hypocarbia in normal man. *Anesthesiology* 29:254–58.
10. Riegle, C.M., Thompson, A.E., Gartner, J.C. and Shaw, B.W. (1984) Intensive care unit course following paediatric hepatic transplantation. *Critical Care Medicine* 12:220.
11. Sealey, M.M. and Gray, T.A. (1985) Severe hypercalcaemia due to a parathyroid type hormone secreting tumour of the liver treated by hepatic transplantation. *Anaesthesia* 40:918–19.
12. Papper, S., Saxon, L., Burg, M.B. et al. (1957) The effect of morphine sulfate upon the renal excretion of water and solute in man. *Journal Laboratory Clinical Medicine* 50:692–704.
13. Noble, W.H. and Severinghaus, J.W. (1972) Thermal and conductivity dilution curves for rapid quantification of pulmonary edema. *Journal of Applied Physiology* 32:770–75.
14. Tew, D. and Park, G. R. (1991) Observations: Low doses of frusemide produce a diuresis. *Clinical Intensive Care* 1:187.
15. Lowe, J., Gray, I., Henry, D. and Lawson, D. (1979) Adverse reactions to frusemide in hospital inpatients. *British Medical Journal* 2:360–62.
16. Johnston, C. D., Nicholls, D. P., Leahe, W. J. and Finch M. B. (1988) The acute non-diuretic effects of frasimide in man: The role of angiotensin II. *Br J Clin Pharmacol* 15:601:–602P.
17. Vargas-Tank, I., Escobar, C., Fernandez, G. et al. (1984) Massive pleural effusions in cirrhotic patients with ascites. *Scandinavian Journal of Gastroenterology* 19:294–98.
18. Lachmann, R., Calne, R.Y. and Park, G.R. (1993) Rhabdomyolysis and bilateral diaphragmatic palsies following abdominal tamponade. *Anaesthesia* 48:914–30.
19. Becker, A., Barak, S., Braun, E. and Meyers, M.P. (1960) The treatment of postoperative pulmonary at-

electasis with intermittent positive breathing. *Surgery, Gynaecology and Obstetrics* 111:517–21.

20. Park, G.R. and Gempeler, F. (1993) *Sedation and Analgesia in the Critically Ill Patient*. London: Bailliere Tindall.
21. Park, G.R. and Fulton, B. *The Management of Acute Pain*. (1991) Oxford University Press.
22. Merriman, H.M. (1981) The techniques used to sedate ventilated patients. *Intensive Care Medicine* 7:217–24.
23. Bion, J.F. and Ledingham, I. McA. (1987) Sedation in the intensive care: A postal study. *Intensive Care Medicine* 13:215–16.
24. Nimmo, W.S., Heading, R.C., Wilson, J. et al. (1975) Inhibition of gastric emptying and drug absorption by narcotic analgesics. *British Journal of Clinical Pharmacology* 2:509.
25. Leaman, D.M., Levenson, L., Zelis, R. and Shiroff, R. (1978) Effect of morphine on splanchnic blood flow. *Br Heart J* 40:569–71.
26. Teverskoy, M., Gelman, S., Fowler, K.C. and Bradley, E.L. (1985) Influence of fentanyl and morphine on intestinal circulation. *Anaesthesia and Analgesia* 64:577–84.
27. Gelman, S., Reves, J.G. and Harris, D. (1983) Circulatory responses to midazolam anaesthesia: Emphasis on canine splanchnic circulation. *Anaesthesia and Analgesia* 62:135–39.
28. Lassen, H.C.A., Bjorneboe, M., Ibsen, B. and Neukirch, F. (1954) Treatment of tetanus with curarisation, general anaesthesia and intratracheal postive pressure ventilation. *Lancet* ii:1040.
29. Lassen, H.C.A., Henriksen, E., Neurkirch, F. and Kristensen, H.S. (1956) Treatment of tetanus severe prolonged bone-marrow depression after prolonged nitrous oxide anaesthesia. *Lancet* i:527–30.
30. Tubaro, E., Borelli, G., Croce, C. et al. (1983) Effect of morphine on resistance to infection. *Journal of Infectious Diseases* 148:656–66.
31. Moudgil, G.C. (1981) Effect of premedicants, intravenous anaesthetic agents and local anaesthetics on phagocytosis in vitro. *Canadian Anaesthetists Journal* 28:597–601.
32. Shelly, M.P., Quinn, K.G. and Park, G.R. (1989) Dihydrocodeine; A cause of renal failure. *European Journal of Anaesthesiology* 6:303–14.
33. Allison, S.P. (1986) Some metabolic aspects of injury. In *The Scientific Basis for the Care of the Critically Ill* (Little, R.A. and Frayn, K.N. eds). Manchester University Press, pp. 169–83.
34. Dundee, J.W., Johnston, H.M.L. and Gray, R.C. (1976) Lorazepam as a sedative-amnesic in an intensive care unit. *Current Medical Research and Opinion* 4:290–95.
35. Lowry, K.G., Dundee, J.W., McClean, E. et al. (1985) Pharmacokinetics of diazepam and midazolam when used for sedation following cardiopulmonary bypass. *British Journal of Anaesthesia* 57:883–85.
36. Dundee, J.W., Samuel, I.O., Toner, W. and Howard, P.J. (1980) Midazolam: A water-soluble benzodiazepine. *Anaesthesia* 35:454–58.

37. Crevoisier, C., Ziegler, W.H., Eckert, M. and Heizmann P. (1983) Relationship between plasma concentration and effect of midazolam after oral and intravenous administration. *British Journal of Clinical Pharmacology* 16:51S–61S.
38. Amrein, R., Leisman, B., Bentzinger, C. and Roncari G. (1987) Flumazenil in benzodiazepine antagonism. *Medical Toxicology* 2:411–19.
39. Klotz, U. and Kanto, J. (1988) Pharmacokinetics and clinical use of flumazenil (Ro15-1788). *Clinical Pharmacokinetics* 14:1–12.
40. Bodenham, A., Brownlie, G., Dixon, J.S. and Park, G.R. (1988) Reversal of sedation by prolonged infusion of flumazenil (Anexate, Ro15-1788). *Anaesthesia* 43:376–78.
41. Pepperman, M. L. (1989) Benzodiazepine sedation and the use of benzodiazepine antagonists in intensive care. *Intensive Therapy and Clinical Monitoring* 10:58–61.
42. Grounds, R.M., Lalor, J.M., Lumley, D. et al. (1987) Propofol infusion for sedation in the intensive care unit: A preliminary report. *British Medical Journal* 42:929–37.
43. Beller, J.P., Pottecher, T., Lugnier, A. et al. (1988) Prolonged sedation with propofol in ICU patients: Recovery and blood concentrations and changes during periodic interruptions in infusion. *British Journal of Anaesthesia* 61:583–88.
44. Aitkenhead, A.R., Pepperman, M.L., Willatts, S.M. et al. (1989) Comparison of propofol and midazolam for sedation in critically ill patients. *Lancet* ii:704–09.
45. Gray, P.A. and Park, G.R. (1989) Chlormethiazole sedation for critical ill patients in renal failure. *Anaesthesia* 44:913–15.
46. Modig, J. (1988) Indications of chlormethiazole as a protective agent in experimental endotoxaemia. *European Surgical Research* 20:195.
47. Kong, K.L., Willatts, S.M. and Prys-Roberts, C. (1989) Isoflurane compound compared with midazolam for sedation in the intensive care unit. *British Medical Journal* 298:1277–79.
48. Burns, A. and Park, G.R. (1989) Serum fluoride after isoflurane sedation. British Medical Journal (1989) 298:1642.
49. Dodson, M.E. (1982) A review of methods for relief of postoperative pain. *Annals of the Royal College of Surgeons* 64:324–27.
50. Shelly, M.P., Cory, E.P. and Park, G.R. (1986) Pharmacokinetics of morphine in two children before and after liver transplantation. *Br J Anaesth* 58:1218–23.
51. Yate, P.M., Thomas, D., Short, S.M. et al. (1986) Comparison of infusions of alfentanil or pethidine for sedation of ventilated patients on the ITU. *British Journal of Anaesthesia* 58:1091–99.
52. Klotz, U., McHorse, T.S., Wilkinson, G.R. and Schenker, S. (1974) The effect of cirrhosis on the disposition and elimination of meperidine in man. *Clinical Pharmacology and Therapeutics* 16:677.
53. Szeto, H.H., Inturrisi, C.E., Houde, R. et al. (1977) Accumulation of normeperidine, an active metabolite of

meperidine, in patients with renal failure or cancer. *Annals of Internal Medicine* 86:738–41.

54. Kaiko, A.J., Foley, K.M., Grabinsky, P.Y. et al. (1983) Central nervous system excitatory effects of meperidine in cancer patients. *Annals of Neurology* 13:180–85.

55. Merriman (1980)

56. Miller-Jones, C.H.M. and Williams, J.H. (1980) Sedation for ventilation. *Anaesthesia* 35:1104–07.

57. Isherwood, C.N., Calvey, T.N., Williams, N.E. et al. (1984) Elimination of phenoperidine in liver disease. *British Journal of Anaestesia* 56:843–46.

58. Alazia, M., Levron, J.C., Quidon, C., and Francois, G. (1987) Pharmacokinetics of fentanyl during continuous infusion in critically ill patients. *Anesthesiology* 67:A665.

59. Shafer, A.A., White, P.F., Schuttler, J. and Rosenthal, M.H. (1983) Use of fentanyl infusion in the intensive care unit. Tolerance to its anaesthetic effects. *Anesthesiology* 59:245–48.

60. Bodenham, A. and Park, G.R. (1988) Alfentanil infusions in patients requiring intensive care. *Clinical Pharmacokinetics* 15:216–26.

61. Sear, J.W., Fisher, A. and Summerfield, R.J. (1987) Is alfentanil by infusion useful for sedation on the ITU? *European Journal of Anaesthesiology* S1:55–61.

62. Van Peer, A., Vercauteren, M., Noorduin, H. et al. (1986) Alfentanil kinetics in renal insufficiency. *European Journal of Clinical Pharmacology* 30:245–48.

63. Engberg, G. (1975) Single dose intercostal nerve blocks with etidocaine for pain relief after upper abdominal surgery. *Acta Anaesthesiologica Scandinavica* 60(s):43–49.

64. Goodchild, C. and Noble, J. (1987) The effects intrathecal midazolam on sympathetic nervous system reflexes in man—a pilot study. *British Journal of Clinical Pharmacology* 23:279–85.

65. Cripps, T.P. and Goodchild, C.S. (1988) Intrathecal midazolam and the stress response to upper abdominal surgery: Adrenocortical, glycaemic and analgesic effects. *Clinical Journal of Pain* 4:125–28.

66. Messmer, K. (1975) Hemodilution. *Surgical Clinics of North America* 55:659–78.

67. Stockwell, M. A., Soni, N. and Riley B. (1992) Colloid solutions in the critically ill. *Anaesthesia* 47:3–9.

68. Polson, R., Park, G.R., Lindop, M.J. et al. (1987) The prevention of renal impairment in patients undergoing liver grafting by infusion of low dose dopamine. *Anaesthesia* 42:15–19.

69. Bennett, W.M. and Pulliam, J.P. (1983) Cyclosporin nephrotoxicity. *Annals of Internal Medicine* 99:851–54.

70. Koppel M.H., Coburn, J.W., Mims, M.M., Goldstein, H., Boyle, J.D., and Rubini, M.E. (1969) Transplantation of cadaveric kidneys from patients with hepatorenal syndrome. *New England Journal of Medicine* 280; 1367–1371.

71. Burns, A.M., Hue, D.P., Wraight, E.P. and Park, G.R. (1993) Creatinine and ^{51}Cr-EDTA clearance after liver transplantation. *Anaesthesia* 48:763–65.

72. Dawson, J.L. (1965) Postoperative renal function in obstructive jaundice: Effect of mannitol enuresis. *British Medical Journal* 1:82–86.

73. Goldberg, L.I. (1972) Cardiovascular and renal actions of dopamine: Potential clinical applications. *Pharmacology Reviews* 24:1–29.

74. Lokhandwala, M.F., Amenta, F. and Jundhyala, B.S. (1991) Renal research of dopexamine hydrochloride. *Clin Intensive Care* 2:12–17.

75. Polson, R.J., Park, G.R., Lindop, M.J. et al. (1987) The prevention of renal impairment in patients undergoing orthotopic liver grafting by infusion of low dose dopamine. *Anaesthesia* 42:15–19.

76. Swygert, T.H., Brajtbord, D., Paulson, A.W. et al. (1988) The effects on renal function of low dose dopamine infusions in liver transplant recipients. *Anesthesiology* 64:499.

77. Gray, P.A., Jones, T. and Park, G.R. (1994) Blood concentrations of dopamine in patients during and after orthotopic liver transplantation. *Br J Clin Pharmac* 37:89–92.

78. Hasselgren, P.O., Biber, B. and Fornander, U. (1983) Improved blood flow and protein synthesis in the post ischaemic liver following infusion of dopamine. *Journal of Surgical Research* 34:44–52.

79. Townsend, M.C., Schirmer, W.J., Schirmer, J.M. and Fry, D.E. (1987) Low dose dopamine improves effective hepatic blood flow in murine peritonitis. *Circulatory Shock* 21:149–53.

80. Trachte, G.J. and Lefer, A.M. (1977) Influence of dopamine on liver dynamics in haemorrhagic shock. *Circulatory Shock* 4:305–15.

81. Hirsch, L.J., Ayabe, T. and Glick, G. (1976) Direct effects of various catecholamines on liver circulation in dogs. *American Journal of Physiology* 230:1394–99.

82. Maestracci, P., Grimaud, D., Livrelli, N. et al. (1981) Increase in hepatic blood flow and cardiac output during dopamine infusion in man. *Critical Care Medicine* 9:14–16.

83. Munglani, R., Gray, P., Park, G.R. (1990) Increases in oxygen consumption during administration of dopexamine in liver failure. *Clin Intensive Care* 1:134–135.

84. Gray, T.A., Buckley, B.M., Sealey, M.M. et al. (1986) Plasma ionised calcium monitoring during liver transplantation. *Transplantation* 41:335–39.

85. Orr, M.D. (1982) Autotransfusion: Intra-operative scavenging. *International Anesthesiology Clinics* 20: 97–119.

86. Ibister, J.P. and Davis, R. (1980) Should autologous blood transfusion be re-discovered? *Anaesthesia and Intensive Care* 8:168–71.

87. Mendel, L., Smith, M.F. and Park, G.R. (1986) Lack of haematological and biochemical consequences following autologus blood transfusion. *Anaesthesia* 41: 1259–60.

88. Knight, A., Bihari, D. and Tinker, J. (1985) Stress ulceration in the critically ill patient. *British Journal Hospital Medicine* 33:216–19.

89. McDougal, B.R.D., Bailey, R.J. and Williams, R. (1977) H_2-receptor antagonists and antacids in the prevention of acute gastrointestinal haemorrhage in fulminant hepatic failure. *Lancet* 617–19.

90. Shapiro, M.J., Wood, R.P., Shaw, B.W. and Grenvik, A. (1986) Postoperative care of liver transplantation patients. In *Hepatic Transplantation* (Winter, P.M. and Kang, Y.G., eds). New York: Praeger Publishers.

91. Henry, D.A., MacDonald, I.A., Kitchingham, G. et al. (1980) Cimetidine and ranitidine: Comparison of effects on hepatic drug metabolism. *British Medical Journal* 281:775–77.

92. Martin, L.E., Bel, J.A., Carey, P.F. et al. (1982) A review of pharmacokinetics of renitidine in animals and man. In Misicweicz and Wormsley (eds.), *The clinical use of ranitidine.* Oxford: Medicine Publishing Foundations, pp. 22–31.

93. Borrero, E., Bank, S., Margolis, I. et al. (1985) Comparison of antacid and sucralfate in the prevention of gastrointestinal bleeding in patients who are critically ill. *American Journal of Medicine* 79:62–64.

94. Driks, M.R., Craven, D.E., Celli, B.R. et al. (1987) Nosocomial pneumonia in intubated patients given sucralfate as compared with antacids or histamine type 2 blockers. *New England Journal of Medicine* 317:1376–82.

95. Tryba, M. (1987) Prevention of stress bleeding and the risk of nosocomial pneumonia in ventilated ICU patients. *Anesthesiology* 67:A124.

96. Editorial (1989) Stress ulcer prophylaxis in critically ill patients. *Lancet* ii:1255–56.

97. Pingleton, S.K. and Hadzima, S.K. (1983) Enteral alimentation and gastrointestinal bleeding in mechanically ventilated patients. *Critical Care Medicine* 11:13–16.

98. Harper, P., Williamson, L., Luddington, R. et al. (1991) The effects of antithrombin supplementation on coagulation and renal function in intensive care patients. *Transfusion Medicine* 1:121–28.

99. van Obberg, L.J., Dangoisse, M., O'Connor, T. et al. (1989) Treatment of severe early postoperative haemorrhage by abdominal binding after liver transplantation. *European Journal of Anaesthesiology and Related Specialties* 1:3.

100. Aberg, T.W. (1989) Pneumatic antishock garments and intraabdominal binding. MD Thesis. University of Lund.

101. Richardson, J.D. and Trinkle, J.K. (1976) Haemodynamic and respiratory alterations with increased intra-abdominal pressure. *Journal of Surgical Research* 20:401–04.

102. Toomasian, J.M., Glavinovich, G., Johnson, M.N. and Gazzaniga, A.B. (1978) Haemodynamic changes following pneumoperitoneum and graded haemorrhage in the dog. *Surgical Forum* 29:32–33.

103. Kashtan, J., Green, J.F., Parsons, E.O. and Holcroft, J.W. (1981) Haemodynamic effects of increased abdominal pressure. *Journal of Surgical Research* 30:249–55.

104. Park, G.R., (1991).

105. Clark, G.A. (1928) Comparison of the effects of adrenaline and pituitrin on the portal circulation. *Journal of Physiology* 66:274–79.

106. Shelly, M.P., Greatorex, R., Calne, R.Y. and Park, G.R. (1988) The physiological effects of vasopressin when used to control intra-abdominal bleeding. *Intensive Care Medicine* 14:526–31.

107. Schroter, G.P.J., Hoelscher, M., Putnam, C.W. et al. (1976) Infections complicating orthotopic liver transplantation. *Archives of Surgery* III:1337–47.

108. Murray, W.R. and MacSween, R.N.M. (1983) Hepatobiliary disturbances. In *Recent Advances in Critical Care Medicine* (Ledingham, I.McA. and Hanning, C.D., eds). Edinburgh: Churchill Livingston, pp 152–56.

109. Fagan, E., Harvey, F., Rolando, N. and Williams, R. (1989) Bacterial and fungal sepsis in acute liver failure. *Care of the Critically Ill* 5:64–66.

110. Cuervas-Mons, V., Martinez, J., Dekker, K. et al. (1986) Adult liver transplantation: An analysis of the early causes of death in 40 consecutive cases. *Hepatology* 6:495–501.

111. Ho, M. (1986) Infections in liver transplant recipients. In *Hepatic Transplantation,* (Winter, P.M. and Kang, Y.G., eds). New York: Praeger Publishers.

112. Park, G.R., Drummond, G.B., Lamb, D. et al. (1982) Disseminated aspergillosis occurring in patients with respiratory, renal and hepatic failure. *Lancet* ii:179–83.

113. Nolan, P.J. (1978) Bacteria and the liver. *New England Journal of Medicine* 299:1069–70.

114. Smith, H.S., Kennedy, D.J. and Park, G.R. (1984) A nomogram for the rapid calculation of metabolic requirements on intubated patients. *Intensive Care Medicine* 10:147–48.

115. Park, G.R. (1980) Rapid calculation of nitrogen losses. *Intensive Care Medicine* 6:242–44.

116. Benjamin, D.R. (1981) Liver dysfunction with parenteral nutrition. *American Journal of Clinical Pathology* 76:276–83.

117. Wolfe, B.M., Walker, B.K., Shaul, D.B. et al. (1988) Effect of total parenteral nutrition on hepatic histology. *Archives of Surgery* 123:1084–90.

118. Kuse, E. R., Kotzerke, J., Kemnitz, J. et al. (1989) Parenteral nutrition after liver transplantation: Influence of MET/LET lipid emulsion on the recovery of the liver RES function and liver tissue fat content. *European Journal of Anaesthesiology and Related Specialities* 1:15.

119. Burgess, P., Hall, R.I., Bateman, D.N. and Johnston, I.D.A. (1987) The effect of total parenteral nutrition on hepatic drug oxidation. *Journal of Parenteral and Enteral Nutrition* 11:540–43.

120. Shelly, M.P. and Church, J.J. (1987) Bowel sounds during intermittent positive pressure ventilation. *Anaesthesia* 42:207–09.

121. Weston, M.J., Talbot, L.C., Howorth, P.J.N. et al. (1976) Frequency of arrhythmias and other cardiac ab-

normalities in fulminant hepatic failure. *British Heart Journal* 38:1179–88.

122. Sinclair, S.B., Greig, P.D., Blendis, L.M. et al. (1989) Biochemical and clinical response of fulminant viral hepatitis to administration of prostaglandin E. A preliminary report. *J Clin Invest* 84:1063–1069.

123. Harrison, P.H., Wendon, J.A., Gimson, A.E.S. et al. (1991) Improvement by acetylcysteine of haemodynamics and oxygen transport in fulminant hepatic failure. *New England Journal of Medicine* 324:1852–57.

Chapter 15
Bacterial Infection and the Liver

S. Kim Jacobson and Roderic E. Warren

The literature on bacterial infection of the liver and its treatment is diffuse but extensive. The literature on infection caused by viruses and other organisms is enormous and, in general, outside the scope of this chapter. We have not attempted to be exhaustive in our coverage and have confined our attention primarily to biliary infection and infections after liver transplantation because these are the areas in which either common or difficult problems in intensive care exist. The effects of changes in hepatic function on pharmacokinetics of antibiotics have been poorly studied, but we address antibiotics that are in common use.

Cholecystitis

Cholecystitis implies inflammation, but not necessarily infection, of the gallbladder. Acute cholecystitis is thought to be caused initially by a chemical inflammation perhaps mediated by lysolecithin.[1] Inflammation may lead to relative ischemia and biliary obstruction. Unobstructed bile yields few organisms on conventional culture, but multiplication of organisms occurs in the stagnant bile in biliary obstruction. In the absence of surgical intervention, the invading organisms are usually from the enteric flora, but there is some debate as to their mode of entry. Gallbladder bile yields organisms in 30–50% of those with cholecystitis. Direct ascending infec-

tion through the cystic duct appears the most likely route in cholecystitis, but there is some evidence to suggest bacteria reach the bile ducts from portal bacteremia and hepatic shedding of organisms,[2] and this may be important in cholangitis and may or may not precede gallbladder colonization. The most common isolate in cholecystitis is *Escherichia coli,* but other *Enterobacteriaceae* may be implicated as may enterococci, streptococci, and anaerobes. The frequency with which anaerobes are isolated is controversial, but they have been isolated from gallbladder bile in both adults and children. *Clostridium perfringens* and *Bacteroides fragilis* are the most common.[3] In one study, isolation rates of 6% were reported,[4] while in contrast, other studies report isolation rates of over 50% in inflammatory biliary disease.[3] Anaerobes are more common in sclerosing cholangitis and other biliary strictures[5] and after intestinal anastomoses to the biliary system.[6] These organisms may be involved in serious complications of biliary tract infection such as sepsis and emphysematous cholecystitis.

The presence of bactobilia is strongly associated with perioperative complications such as wound infection; subphrenic, peritoneal, and liver abscesses; peritonitis; and cholangitis as well as empyema of the gallbladder and pericholecystic abscess. Lykkard Nielsen and colleagues reported finding a postoperative wound infection rate of 15% in elective cholecystectomies, but one-third of their patients were over 60 years old or had previously had an attack of acute cholecystitis.[4] Half of their patients had bactobilia at operation and 86% of all wound infections occurred in this group. Hambraeus and coworkers further substantiated the risk of wound infection secondary to biliary tract surgery as being associated with bactobilia.[7] In patients who had sterile bile at operation, the postoperative infection rate was 3.7%, similar to the rate for other clean operations, whereas the infection rate in the presence of bactobilia was 16.5%. They also noted a massive transfer of bacteria at operation from bile to the liver bed and subcutaneous fat in 81% of cases who had bactobilia. In their series six of 19 infections were classified as exogenous with *Staphylococcus aureus* predominating. Chetlin and Elliot reported their experience of more than 1400 biliary operations and postoperative complications were 40 times greater in patients with positive bile cultures than in cases with sterile bile.[8] Ten of the 22 fatalities reported in this series were caused by septicemia.

The frequency of bactobilia in cholecystitis varies in different centers and also varies with different risk factors. Thompson and coworkers reported predictive factors for bactobilia at operation in acute cholecystitis as preoperative temperature $>37°C$, a total serum bilirubin level >8.6 μ/mol/L, and a white cell count $>14.1 \times 10^9$/L.[9] Of patients with two or three of these risk factors, 63% had bactobilia. However, this study excluded patients with common bile duct stones which are also an established risk factor with bactobilia occurring in 15–30% of such patients with cholelithiasis and chronic cholecystitis.[9,10] Other risk factors for bactobilia include previous attacks of cholecystitis in those aged over 60 years, early or emergency surgery, diabetes mellitus, hypertension, and atherosclerosis.[9,11] In the presence of obstruction of bile drainage from common bile duct stone, strictures, and strictures of biliary intestinal anastomoses, the percentage of patients with common bile duct bactobilia increases to 60–100%,[4] although this incidence is much lower in patients when bile duct obstruction is caused by carcinoma of the pancreas or ampulla.[12]

Cholangitis

Cholangitis implies a similar process to cholecystitis but occurring in the hepatic and common bile ducts. It is more likely to occur as a consequence of other pathologies such as pancreatic and biliary tumors or flukes and after biliary surgery, percutaneous transhepatic biliary drainage (PTBD), cholangiography (PTC) or endoscopic retrograde cholangiopancreatography (ERCP).[13] The organisms associated with cholangitis again usually originate from the gut, but patients who have a T-tube in situ acquire organisms also from the skin or the drainage bag. It is more difficult to treat cholangitis and eradicate organisms in patients with a T-tube or biliary stent, perhaps because the organisms colonize the foreign material and form biofilms on the surface. Cholangiography or irrigation to clear sludge or blockage increases the risk of introducing organisms further.[14] PTBD has a high incidence of cholangitis as a complication, with rates from 14 to 47%,[15] and sepsis of the biliary tract is considered the main contributory factor in the death of such patients. This is also the case with endoscopic drainage.[16] Audisio and colleagues report the finding of microorganisms in all subjects post PTBD within 15 days of operation, although not all patients developed cholangitis and there was no relation to whether drainage was internal or external.[15] Fifteen patients developed cholangitis and survived a median of 21 days: 24 without cholangitis survived for a median of 89 days. The factors most obviously associated with sepsis were preexisting neoplastic strictures and the presence of multiple intrahepatic biliary obstructions.

Bacteremia is said to occur in up to 50% of patients with cholangitis. Raised pressure owing to obstruction in the biliary tree, with or without instrumentation, is an important factor in the etiology of bacteremia.[17,18] Low-pressure systems with inevitable presence of intestinal bacterial flora are not at great risk of cholangitis; for example, there does not seem to be an increased incidence of cholangitis in pediatric patients after liver transplantation where there is a Roux-en-Y loop without functional sphincter of Oddi,[14] but this may be because biliary stricture, sludging, leakage, and T-tube obstruction are rarer after this anastomosis.[19]

Liver Abscess

Primary pyogenic liver abscesses are uncommon, accounting for one in 5,000 hospital admissions. Amoebic liver abscesses are much more commonly acquired in tropical climes. Pyogenic abscesses commonly involve *Streptococcus milleri,* which commonly carries the Lancefield group F antigen, alone, although nonsporing anaerobes are also common,[20] and in some series appear to be present frequently with coliforms in the absence of *S. milleri.*[21] Interesting recent taxonomic work indicates that the *S. milleri* strains are usually *Streptococcus intermedius* sensu stricto, a species also responsible for brain abscess and found on dental plaque, whereas the different species within the *S. milleri* group, *Streptococcus constellatus* and *Streptococcus anginosus,* are more frequent in other abdominal sites.[22] It is not yet clear how such liver and brain abscesses arise. Although treatment by a single aspiration and antimicrobial therapy has been advocated,[23,24] others have found this approach unsuccessful.[25] Our hospital, like others, now treats such pyogenic abscesses by ultrasound-guided, pigtail catheter drainage.[26] Appropriate starting therapy for a liver abscess includes metronidazole, which in increased dose (800 mg tds) provides anti-amoebic as well as anti-anaerobic activity, and a cephalosporin active against both *S. milleri* and coliforms that may be present. Alternatively penicillin, metronidazole, and an aminoglycoside such as gentamicin may be preferred. When culture and gas–liquid chromatography results for volatile fatty acids associated with anaerobic infection are available, then the initial empirical treatment can be modified and the spectrum narrowed. It is important to obtain diagnostic material for culture to ensure that chemotherapy is correct. Amoebiasis should be suspected, even in the absence of tropical travel, if the abscess is "sterile" and contains amorphous debris and no pus cells. Tests for antibody to *Entamoeba histolytica* should be part of the diagnostic workup in all cases of nonbiliary liver abscess as this infection may disseminate if not treated.

Secondary liver abscesses after resection for hepatic malignancy are not uncommon (13%), and they also occur after packing the abdomen after liver trauma. They may be caused by a wide variety of organisms.[27] After major hepatic resection such sepsis often precipitates liver failure. Culture of subhepatic drainage fluid after hepatectomy permits early treatment. With such a high incidence of sepsis and serious sequelae, antibiotic prophylaxis would be justified, although there are no trials to this effect, and it would seem sensible to follow the guiding principles of liver transplantation prophylaxis.

Infection in Liver Allograft Recipients

Infections with certain organisms, which are usually considered a hallmark of immunocompromised patients, are not common after liver transplantation except in restricted situations. Peculiar patterns of infection after liver transplantation are unusual except vanishing bile-duct syndrome, which may be associated with cytomegalovirus (CMV) infection.[28] The degree of immunosuppression may be critical to some opportunistic organisms. This is suggested by the level of CD4 counts in patients with AIDS at which certain infections become prevalent. Some correlation with the duration of sustained immunosuppression is likely as an explanation for the timing of some infections after transplantation. There are no quantitative data for CD4 counts and prevalence of particular infections in the context of liver transplantation. *Pneumocystis carinii* pneumonia is rare,[29] is not seen in the first 20 days after transplantation,[30,31] but is associated with the use of augmented immunosuppression with antilymphocyte globulin (OKT3 sera)[30] and lymphopenia. Liver transplant recipients are susceptible to listeria and salmonella infections from an early time after operation. These organisms originate from dietary sources and can be reduced in incidence by appropriate dietary advice and perhaps by concurrent prophylaxis with cotrimoxazole if this is given to prevent *Pneumocystis carinii* infection in augmented immunosuppression or lymphopenia. Toxoplasmosis caused by reactivation does not appear to occur in liver transplantation, unlike in AIDS. It is often difficult to clearly associate specific clinical features of infection with donor-transmitted primary *Toxoplasma gondii* infection.[32,33] Cryptococcosis is very rare after liver transplantation,[34] although a common disease in advanced lymphopenia in AIDS. *Aspergillus* spp. appear, in our unit's autopsy experience, relatively rarely after liver transplantation compared with patients with neutropenia. Claims to the contrary, and reports of a very high incidence, often represent nosocomial outbreaks caused by inadequate accommodation and air quality with clustering in time and space which sometimes are only recognizable in retrospect.[35–38] Sporadic cases of aspergillosis do occur, usually in patients who have breathed room air that has not passed through high-efficiency particulate air (HEPA) filters, rather than in patients receiving ventilatory support with compressed gases. Such infection does not usually occur in accommodation with HEPA filters. Abrogation of B-cell responses by immunosuppression is unusual after liver transplantation, and infections with *Streptococcus pneumoniae, Haemophilus influenzae* type b, and *Neisseria meningitidis* are no more common than in the general population, but infections with *S. pneumoniae* are seen 3–6 months after transplantation,[31] and patients who also undergo splenectomy at the time of operation are at increased risk of infection by these organisms.

Viral Infections in the Post Transplant Period

Donor-transmitted CMV infection from seropositive donors is frequent, and seronegative recipients often have pneumonia or disseminated disease. Such CMV infection however is very rare within 3 weeks of receipt of the allograft unless this is a retransplant and infection has arisen from a previous allograft.[33] Reactivation of herpes virus infection with herpes simplex [30] and varicella zoster are common, and primary infections are more severe in liver transplant recipients. Varicella zoster is rarely overlooked and usually responds to acyclovir in an appropriately high dose,[19] but this is not invariable and deaths do occur in large series.[39] In intensive care units looking after such patients, the risk of seronegative staff acquiring the infection, and perhaps transmitting it in the incubation period to other immunocompromised patients, is high and justifies serologic screening of staff. Herpes simplex infections may disseminate in liver transplant patients and cause fatal pneumonitis or hepatitis, and appropriate culture samples should be taken regularly from seropositive patients unless they are receiving acyclovir. Measles infections are to be feared as a cause of pneumonia without rash in the immunocompromised patient but were surprisingly rare even in the era before high vaccination rates. Pulmonary and disseminated adenovirus infection is not uncommon and often severe in children with liver transplants.[33] Children often have unusually persistent respiratory syncytial virus and rotavirus infection as in other causes of immunosuppression.[40]

Bacterial Infections in the Post Transplant Period

The usual causative organisms of infection after liver transplantation are those more associated with other major abdominal and liver surgery and vary with the time elapsed since transplantation. Infection remains the major cause of death in intensive care after liver transplantation.[41] In the case of bacterial and yeast infection, events at the site of the graft predispose to subsequent infection. Vascular occlusion, hemorrhage, and local sepsis, which may itself be associated with the earlier complications, are major causes for further operations, delay in extubation of the trachea and, perhaps, prolongation of ICU stay. Therefore, it is not surprising that in intensive care, local sepsis is often associated with nosocomial pneumonia. Pneumonia caused by gram-negative bacilli appears common and serious.[30] It is not surprising that intra-abdominal and pulmonary infections are often found in those patients with multiorgan and particularly renal failure, often with a background of poor hemostasis. After transplantation, successive infective episodes may be caused by relapses or reinfection with the same organism as in previous episodes, but it is also common for successive episodes to involve new organisms resistant to recent antimicrobial chemotherapy. Choice of empirical chemotherapy at each successive infective episode almost inevitably involves the use of multiple agents and needs to be comprehensively broad spectrum, including activity against any likely pathogens including those previously present in the patient or those present in the ICU.

The acquisition of resistance in each episode may not imply the acquisition of a greater number of resistances to multiple antibiotics. Resistances to particular antibiotics are more common in particular species, and the prevalence of particular resistant species varies in different environments. For each antibiotic-resistant species, the pattern of antibiotic resistance linkage varies. New organisms acquired in successive episodes may be resistant only to the last antibiotic used rather than to all antibiotics to which the patient has been exposed. Within classes of antibiotics, cross-resistance because of a common bacterial resistance mechanism can sometimes be assumed (Table 15-1), and reports of unexpected susceptibility in in vitro tests should call these tests and the laboratory into suspicion. Such tests should be reviewed for compliance with international standards of performance and repeated. Cross resistance is a feature of resistance to penicillins and cephalosporins (mediated by β-lactamases), aminoglycosides (mediated by bacterial membrane impermeability or cytoplasmic aminoglycoside modifying enzymes), fluoro-

Table 15-1. Predictable Cross-Resistances of Antibiotics

Resistance	Organism	Predictable Cross-Resistance
Cefotaxime Aztreonam Ceftriaxone	Enterobacteriaceae	All cephalosporins except cefoxitin
Piperacillin	Enterobacteriaceae	Cross resistance and ampicillin
Azlocillin Mezlocillin	Pseudomonas	
Cefuroxime	Enterobacteriaceae	Cefazolin, cephradine and sometimes cefotaxime
Imipenem	All	Meropenem
Gentamicin	Enterobacteriaceae	Tobramycin (in the UK—varies elsewhere)
	Enterococci	also reduced netilmicin activity
Methicillin	Staphylococci	All penicillins, cephalosporins, imipenem
Ampicillin	Enterococci	Azlocillin, piperacillin, benzylpenicillin
Ciprofloxacin	Enterobacteriaceae	Ofloxacin

quinolones (mediated by bacterial permeability changes or mutations in bacterial DNA gyrase), and high-level resistance to glycopeptides (mediated by a change in the vancomycin/teicoplanin target).

Antimicrobial Prophylaxis in Liver Transplant Recipients

In the context of bacterial infection, patients coming to transplantation fall into three groups. Patients with parenchymal liver tumors without underlying hepatic disease usually have a relatively acute and short period of hospitalization before diagnosis and few other conditions that predispose them to pretransplantation infection requiring antibiotic therapy. Their gastrointestinal flora is relatively antibiotic susceptible, and it may be reasonable to give narrow-spectrum antibiotics as operative prophylaxis. Many centers use cefotaxime and ampicillin perioperatively. This may be reasonable with this subgroup of patients omitting cover for nosocomial pathogens such as *Pseudomonas aeruginosa* and *Enterobacter spp.* The postoperative course for this patient group is seldom complex and infectious episodes are fewer.

The second group are those with preoperative chronic liver disease including cirrhosis and biliary atresia. Cirrhosis is associated with depletion of Kupffer cell numbers,[42] a predisposition to bacteremia, and spontaneous bacterial peritonitis and endotoxemia. The predisposition to bacteremia includes staphylococcal infection as well as organisms that travel via the portal vein from the gastrointestinal tract, since the liver macrophage is a major removal site of all particulate antigens such as organisms.[43] Patients with cirrhosis and biliary atresia have often received antibiotics for infection and have previously been in the hospital for long periods. Patients with secondary nonmalignant biliary cirrhosis, biliary strictures including sclerosing cholangitis, and biliary atresia after Kasai operations or who have been transplanted previously, usually have abnormal flora in their biliary tree. In nontransplanted patients this includes anaerobes in some 30% of cases. Use of neomycin, as in the treatment of hepatic encephalopathy, often selects for resistant organisms in the gut flora,[44,45] and ciprofloxacin may be preferable since fecal levels exceed the maximum (MIC) so far described in resistant *Enterobacteriaceae* and pseudomonads. For all such patients who are likely to have abnormal flora, a wider spectrum of antibacterial cover as prophylaxis for surgery is prudent and this should cover Pseudomonas, *Enterobacter,* spp. and anaerobes. Here the use of imipenem alone or a combination of ciprofloxacin, vancomycin, and metronidazole may be considered. The need for vancomycin, rather than a beta-lactam, is arguable but provides activity against methicillin-resistant *S. aureus* (MRSA), methicillin-resistant coagulase-negative staphylococci, and ampicillin-resistant *Enterococcus faecium,* all of which are common pathogens and colonists in tertiary referral centers.

The third group of patients needing transplantation are those in acute hepatic failure, including those whose previous grafts have become infarcted through vascular occlusion and those with acute Budd-Chiari syndrome. In these patients an episode of septicemia is frequently fatal before acute transplantation can be arranged. Such patients, in addition to bacterial infection, are predisposed to yeast infection. Although there are no supporting controlled clinical trial data, we manage these patients with systemic antibacterial and antifungal prophylaxis until transplantation can take place or until liver recovery occurs. We prefer a regimen of ciprofloxacin (6mg/kg/day), vancomycin (15 mg/kg/day), metronidazole, and amphotericin B (0.5mg/kg/day) but will modify the ciprofloxacin component if ciprofloxacin-resistant Gram-negative strains including *P. aeruginosa* or *Xanthomonas maltophilia* colonize the patient. In these patients, who are usually under intensive microbiological surveillance and are transplanted within a week of starting the systemic prophylaxis, we usually continue the same antibiotics over the operation and for 48 hours postoperatively. Only if prophylaxis has lasted more than 7 days or resistant organisms are detected do we change the operative prophylaxis.

In general, perioperative prophylaxis in liver transplantation is usually now given for 48 hours rather than the 5–7 days that was initially the norm. A high proportion of patients develop pyrexia at 4–5 days, and it is important to be confident that negative cultures taken at this time represent the absence of infection rather than antimicrobial suppression of growth. If the patient has received no antibiotics for 48 hours, initial antibiotics started empirically for fever should be stopped promptly if cultures are negative, avoiding selection for resistant organisms and yeasts. In general, as in neutropenic patients, fever demands urgent empirical antimicrobials. Bacteremia in the first 2 weeks after transplantation is often associated with line infection with coagulase-negative staphylococci, and despite operative prophylaxis, *S. aureus* bacteremia associated with deep wound infection is not unknown. In most ICUs 30–60% of coagulase-negative staphylococci are resistant to methicillin, and all other beta-lactam antibiotics and a glycopeptide antibiotic such as vancomycin or teicoplanin is usually required in empirical regimens in this first 2-week period. If this is omitted our experience is that failure of the initial regimens will lead clinicians to also introduce extended spectrum Gram-negative antimicrobials despite the growth of coagulase-negative staphylococci from blood cultures.

Antimicrobial Treatment in the Post Transplant Period

Only some 14% of patients have Gram-negative colonization of the bile in the first 10 days after transplantation,[14] but Gram-negative respiratory colonization and infection is much more common (if selective digestive decontamination [SDD] is not used). For this reason broad spectrum antibacterial cover against Gram-negative organisms is normally required in addition to glycopeptides for fever in this initial period. If SDD is being used the use of such Gram-negative cover is less critical, and from experience in neutropenia this is especially true if ciprofloxacin is being used in decontamination, since this antibiotic is probably more effective in decontamination. Certainly the spectrum of breakthrough organisms is different if either of the decontaminating approaches of ciprofloxacin or topical nonabsorbed aminoglycoside, colistin, and amphotericin is used at least in neutropenia.[46,47] SDD has proved controversial in other ICU areas. In liver transplantation, despite extensive use,[31,48–50] SDD has not been subject to a rigorous large-scale comparative clinical trial with simultaneous controls. The assumption that it is helpful and that other factors such as selection criteria, antibiotic policy, and exclusion of patients requiring retransplantation are not responsible for diminished sepsis rates needs validation. Early experimental studies also involved changes in other aspects of perioperative management.[51] In some studies, using oral aminoglycosides, resistance selection in Gram-positive cocci has been noted.[52,53] High-level gentamicin-resistant enterococci are a particularly noteworthy problem in many liver centers. In one unit vancomycin, gentamicin, and β-lactam–resistant enterococci have emerged as pathogens.[54] Vancomycin-resistant enterococci have also been reported from another transplant unit as colonizing organisms and in rare infections.[55] The emergence of vancomycin resistance is an alarming trend. The influence of oral aminoglycosides in selecting these organisms has not been studied.

In the later posttransplant period, until the withdrawal of the T-tube or stent, enterococci are important pathogens. In our experience, despite not using selective decontamination, they are the most common single genus, other than staphylococci, responsible for bacteremia,[56] although this seems to have diminished with a reduction in the use of T-tubes. Wide spectrum antibacterial cover is needed for fever because of the likelihood of nosocomial infection with antibiotic-resistant species. Overuse of β-lactam antibiotics, particularly cephalosporins, is associated with emergence of *Enterobacter cloacae* with stable-derepression of chromosomal class 1 β-lactamase[14] or *Klebsiella spp.* with extended spectrum plasmid-mediated β-lactamases, both resistant to cephalosporins and ureidopenicillins. Resistant strains of *X. maltophilia* can also be selected both by imipenem and by quinolones. In the presence of a T-tube many bacteremias can be shown to be of biliary origin, but if bile cannot be sampled the source of many bacteremias is occult.[57] Liver pain is not a feature of cholangitis after liver transplantation, but elevated alkaline phosphatase with fever suggests a diagnosis of cholangitis and there are suggestive features on Doppler examination.[58] Appropriate components of combination empirical therapy for fever after the initial 2 weeks include third-generation cephalosporins, ureido-or aminopenicillins, aminoglycosides, and quinolones. If MRSA or ampicillin-resistant enterococci are prevalent, glycopeptides may also be needed.

Yeast Infections in the Post Transplant Period

The incidence of disseminated candidosis is increased in liver transplant recipients.[34,57] Its associations are less with immunosuppression than with prolonged operative procedures associated with hemorrhage and the use of prolonged antibiotic prophylaxis and treatment, although preoperative and postoperative steroid use is a factor. Candidosis is positively associated with preoperative thrombocytopenia and operative transfusion requirements, long periods in the operating room, and prolonged postoperative intravenous antibiotics.[59] Retransplantation and previous sclerosing cholangitis also appear to be risk factors,[60] although the former has not been confirmed as an independent risk factor. Some centers use low-dose (10mg/day) intravenous amphotericin B prophylaxis in the early days after transplantation and have reported a low incidence of fungal infection, but a causal association has not been proved.[61] It is interesting to note that chronic disseminated (hepatosplenic) candidosis, which is increasingly recognized as an accompaniment of neutrophil recovery in neutropenia, has not been described after the Kupffer cell depletion that follows hepatic transplantation.[62] Candida infection of the intestinal or biliary conduit is difficult to distinguish from colonization. Treatment is also difficult as amphotericin B penetrates bile poorly, and triazole antifungals may select for superinfection with resistant yeasts such as *Candida glabrata* (seldom invasive) or *Candida krusei* (usually fluconazole resistant and itraconazole susceptible).[63] There is a theoretical risk of imidazoles or triazoles antagonizing the action of amphotericin B by blocking ergosterol formation if these antifungal agents are used with amphotericin B, but it is difficult to see how amphotericin would clear mucosal candidosis in the conduit. Conduit candidosis may lead to anastomotic leakage.

Antimicrobial Treatment and Prophylaxis of Cholangitis and Cholecystitis in the Nontransplant Patient

The efficacy of antibiotics in the prophylaxis or treatment of such infections depends less on the extent to which they are excreted in the bile and more on effective levels of an appropriate antibiotic in the serum and tissues where bacteremia and wound sepsis actually occur. These tissue (e.g., gallbladder wall) and serum levels are easier to achieve.[64] If surgery or intervention removes the obstruction, the washout phenomenon of restoration of flow would be anticipated to reduce bacterial numbers in bile even without antibiotic intervention, and complete eradication of microorganisms from the gallbladder and biliary tree is not necessary. Caution is needed in extrapolating this situation to one where obstruction remains or T-tubes or stents are in place, as an important issue may be the frequency and cause of further infection when antibiotics are stopped. The occurrence of the syndrome of septic hepatic infarction, which is seen only after liver transplantation,[65] and of some primary hepatic diseases where there are decreases in Kupffer cell numbers or function may also demand a more cautious approach. In cholecystitis there is no evidence to suggest that postoperative complications in patients with obstruction are any higher than those without, again suggesting that the concentration of antibiotic in the bile is irrelevant.[64]

Nevertheless, the presence of antibiotics in the bile may be helpful perioperatively as the infectivity of spilled material may be reduced. The factors that influence the biliary excretion of antibiotics include molecular weight, polarity, and hepatic metabolism although the role of each of these has not been clearly elucidated. The fraction of antibiotic excreted in bile may be an insensitive and misleading way of suggesting efficacy in producing antibiotic effects in bile as daily bile volume is low (approximately 1/L.). Only around 1% of a 1 Gml dose of an antibiotic need enter the bile to attain a mean concentration of 10 μ/mL,[66] and it is biliary concentration and antibacterial potency as measured by MIC, not the excreted fraction, that will determine the likely effects. No antibiotic is known to enter bile when there is complete biliary obstruction, and biliary levels are lower in the gallbladder with cystic duct obstruction. Biliary levels of antibiotics in unobstructed gallbladder bile are higher than in common-duct bile due to concentration. The effects of chronic rather than acute intubation of the common duct on biliary concentrations are not known, although reduced excretion after obstruction may be prolonged.

The Effects of Liver Disease on Antibiotic Pharmacokinetics

Liver disease may have a profound effect on the pharmacokinetics of antibiotics as well as other drugs, although there are few definitive examples of this. Changes in intrinsic hepatic clearance may occur by either reduction in hepatic metabolism or bypassing the liver by shunting. Drug metabolism occurs predominantly in the pericentral area of the hepatic lobule, which is more affected in acute hepatitis than, for example, primary biliary cirrhosis. The protein binding may be altered by reduction in plasma levels of albumin (acidic drugs, e.g., sulphonamides) or α1-acid glycoprotein (basic drugs, e.g., trimethoprim).[67] This affects both hepatic and renal clearance. Hepatic blood flow also affects clearance. The relative importance of protein binding and blood flow theoretically varies by drug, but the practical application of this is limited.[67] The volume of distribution of any drug may change profoundly in chronic liver disease and the presence of ascites may affect this. Drugs such as rifampicin, which normally undergo first-pass metabolism in the liver, have increased systemic concentrations.[68] Some antibiotics such as clindamycin have enterohepatic circulations and the effects of liver disease on clearance may be unpredictable. Antibiotic problems can be unpredictable. Drug interactions caused by P450 cytochrome induction or inhibition by antibiotics such as rifampicin, griseofulvin,

and tetracyclines are well known. The effects of cephems, such as latamoxef, with 4 methyl-tetrazole side chains in clotting function were not predicted and have severely reduced their use. Similarly, metronidazole interactions with alcohol are often forgotten. On a practical management point, hyperbilirubinemia may cause a falsely low result in gentamicin assays if photometric immunoassays rather than bioassays are used.[69]

A wide variety of prophylactic antibiotics have been assessed in biliary surgery, including ampicillin,[70] gentamicin,[71] cotrimoxazole,[72] cephaloridine,[73] cefazolin,[74] cephradine,[75] cefoxitin,[76] cefamandole,[75] cefuroxime,[77] and cefotaxime.[78] All reduced subsequent wound sepsis. In the absence of jaundice, duct stones, cholecystitis, or antibiotic use in the recent past, the incidence of sepsis is low and some authors consider prophylaxis unnecessary. Audit data suggest that such risk factors cannot be relied on and prophylaxis is required for all.[79] Postoperative sepsis is often staphylococcal as in clean surgery, and prophylactic effects may be important for infections caused by this organism. There is little evidence that later cephalosporins are more useful than earlier compounds, providing that antibiotic resistance is rare. However, old trials must be interpreted with caution because resistance rates tend to increase with time after the introduction of an antibiotic.

Use of Penicillins in Biliary Disease

Of the penicillins, ampicillin is actively excreted in bile and levels are found to be greater than those in serum in an unobstructed biliary tree.[66] Treatment results are good if ampicillin is active in vitro against the biliary pathogens isolated[80] and bad if they are resistant.[81] The ureidopenicillins, mezlocillin, azlocillin, and piperacillin, have a broader spectrum of activity and are active against *P. aeruginosa,* but β-lactamases that destroy these compounds and make the organisms resistant are common in *E. coli* and *Klebsiella spp.* among other Gram-negative species, and consequently they cannot really be considered broad spectrum.[82] Initial results with mezlocillin in a comparative trial against ampicillin with gentamicin suggested it was better,[83] but the advantages of ureidopenicillins over cephalosporins must be reconsidered in the light of the common resistance of *E. coli* and *Klebsiella spp.* to the former. Piperacillin is well excreted in bile,[84] unless there has been prolonged biliary obstruction when, even after relief by PTBD, biliary levels may remain low for long periods.[85] Azlocillin shows greater dosage-dependent pharmacokinetics than piperacillin or mezolocillin, suggesting a saturable renal excretion. Biliary levels of azlocillin can be very high and as with piperacillin remain high after serum levels have decreased. Biliary excretion of mezlocillin increases if hepatic function is impaired, but the stability of ureidopenicillins in stored bile is poor and the effects of this have not been examined in vivo in the presence of biliary pathology.[86]

Use of Cephalosporins and Carbapenems in Biliary Disease

Cephalosporins produce serum and biliary concentrations that are equivalent in the unobstructed biliary tree, but there are substantial variations in potency between first- and third-generation compounds in activity against *E. coli* and other *Enterobacteriaceae*. Most have the disadvantage of not including *Enterococcus faecalis* in their spectrum. Cefoperazone is often recommended because of its active excretion in bile and modest activity against enterococci. In a comparative clinical trial it was more effective in preventing bacteremia and curing infection than an ampicillin–tobramycin combination,[81] and this was associated with rarer resistance to the β-lactam component. However, French and colleagues showed that in the obstructed biliary tree at the time of operation there was no detectable drug in the bile after prophylactic administration for 24 hours.[82] Both cefoperazone and ceftazidime, which is not actively excreted, reached similar concentrations 24 hours after decompression, and the active excretion of cefoperazone had not recovered by this time. They concluded that there was no advantage in giving drugs that are actively excreted in bile in the presence of obstruction. Ceftazidime does reach adequate levels in the common bile duct in the absence of obstruction, although tissue levels in the gallbladder are reported occasionally to be low.[87] Its extended spectrum, which includes *P. aeruginosa,* is seldom needed in the absence of this organism. Cefotaxime is metabolized in the liver to its de-

sacetyl form which has different potency and activity and more closely resembles cefuroxime in spectrum. The proportion that is excreted in the bile as the desacetyl form becomes significant only in renal failure when the desacetyl metabolite accumulates. In other circumstances the more potent parent compound is the major biliary product. It has been suggested that the combination of cefotaxime and its desacetyl metabolite together have synergic activity against *Bacteroides spp.,* but the relevance of this to biliary infection has not been assessed. For unknown reasons clearance of cefotaxime is reduced in patients after liver transplantation without evidence of renal dysfunction and dosage can be reduced.[88]

Ceftriaxone is a third-generation cephalosporin with a similar spectrum to cefotaxime. Its serum half-life is considerably longer than that of cefotaxime which permits once daily dosage. Its biliary excretion is much higher with as much as 40% of the parent compound excreted in the bile.[89] Such high delivery of active compound to the gut may disturb the flora and lead to elimination of susceptible coliforms and colonization with resistant organisms including *Clostridium difficile*. In liver transplant recipients the total body clearance of ceftriaxone has been shown to be only approximately one-fifth that of normal subjects.[90] A similar alteration in the pharmacokinetics of ceftriaxone has been reported in patients with liver failure owing to other causes[91] and in patients undergoing cholecystectomy.[92] High biliary concentrations of ceftriaxone can cause the transient appearance of sludge in the biliary tree, probably because ceftriaxone secretion causes a passive flow of calcium into the bile ducts and thus the solubility product of calcium ceftriaxone is exceeded and results in precipitation in the bile.[93] Whether or not this is a problem in patients with reduced liver function, in whom secretion would be presumed to be lower, is unknown.

Imipenem is a beta-lactam carbapenem with very broad spectrum activity including *P. aeruginosa, Enterobacter spp.*, and *Klebsiella spp.* that are cephalosporin resistant, methicillin-susceptible staphylococci and anaerobes but not all enterococci, coagulase-negative staphylococci or *X. maltophilia*. It is hydrolyzed by dehydropeptidase-1, a renal tubular brush border enzyme, to a metabolite and this process is associated with increased nephrotoxocity. Coadministration with a reversible inhibitor of this enzyme, cilastatin, is essential to prevent toxicity and provide active concentrations of this drug in urine. Imipenem is not actively excreted in the bile and levels are only 1–8 mg/L, much lower than the other beta-lactams we have discussed which may be actively transported into bile.[94] This may reduce gastrointestinal levels and selection for resistant *Enterobacteriaceae* and pseudomonads in the gut flora. In the presence of renal dysfunction imipenem is cleared to some extent via nonrenal pathways, however cilastatin is not and accumulates,[95] although there are no reports associated with toxicity involving this agent.

Use of Aminoglycosides in Biliary Disease

Aminoglycosides, even in normal patients, reach only half the serum concentration in the bile,[96] and although the levels reached are still higher than the MIC, for most pathogens bacterial counts are seldom reduced by gentamicin.[97] Quinolones reach very high levels in the bile of a functioning gallbladder, and the concentration may be as high as 50 times that in serum in the case of ciprofloxacin.[98] Norfloxacin also reaches very high levels in the wall of the gallbladder and bile, but these are markedly reduced in the nonfunctioning gallbladder and may not exceed the MIC of common biliary organisms.[99] The advantages of using the quinolones are their broad spectrum with the exception of streptococci, enterococci, and anaerobes, and at present low resistant rates except in staphylococci. Their lack of renal toxicity and oral availability are also advantages.

Other Antibiotics and Biliary Disease

For infections with anaerobes metronidazole remains the drug of choice, but dosage should be reduced in patients with liver failure. In alcoholic liver disease with ascites and prolonged prothrombin time the mean elimination half-life increases to some 20 hours compared with 8 hours, systemic clearance and metabolism decreases,[100] and the incidence of neurological adverse drug reactions increases.[101] There are few data on metronidazole's biliary excretion. Most is excreted in urine in the unchanged form although approximately 30% is metabolized in the liver and there is dispute as to whether or not hepatic failure affects excretion.

Its efficacy in biliary infection with *Bacteroides spp* is unassessed.

Biliary excretion of vancomycin and teicoplanin is poor and has not been studied in modern trials. This can pose problems in the clearance of MRSA and *Streptococcus faecium* from biliary sites, although these antibiotics are useful for treating systemic spread or hepatic infection. Some patients with diminished hepatic function in the presence of minimal or no renal dysfunction have greatly prolonged serum half-lives for vancomycin. The reason for this unpredictable effect is not known.[102] Chloramphenicol and fusidic acid are excreted in bile largely as microbiologically inactive metabolites.[103,104]

Summary

Initial treatment of cholangitis and cholecystitis is and should be started empirically, although blood and bile (if available) should be cultured. If there is previous information on biliary organisms this should be taken into account, although coagulase-negative staphylococci can almost always be ignored in the presence of a chronic T-tube drainage. Local patterns of antibiotic susceptibilities properly determined by recognized laboratory methods and knowledge of the organisms responsible in the local environment should otherwise govern the initial empirical choice of antibiotics. Although combinations may occasionally be needed, few of these have been assessed formally, synergy has not been shown to be of any advantage, and alternative single-agent regimens should be sought.

References

1. Lykaard-Nielsen, M. and Justesen T. (1976) Anaerobic and aerobic bacteriological studies in biliary tract disease. *Scandinavian Journal of Gastroenterology* 11:437–46.

2. Bjorvatn, B. (1984) Cholecystitis–Etiology and Treatment Microbiological Aspects. *Scandinavian Journal of Gastroenterology,* 90(Suppl): 65–70.

3. Brook, I. (1989) Aerobic and anaerobic microbiology of biliary tract disease. *Journal of Clinical Microbiology* 27:2373–75.

4. Lykkegaard-Nielsen, M., Moesgaard, F., Justesen, T., Scheibel, J.H. and Lindenberg, S. (1981) Wound sepsis after elective cholecystectomy. Restriction of prophylactic antibiotics to risk groups. *Scandinavian Journal of Gastroenterology* 16:937–40.

5. Bourgault A.M., England, D.M., Rosenblatt, J.E., Forgacs, P. and Bieger, C. (1979) Clinical characteristics of anaerobic bactibilia. *Archives of Internal Medicine* 139:1346–49.

6. Brook, I. and Altman, R.P. (1983) The significance of anaerobic bacteria in biliary tract infection after hepatic portoenterostomy for biliary atresia. *Surgery* 95:281–83.

7. Hambraeus, A., Laurell, G., Nybacka, O. and Whyte, W. (1990) Biliary tract surgery: A bacteriologic and epidemiologic study. *Acta Chirurgica Scandinavica* 156:155–62.

8. Chetlin, S.H. and Elliot, D.W. (1971) Biliary Bacteraemia. *Archives of Surgery* 102:303–06.

9. Thompson, J.E., Bennion, R. S., Doty, J.E., Muller, E.L. and Pitt, H.A. (1990) Predictive factors for bactibilia in acute cholecystitis. *Archives of Surgery* 125:261–64.

10. Kaufman, H.S., Magnuson, T.H., Lillemoe, K.D., Frasca, P. and Pitt, H.A. (1989) The role of bacteria in gallbladder and common duct stone formation. *Annals of Surgery* 209:584–92.

11. Truedson, H., Elmros, T. and Holm, S. (1983) The incidence of bacteria in gallbladder bile at acute and elective cholecystectomy. *Acta Chirurgica Scandinavica* 149:307–13.

12. Flemma, R.J., Flint, L.M., Osterhout, S. and Shingleton, W.W. (1967) Bacteriological studies of biliary tract infection. *Annals of Surgery* 166:563–70.

13. Bilbao, M.K., Dotter, C.T., Lee, T.G. and Katon, R.M. (1976) Complications of Endoscopic Retrograde Cholangiopancreatography. A study of 10000 cases. *Gastroenterology* 70:314–20.

14. Warren, R.E. (1987) *Bacterial and Fungal Infections in Liver Transplantation.* Grune and Stratton, London, Chapter 29. 2nd edn. (Calne, R. ed.).

15. Audisio, R.A., Bozzetti, F., Severini, A., et al. (1988) The occurrence of cholangitis after percutaneous biliary drainage: Evaluation of some risk factors. *Surgery* 1988 103:507–12.

16. Leung, J.W.C., Chung, S.C.S., Sung, J.J.Y., Banez, V.P. and Li, A.K.C. (1989) Urgent endoscopic drainage for acute suppurative cholangitis. *Lancet* i:1307.

17. Huang, T., Bass, T.A. and Williams, R.D. (1969) The significance of biliary pressure in cholangitis. *Archives of Surgery* 98:629–32.

18. Lygidakis, N.J. and Brummelkamp, W.H. (1985) The significance of intrabiliary pressure in acute cholangitis. *Surgery, Gynecology and Obstetrics* 161:465–69.

19. Salt, A., Noble-Jamieson, G., Barnes, N.D. et al. (1992). Liver transplantation in 100 children: Cambridge and Kin's College Hospital series. *British Medical Journal* 304:416–21.

20. Moore-Gillon, J.C., Eykyn, S.J., and Phillips, I. (1981) Microbiology of pyogenic liver abscess. *British Medical Journal* 283:819–31.

21. Perera, M.R., Kirk, A. and Noone, P. (1980) Presentation, diagnosis and management of liver abscess. *Lancet* ii:629–32.

22. Whiley, R.A., Fraser, H., Hardie, J.M. and Beighton, D. (1990) Phenotypic differentiation of *Streptococcus intermedius, Streptococcus constellatus,* and *Streptococcus anginosus* within the "*Streptococcus milleri* Group." *Journal of Clinical Microbiology* 28:1497– 1501.

23. Herbert, D.A., Fogel, D.A., Rothman, J., Wilson, S., Simmons, F. and Ruskin J. (1982) Pyogenic liver abscesses: successful non-surgical therapy. *Lancet* i:134–36.

24. Berger, L.A. and Osborne, D.R. (1982) Treatment of pyogenic liver abscesses by percutaneous needle aspiration. *Lancet* i:132–36.

25. McCorkell, S.J. and Niles, N.L. (1985) Pyogenic liver abscesses: another look at medical management. *Lancet* i:803–06.

26. Shpitz, B., Kaufman, Z.V.I., Kantarovsky, A., Freund, U. and Dinbar, A. (1990) Pyogenic liver abscess. *Israel Journal of Medical Sciences* 26:564–67.

27. Yanaga, K., Kanematsu, T., Sugimachi, K. and Takenaka, K. (1986) Intraperitoneal septic complications after hepatectomy. *Annals of Surgery* 203:148–52.

28. O'Grady, J.G., Alexander, G.J.M., Sutherland, S. et al. (1988) Cytomegalovirus infection and donor/recipient HLA antigens: Interdependent infections in the pathogenesis of vanishing bile duct syndrome after liver transplantation. *Lancet* ii:302–05.

29. Schroter, G.P.J., Hoelscher, M., Putnam, C.W., Porter, K. A., Hansbrough, J. F. and Starzl, T. E. (1976) Infections complicating orthotopic liver transplantation: A study emphasizing graft-related septicaemia. *Archives of Surgery* 111:1337–47.

30. Kusne, S., Dummer, J.S., Singh, N. et al. (1988b) Infections after liver transplantation. An analysis of 101 consecutive cases. *Medicine (Baltimore)* 67:132–43.

31. Paya, C.V., Hermans, P.E., Washington, J. et al. (1989) Incidence, distribution, and outcome of episodes of infection in 100 orthotopic liver transplantations. *Mayo Clinic Proceedings* 64:555–64.

32. Wreghitt, T.G. (1987) Viral and *Toxoplasma gondi* Infections in Liver Transplantation, (Calne, R. ed) Grune and Stratton, London, Chapter 30.

33. Salt, A., Sutehall, G., Sargaison, M. et al. (1990) Viral and *Toxoplasma gondii* infections in children after liver transplantation. *Journal of Clinical Pathology* 45:63–67.

34. Schroter, G.P.J., Hoelscher, M., Putnam, C.W., Porter, K.A. and Starzl, T.E. (1977) Fungus infections after liver transplantation. *Annals of Surgery* 106:115–22.

35. Wajszczuk, C.P., Dummer, J.S., Ho, M. et al. (1985) Fungal infections in liver transplant recipients. *Transplantation* 40:347–53.

36. Boon, A.P., Adams, D.H., Buckels, J. and McMaster, P. (1990) Cerebral aspergillosis in liver transplantation. *Journal of Clinical Pathology* 43:114–18.

37. Boon, A.P., O'Brien, D. and Adams, D.H. (1991) Ten year review of invasive aspergillosis detected at necropsy. *Journal of Clinical Pathology* 44:452–54.

38. Ayliffe, G.A.J., Elliot, T.S.J., Babb, J.R. and Davies, J. (1990) Environmental investigations for Aspergillus. Abstract P11/4 Programme & Abstracts *2nd International Conference of the Hospital Infection Society,* Kensington, London 1990.

39. McGregor, R.S., Zitelli, B.J., Urbach, A.H., Malatack, J.J. and Gartner, J.C. (1989) Varicella in pediatric orthotopic liver transplant recipients. *Pediatrics* 83: 256–61.

40. Booth, I.W., Chrystie, I.L., Levinsky, R.J., Marshall, W.C., Pincott, J. and Harries, J.T. (1982) Protracted diarrhoea immunodeficiency and viruses. *European Journal of Paediatrics* 138:271–72.

41. Park, G.R., Gomez-Arnau, J., Lindop, M.J., Klinck, J.R., Williams, R. and Calne, R.Y. (1989) Mortality during intensive care after orthotopic liver transplantation. *Anaesthesia* 44:959–63.

42. Manifold, I. H., Bishop, F.M., Cloke, P., Underwood, J.C.E. and Triger, D.R. (1982) Lysozyme in chronic liver disease, a biochemical and histological study. *Journal of Clinical Pathology* 35:815–19.

43. Thomas, H.C., McSween, R.N.M. and White, R.G. (1973) Role of the liver in controlling the immunogenicity of commensal bacteria in the gut. *Lancet* i:1288–91.

44. Lal, D., Gorbach, S. and Levitan R. (1972) Intestinal microflora in patients with alcoholic cirrhosis: urea-splitting bacteria and neomycin resistance. *Gastroenterology* 62:275–79.

45. Valtonen, M.V., Suomalainen, R.J., Ylikahri, R.H. and Valtonen, V.V. (1977) Selection of multiresistant coliforms by long term treatment of hypercholesterolaemia with neomycin. *British Medical Journal* i:683–84.

46. Warren, R.E. (1991) Protecting neutropenic patients from bowel-derived organisms. *Journal of Hospital Infection* 19(Suppl C):43–58.

47. Warren, R.E., Wimperis, J.Z., Baglin, T.E., Constantine, C.E. and Marcus, R. (1990) Prevention of infection by ciprofloxacin in neutropenia. *Journal of Antimicrobial Chemotherapy* 26(Suppl F):109–23.

48. Wiesner, R.H., Hermans, E., Rakela, J. et al. (1988) Selective bowel decontamination to decrease Gram-negative aerobic bacterial and Candida colonisation and prevent infection after orthotopic liver transplantation. *Transplantation* 45:570–74.

49. Wiesner, R.H. (1990) The incidence of Gram-negative bacterial and fungal infections in liver transplant patients treated with selective decontamination. *Infection* 18(Suppl 1):S19–S21.

50. Badger, I.L., Crosby, H.A., Kong, K.L. et al. (1991) Is selective decontamination of the digestive tract beneficial in liver transplant patients? Interim results of a prospective randomized trial. *Transplantation Proceedings* 23:1460–61.

51. Schalm, S.W., Popescu, D.T., Van der Waay, D. et al. (1975) Orthotopic liver transplantation: an experimental study on the prevention of infections with Gram-negative organisms. *British Journal of Surgery* 62: 513–17.

52. Nau, R., Ruchel, R., Mergerian, H., Wegener, U., Winkelmann, T. and Prange, H.W. (1990) Emergence of antibiotic-resistant bacteria during selective decontamination of the digestive tract. *Journal of Antimicrobial Chemotherapy* 24:881–83.

53. Blair, P., Rowlands, B.J., Lowry, K., Webb, C.H., Armstrong, P. and Smilie, J. (1991) Selective decontamination of the digestive tract: A stratified randomized prospective study. *Surgery* 110:303–10.

54. Wade J., Rolando, N. and Casewell, M. (1991) Resistance of *Enterococcus faecium* to vancomycin and gentamicin. *Lancet* i:1616.

55. Green, M., Barbadora, K. and Michael, M. (1991) Recovery of vancomycin-resistant Gram-positive cocci from pediatric liver transplant recipients. *Journal of Clinical Microbiology* 29:2503–06

56. Warren, R.E. (1988) Difficult streptococci. *Journal of Hospital Infection* 11(Suppl A):352–57.

57. Ho, M., Wajszczuk, C.P., Hardy, A. et al. (1983) Infections in kidney, heart and liver recipients on cyclosporine. *Transplantation Proceedings* XV(Suppl 1):2768–72.

58. Coulden, R.A., Britton, P.D., Farman, P., Noble-Jamieson, G. and Wight, D.G.D. (1990) Preliminary report: hepatic vein doppler in the early diagnosis of acute liver transplant rejection. *Lancet* 363:273–75.

59. Kusne, S., Dummer, J.S., Singh, N. et al. (1988) Fungal infections after liver transplantation. *Transplantation Proceedings* XX(Suppl 1):650–51.

60. Castaldo, P., Stratta, R.J., Wood, R.P. et al. (1991) Fungal disease in liver transplant recipients: a multivariate analysis. *Transplantation Proceedings* 23:1517–19.

61. Mora, N.P., Cofer, J.B., Solomon, H. et al. (1991) Analysis of severe infections after 180 consecutive liver transplants: the impact of amphotericin B prophylaxis for reducing the incidence and severity of fungal infections. *Transplantation Proceedings* 23:1528–30.

62. Gouw, A.S.H., Houthoff, H.J., Huitema, S., Beelen, J.M., Gips, C.H. and Poppema, S. (1987) Expression of major histocompatibility complex antigens and replacement of donor cells by recipient ones in human liver grafts. *Transplantation* 43:291–96.

63. Wingard, J.R., Merz, W.G., Rinaldi, H.G. et al. (1991) Increase in *Candida krusei* infection among patients with bone marrow transplantation and neutropenia treated prophylactically with fluconazole. *New England Journal of Medicine* 325:1274–77.

64. Thomas, M. (1983) Antibiotics in bile. *Journal of Antimicrobial Chemotherapy* 12:419–22.

65. Starzl, T.E., Porter, K.E., Putnam, C.W. et al. (1976) Orthotopic liver transplantation in ninety three patients. *Surgery Gynecology and Obstetrics* 142:487–525.

66. Dooley, J.S., Hamilton Miller, J.M.T., Brumfitt, W. and Sherlock, S. (1984) Antibiotics in the treatment of biliary infection. *Gut* 25:988–98.

67. Davey, P.G. (1986) Pharmacokinetics in liver disease. *Journal of Antimicrobial Chemotherapy* 21:1–8.

68. Secor, J.W., and Schenker, S. (1987) Drug metabolism in patients with liver disease. In: *Advances in Internal*

Medicine, Vol 32, (Stollerman, G.H., Harrington, W.J., Lamont, J.T., Leonard, J.L. and Siperstein, M.D. eds). Yearbook Medical Publishers, Chicago, pp. 379–405.

69. Jolley, M.E., Stroupe, S.D., Wang, C.H.J., Panas, H.N., Keegan, C.L. and Schmidt, R.L. (1981) Fluorescence polarization immunoassay 1. Monitoring aminoglycoside antibiotics in serum and plasma. *Clinical Chemistry* 27:1190–97.

70. Keighley, M.R.B. (1977) Microorganisms in the bile-a preventable cause of sepsis after biliary surgery. *Annals of the Royal College of Surgeons of England* 59:328–43.

71. Keighley, M.R.B., Drysdale, R.B., Quoraishi, A.H., Burdon, D.W. and Alexander-Williams, J. (1975) A controlled trial of parenteral prophylactic gentamicin therapy in biliary surgery. *British Journal of Surgery* 62:275–79.

72. Morran, C., McNaught, W. and McArdle, C.S. (1978) Prophylactic co-trimoxazole in biliary surgery. *British Medical Journal* 2:462–64.

73. Chetlin, S.H. and Elliot, D.W. (1973) Preoperative antibiotics in biliary surgery. *Archives of Surgery* 107:319–23.

74. Strachan, C.J.L., Black, J., Powis, S.J.A. et al. (1977) Prophylactic use of cephazolin against wound sepsis after cholecystectomy. *British Medical Journal* 1:1254–56.

75. Karran, S.J., Lewington, V., Allen, S. and Cooper, A. (1981) Prospective double blind evaluation of single dose intravenous prophylaxis using three cephalosporins in biliary surgery. *Proceedings of the XV Congress ESSR,* Garmish-Pattenkirchen.

76. Hansbrough, J.F. and Clark, J.E. (1982) Concentrations of cefoxitin in gallbladder bile of cholecystectomy patients. *Antimicrobial Agents and Chemotherapy* 22:709–10.

77. Karran, S.J., Allen, S., Levington, V., Seal, D. and Reeves, D. (1980) Cefuroxime prophylaxis in biliary surgery. Cefuroxime Update. *Royal Society of Medicine International Congress* No. 38, pp. 27–34.

78. Sykes, D. and Basu, P.K. (1984) Prophylactic use of cefotaxime in elective biliary surgery. *Journal of Antimicrobial Chemotherapy* 14(Suppl B):237–39.

79. Wells, G.R., Taylor, E.W., Marin, L. and the West of Scotland Surgical Infection Study Group. (1989) Relationship between bile colonisation high risk factors and postoperative sepsis in patients undergoing biliary tract operations while receiving prophylactic antibiotics. *British Journal of Surgery* 76:374–77.

80. Chacon, J.P., Criscuolo, P.D., Kobata, C.M., Ferraro, J.R., Saad, S.S. and Reis, C. Prospective randomized comparison of pefloxacin and ampicillin plus gentamicin in the treatment of bacteriologically proven biliary tract infections. *Journal of Antimicrobial Chemotherapy* 26(Suppl B):167–72.

81. Bergeron, M.G., Mendelson, J., Harding, G.K. et al. (1988) Cefoperazone compared with ampicillin plus tobramycin for severe biliary tract infections. *Antimicrobial Agents and Chemotherapy* 32:1231–36.

82. French, G.L., Chan, R.C.Y., Chung, S.C.S. and Leung, J.W.C. (1989) Antibiotics for cholangitis. *Lancet* ii:1271–72.

83. Gerecht, W.B., Henry, N.K., Hoffman, W.W. et al. (1989) Prospective randomized comparison of mexlocillin therapy alone with combined ampicillin and gentamicin therapy for patients with cholangitis. *Archives of Internal Medicine* 149:1279–84.

84. Giron, J.A., Meyers, B.R. and Hirschman, S.Z. (1981) Biliary concentrations of piperacillin in patients undergoing cholecystectomy. *Antimicrobial Agents and Chemotherapy* 19:309–11.

85. Blenkharn, J.I., Habib, N., Mok, D. et al. (1985) Decreased biliary excretion of piperacillin after precutaneous relief of extrahepatic obstructive jaundice. *Antimicrobial Agents and Chemotherapy* 28:778–80.

86. Bergan, T. (1981) Overview of acylureidopenicillin pharmacokinetics. *Scandinavian Journal of Infectious Diseases* (suppl 29):33–48.

87. Shiramatsu, K., Hirata, K., Yamada, T. et al. Ceftazidime concentration in gallbladder tissue and excretion in bile. *Antimicrobial Agents and Chemotherapy* 32:1588–89.

88. Burckart, G.J., Ptachcinski, R.J., Jones, D.H., Howrie, D.L., Venkataramanan, R. and Starzl, T.E. (1987) Impaired clearance of ceftizoxime and cefotaxime after orthotopic liver transplantation. *Antimicrobial Agents and Chemotherapy* 31:323–24.

89. Stoeckel, K., McNamara, P.J., Brandt, R., Plozza-Nottebrock, H. and Ziegler, W.H. (1981) Effects of concentration-dependent plasma protein binding on ceftriaxone kinetics. *Clinical Pharmacology and Therapeutics* 29:650–57.

90. Toth, A., Abdullah, H.Y., Venkataramanan, R. et al. (1991) Pharmacokinetics of ceftriaxone in liver transplant recipients. *Journal of Clinical Pharmacology* 31:722–28.

91. Stoeckel, K., Tuerk, H., Trueb, V. and McNamara, P.J. (1984) Single-dose kinetics in liver insufficiency. *Clinical Pharmacology and Therapeutics* 36:500–09.

92. Hayton, W.L., Schandlik, R. and Stoeckel, K. (1986) Biliary excretion and pharmacokinetics of ceftriaxone after cholecystectomy. *European Journal of Clinical Pharmacology* 30:445–51.

93. Xia, Y., Lambert, K.J., Schteingart, C.D., Gu, J.J. and Hofmann, A.F. (1990) Concentrate biliary secretion and precipitation of calcium ceftriaxone in bile. *Gastroenterology* 99:454–65.

94. Graziani, A.L., Gibson, G.A. and MacGregor, R.R. (1987) Biliary excretion of imipenem-cilastatin in hospitalized patients. *Antimicrobial Agents and Chemotherapy* 31:1718–21.

95. Drusano, G.L. (1986) An overview of the pharmacology of imipenem/cilastatin. *Journal of Antimicrobial Chemotherapy* 18(Suppl E):79–92.

96. Pitt, H.A., Roberts, R.B. and Johnson, W.D. (1973) Gentamicin levels in the human biliary tract. *Journal of Infectious Diseases* 127:299–303.

97. Wacha, H. and Helm, E.B. (1982) Efficacy of antibiotics in bactobilia. *Journal of Antimicrobial Chemotherapy* 9(Suppl A):131–37.

98. Dan, M., Verbin, N., Gorea, A., Nagar, H. and Berger, S.A. (1988) Concentrations of ciprofloxacin in human liver, gallbladder and bile following oral administration. *Reviews of Infectious Diseases* 10(Suppl 1):S125.

99. Stewart, J.S.S., Roy, A., Shrivastava, R.K. and Kelly, J.G. (1988) Norfloxacin levels in human bile, serum, and tissues. *Reviews of Infectious Diseases* 10(Suppl 1):S125–S126.

100. Farrell, G. Baird-Lambert, J., Cvejic, M. and Buchanan, N. (1984) Disposition and metabolism of metronidazole in patients with liver failure. *Hepatology* 4:722–26.

101. Farrell, G., Zaluzny, L., Baird-Lambert, J., Cvejic, M. and Buchanan, N. (1983) Impaired elimination of metronidazole in decompensated chronic liver disease. *British Medical Journal* 287:1845.

102. Brown, N., Ho, D.H.W., Fong, K.L. et al. (1983) Effects of hepatic function on vancomycin clinical pharmacology. *Antimicrobial Agents and Chemotherapy* 23:603–09.

103. Kunin, C.M., Glazko, A.J. and Finland, M. (1959) Persistence of antibiotics in blood of patients with acute renal failure. II. Chloramphenicol and its metabolic products in the blood of patients with severe renal disease or hepatic cirrhosis. *Journal of Clinical Investigation* 38:1498–1508.

104. Godtfredsen, W.O. and Vangedal, S. (1966) On the metabolism of fusidic acid in man. *Acta Chimica Scandinavica B* 20:1599–1607.

Chapter 16
The Perioperative Care of Patients with Hepatitis B

David H. Van Thiel, Vincents J. Dindzans,
Robert R. Schade, and Mordechai Rabinovitz

The Hepatitis B Virus

The hepatitis B virus (HBV) is one of the Hepadna viruses, which are hepatotropic and produce persistent disease in their respective hosts.[1] A relationship between chronic infection and hepatocellular carcinoma has been established for several of the Hepadna viruses, particularly HBV. All of the Hepadna viruses have a characteristic and unusual genomic structure consisting of a small, partly double-stranded circular DNA molecule. The long strand ($-$) is of fixed length, whereas the short strand ($+$) varies in length. The HBV genome is about 3200 base pairs long. The maintenance of the circular structure of the genome is guaranteed by base pairing of the two $5'$ ends of the strands. Currently, 10 complete HBV nucleotide sequences have been reported. Analyses of these show that the divergence between each is small (about 10%).[2] Large open reading frames (ORF) have been conserved among all the sequenced genomes and are thought to represent coding regions for individual viral proteins. The long strand carries four ORFs and, therefore, carries all of the protein coding capacity of the virus. These four ORFs are termed *S/pre S*, *C*, *P* and *X*. Each overlaps with at least one other, and the P ORF overlaps with each of the other three. By emphasizing overlapping ORFs, the HBV genome can encode for many different proteins, and yet it is the smallest known animal viral genome. The S/pre S region codes for the proteins of the viral envelope and is divided into the S gene, the pre S, and pre S_2 regions, which code for a protein that contains the receptor for polymerized human serum albumin and may play a role in HBV binding to hepatocytes. The pre S_1 region appears to be essential for hepatocyte binding. The C gene codes for a large core protein, from which the e-antigen (HBeAg) appears to be a proteolytic cleavage product. The P region codes for a basic protein that appears to have both DNA polymerase and reverse transcriptase activity. Finally, the X region codes for a large polypeptide whose function is unknown.

Two major HBV-specific poly A+ RNAs have been characterized from the liver of infected chimpanzees.[3,4] The first is 2.1 kb long; the second, 3.5 kb long. The 2.1 kb RNA is the messenger for the envelope, and the 3.5 kb RNA is the messenger for the core and DNA polymerase proteins. Two promoter regions and an enhancer region have been identified. Liver-specific and sex-linked expression of the S gene have been reported. The 2.1 kb RNA and hepatitis B surface antigen (HBsAg) production occur in parallel in boys and girls before puberty, whereas the S gene is expressed 5 to 10 times greater in males than in females after puberty. HBV DNA also has a glucocorticoid-responsive element that may mediate expression of HBV genes in infected hepatocytes.[6]

The Incidence and Prevalence of HBV Infection

Current statistics suggest that 16,000 new cases of HBV infection occur annually in the United States. At least 600,000 chronic carriers of HBV are estimated to live in the United States, of whom 250,000 are thought to have chronic liver disease.[7] These statistics suggest that 0.5% of the American population has been infected with HBV. The figures are rather low compared with those for other parts of the world, particularly the more heavily populated areas such as the Far East and Black Africa, where 5–20% of the population is known to be infected and the death rates from postnecrotic cirrhosis and its complications, particularly hepatocellular carcinoma, are quite high.[7] There are few data to suggest that the prevalence of the disease is falling. Worse yet, a steadily increasing number of patients with HBV are referred to transplantation centers.

Modes of Transmission of HBV Infection

The major mechanisms responsible for transmission of HBV from infected carriers to susceptible hosts are through puncture wounds contaminated with serum, through abrasions or cuts contaminated with either serum or infected secretions, by introduction of the virus at a mucosal surface (oral, gastrointestinal, anal, or vaginal), and by introduction of virus-containing saliva, semen, or vaginal secretions to an abrased cutaneous or mucosal surface.[8] Thus, the use of blood and blood products, contaminated needles (as in illicit drug use), syringes or dental and surgical instruments, hemodialysis, tattooing, ear piercing, acupuncture, pin pricks administered during a neurologic examination, and insect bites can all transmit HBV from infected to uninfected persons. The major reservoirs of infection in the United States are shown in Table 16-1.

Persons at increased risk to acquire a HBV infection include those who live in closed institutions (prisons, mental institutions, institutions for the handicapped and retarded, and military institutions). Those with impaired immune systems are also susceptible, including patients receiving hemodialysis, transplant recipients, and those taking chronic immunosuppressive agents, particularly steroids, azathioprine, and cyclosporine but also

Table 16-1. Main Reservoirs of HBV Infection Present in the USA and Their Relative Abundance

Homosexuals	21%
Drug users	15%
Heterosexual contacts	15%
Unknown source	39%
Miscellaneous causes	4%

including a large number of chemotherapeutic agents for cancer. Obviously, hemophiliacs, persons with chronic hemolytic anemias, and those who require chronic or recurrent blood or blood product administration are highly susceptible to HBV infection. The sexually promiscuous (homosexuals, prostitutes, and bisexuals) are very liable to acquire and transmit the disease. Newborns of HBsAg-positive mothers are at very high risk of acquiring a HBV infection and are even more likely to become chronic carriers.

A hospital survey of more than 6,000 adult patients revealed a hepatitis "carrier" rate of approximately 1% in hospitalized adults.[9] That is, 1% of these patients tested positive for HBsAg and were, therefore, potential transmitters of HBV. In only 17% of these HBV-carrier patients was a diagnosis of hepatitis known or suspected. Therefore, if not for the study, 83% of these potentially infective patients would likely have remained unidentified, posing an unrecognized hazard of hepatitis B transmission.

A lower but real risk of acquiring HBV infection exists for individuals who share a household with a chronic carrier, particularly if they are a sexual partner of the carrier. Similarly, immigrants from an area where HBV is endemic are highly likely to acquire the infection and become chronic carriers.

Finally, health care workers are vulnerable to HBV infection, particularly early in their careers. Several important facts about the occupational hazard of HBV infection have emerged:

1. The incidence of HBV among physicians is approximately five times that of volunteer blood donor "controls."[10,11]

2. HBV exposure for physicians is greatest in the early years of their clinical experience, including hospital-based postgraduate training.[12]

3. Exposure to blood and body fluids, rather than patient contact per se, appears to be the principal risk factor in acquiring HBV. Therefore, susceptibility is especially high in specialties such as surgery and pathology, in which percutaneous or "splash"

exposures by blood or body fluids are more likely to occur.[13]

4. The risk of HBV infection for any health professional is further increased when HBV carriers represent a high percentage of the patient population. These carrier groups include renal dialysis patients,[14] residents of prisons and institutions for the mentally retarded,[15] intravenous drug users, male homosexuals, Alaskan Eskimos, and Southeast Asian immigrants.[16–19]

The calculated risk of acquiring a HBV infection from a needle stick is 5% if the needle was used on a patient who is HBsAg positive but is only 0.1% if the patient is HBsAg negative.[20]

The risk to a neonate born of a HBsAg-positive mother is a function of the immune response of the infected mother. Essentially 100% of infants born of HBsAg-positive and HBeAg-positive mothers become infected.[21,22] More than 50% of infants born to mothers who are HBsAg positive, but hepatitis B core antigen (HBcAg) and antibody (HBcAb) negative, become infected. Those whose mothers are HBeAb positive at birth have a lower risk (25% or less) of becoming infected. Infants who become infected are highly likely to become chronic carriers and to be unable to clear the virus. Such an infant has a 90–95% risk of becoming a carrier, whereas the risk for a child over 2 years of age is only 20% and that of an adult varies from 1–10% depending on the gender, environment, health status, and occupation.[8,21,22]

HBV outbreaks among patients have been linked to infected health care personnel, but these appear to be isolated instances, and the overall risk of this type of transmission remains unknown.[23–25] In a recent prospective study, no evidence of hepatitis transmission was found in 246 patients who had been exposed a total of 483 times to nine health care workers with either acute or chronic hepatitis B.

Once acquired as a chronic infection, the rate of seroconversion from HBeAg positive to HBeAb positive is 10% per year, whereas the conversion rate for HBsAg positive to HBsAb positive is only 1–2% per year.

Hepatitis B Virus Infection

Hepatitis B virus has been found in every population studied. Unlike most other viral infections, a proportion of those become chronic carriers be-cause they fail to eliminate HBV. These people serve as permanent reservoirs of HBV infection in the community. The risk of becoming a chronic carrier is greatest if the HBV infection is acquired early in life, particularly during the first year.[22]

In both Europe and the United States, the prevalence of hepatitis B infection ranges between four and 30 persons per hundred thousand per year. Serologic evidence of past infection with HBV is seen in less than 10% of the population in these same areas, and a chronic carrier state afflicts about 0.1% of the population. On a global scale, early childhood infection, acquired from an infected mother, is the predominant form of the disease.[21,22] In areas of Southeast Asia, 5–15% of the women of childbearing age are chronic carriers of HBsAg and many of these are also HBeAg positive. Eighty-five percent of their children, if not given specific immunoglobulin at birth, are likely to acquire the infection and become lifetime carriers of the virus.[26]

Although frequently asymptomatic, the chronic carrier state for HBV is not a trivial affair. Fifty percent of all carriers are expected to die of liver-related disease. Of these, 10% will have hepatocellular carcinoma.[27] The presence of HBeAg in the circulation is important because it indicates infectivity and is associated with inflammatory liver disease. Both HBcAg and HBeAg are present on the surface membrane of infected cells and are thought to be important targets for cytotoxic T cells in the elimination of virus-infected cells.

The hepatitis B virus is not cytopathic. The host eliminates the infection by destroying infected cells. The defense against the virus can be divided into two stages. The early nonspecific defense inhibits the replication of virus and destroys virus-infected cells indiscriminately. A later, specific immunity is directed selectively against both circulating free virions and cells infected with the virus. A suboptimal initial response to infection may allow for a greater spread of virus before specific immunity can develop. It has been found that 5% of the world population has a reduced production of interferon and that HBV carriers have defective alpha interferon production.

Therapy of HBV Infection

Adenine arabinoside (Ara-A) is a purine analog; when given to HBsAg and HBeAg carriers, 40%

undergo HBeAg to HBeAb seroconversion fol-lowed by a reduction in the inflammatory activity in the liver.[28] Ara AMP is a water-soluble monophos-phate derivative of Ara A that can be given both by intravenous and intramuscular injection.[29,30] Using a 5-day introductory course of daily Ara AMP, fol-lowed by maintenance therapy at half the introduc-tory dose, seroconversion rates up to 40% have been observed, as with Ara A. Homosexuals do not appear to responsed to Ara AMP.[31] This may be be-cause the drug inhibits both host and viral DNA replication and is immunosuppressive. Unfortu-nately, Ara AMP has considerable toxicity, limiting duration of therapy possible in any given patient.

Alpha interferon has been used to treat HBV in-fections, with reported response rates of approxi-mately 50% for the loss of HBV DNA and HBeAg from the serum of patients treated for long periods. This response has coincided with a reduction in the inflammatory activity in the liver.[32,33]

Prednisone has been shown to increase viral replication, and the withdrawal of prednisone is often followed by exacerbation of acute hepatitis, presumably because there is a rebound of immu-nity associated with the cessation of immunosup-pression.[29] Such exacerbations frequently are followed by either viral clearance or a fulminant course of the hepatitis.

The Care of the HBsAg-Positive Patient

As previously discussed, the blood and all body se-cretions of persons who are HBsAg positive must be considered to be infectious. Thus, those examin-ing such patients should be aware of the potential risks and should be fully protected. Usually, only gloves are required for patient care involving per-sonal contact. When endoscopic procedures and other invasive procedures are to be performed, ap-propriate gowns, caps, goggles, and gloves are rec-ommended. Moreover, such patients should be scheduled for appointments late in the day or as the last operation of the day to prevent passive in-fection of other patients using the same room or equipment before appropriate gas sterilization can be performed. All instruments should be washed and then sterilized before reuse. All bed-ding, pajamas, gowns, towels, and other equipment used in the care of such patients should either be disposed of or, if reused, be autoclaved. Surgeons performing operative procedures may wish to wear double gloves and/or gowns when attending such patients, as may intensive care unit personnel. The use of goggles and caps may also be wise, de-pending on the individual circumstances and proce-dures anticipated.

Protection of the Health Care Workers Attending HBV-Positive Patients

Currently, the ideal method of protecting all health care workers from HBV infection and disease is to immunize them with either the Merck pooled sera preparation or the more recent recombinant prepa-rations.[8] Both vaccines have been proved effective, but the pooled serum preparation is somewhat bet-ter than the current recombinant preparations. Both are best administered intramuscularly in the deltoid area (1 mL), twice at monthly intervals followed by a booster 6 months after the second dose. Recent data indicate that three monthly injections are equally effective, and data from Third World coun-tries suggest that immunity can be produced and costs reduced by a factor of 10 by simply adminis-tering 0.1 mL intradermally, three times at monthly intervals. Whether a booster dose of vaccine is nec-essary 5 or more years after initial vaccination has not been resolved. If in doubt, a booster can be given either to guarantee immunity or to produce an amnestic response.

If an unvaccinated health care worker experi-ences a pin prick or other type of contamination, the simultaneous administration of HBIG (3 mL) at each of two different sites and a series of vaccina-tions is warranted (combined passive–active pro-tection). The vaccination in such cases is admin-istered exactly as if an elective immunization-series were being given.

Those currently recommended to receive HBV vaccinations include all physicians, nurses, bio-chemistry and serologic laboratory personnel, blood bank personnel, and family members and sexual partners of HBsAg-positive individuals. It is anticipated that universal vaccination of individuals at risk to acquire HBV infection and disease will dramatically reduce the burden of the number of cases, chronic carriers, and deaths related directly and indirectly to HBV infection.

References

1. Robinson, W.S. and Marion, L.P. (1988) Biological features of hepadna viruses. In: *Viral Hepatitis and Liver Disease*, (Zuckerman, A.J. ed.). A.R. Liss Inc., New York, pp. 449–58.
2. Tiollais, P., Buendia, M., Brechot, C., Dejean, A., Michel, M.-L. and Pourcel, C. (1988) Structure, genetic organization and transcription of hepadna viruses. In: *Viral Hepatitis and Liver Disease*, (Zuckerman, A.J., ed.). A.R. Liss Inc., New York, pp. 295–300.
3. Standring, D.N., Rutter, W.J., Varmus, H.E. and Ganem, D. (1986) Transcription of the hepatitis B surface antigen gene in cultured marine cells initiates within the presurface region. *J Virol* 50:563–71.
4. Will, H., Reiser, W., and Weimer, T. et al. (1987) Replication strategy of human hepatitis B virus. *J Virol* 61:904–11.
5. Farza, H., Salmon, A.M., Hadchouel, M. and Morcan, J.L. (1984) Hepatitis B surface antigen gene expression is regulated by sex steroids and glucocorticoids in transgenic mice. *Proc Natl Acad Sciences, USA* 84:1187–91.
6. Tur-Kaspa, R., Burk R.D., Shaul, Y. and Shafritz, D.A. (1986) Hepatitis B virus DNA contains a glucocorticoid responsive element. *Proc Natl Acad Sci USA* 83:1627–31.
7. Gust, I. and Crowe, S. (1986) The global importance of viral hepatitis. In: *Clinics in Tropical Medicine and Communicable Diseases*, (Zuckerman, A.J. ed.), A.R. Liss Inc., New York, pp. 281–302.
8. Maynard, J.E., Kane, M.A., Alter, M.J. and Hadler, S.C. (1988) Control of hepatitis B by immunization. In: *Viral Hepatitis and Liver Disease*, (Zuckerman, A.J. ed.), A.R. Liss Inc., New York, pp. 967–69.
9. Maynard, J.E. (1981) Nosocomial viral hepatitis. *Am J Med* 70:439.
10. Smith, J.L., Maynard, J.E., Berquist, K.R., Doto, I.L., Webster, H.M., and Sheller, M.J. (1976) Comparative risk of hepatitis B among physicians and dentists. *J Infect Dis* 133:705–6.
11. Steinbuch, M. and Gaeuman, J.V. (1986) Risk of hepatitis B in hospital personnel. *J Occup Med* 28:276–81.
12. Guillen-Solvas, J., delCastillo, J.L., Maroto Vela, M.C., Espinar, A.C. and Galvez Vargas, R. (1987) The risk of infection with hepatitis B virus in relation to length of hospital employment. *J Hospital Infection* 9:43–7.
13. Palmer, D.L., Barash, M., King, R. and Neil, F. (1983) Hepatitis among hospital employees. *West J Med* 138:519–23.
14. Mayor, G.H., Hourani, M.R., Greenbaum, D.S., and Patterson, M.J. (1979) Prevalence of hepatitis B in 27 Michigan hemodialysis centers. *Am J Public Health* 69:581–84.
15. Jeffrey, P., Koplan, J.P., Walker, J.A. and Bryan, J.A. (1978) Prevalence of hepatitis B surface antigen and antibody in a state prison in Kansas. *J Infect Dis* 137:505–6.
16. Luzzio, A.J., Camp, F.R., Blumberg, B.S., Conte, N.F. and Coley, V.R. (1975) Prevalence of Australia antigen in military populations. *Milit Med* 140:41–3.
17. Schreeder, M.T., Thompson, S.E., Hadler, S.C. et al. (1980) Epidemiology of hepatitis B in gay men. *J Homosex* 5:307–10.
18. Barrett, D.H., Burks, J.M., McMahon, B. et al. (1977) Epidemiology of hepatitis B in two Alaskan communities. *Am J Epidemiol* 105:118–22.
19. Chaudhary, R.K., Nicholls, E.S. and Kennedy, D.A. (1981) Prevalence of hepatitis B markers in Indochinese refugees. *Can Med Assoc J* 125:1243.
20. Dienstag, J.L. (1982) Nosocomial hepatitis: The risk of hepatitis B in health care personnel. In: *Viral Hepatitis*, (Overby, L.R., Deinhardt, F. and Deinhardt, J. eds). M. Dekker, New York, pp. 177–79.
21. Chin, K.C., Chandhuri, A.K.R. and Follett, E.A.C. (1981) Materno-factal transmission of HBsAg by asymptomatic carrier mothers in Glasgow. *J Infection* 3:246–52.
22. Stevens, C.E., Toy, P.T., Tong, M.J. et al. (1985) Perinatal hepatitis B virus transmission in the United States. *Journal of the American Medical Association* 253:2740–1745.
23. Snyman, D.R., Hindman, S.H., Wineland, M.D., Bryan, J. and Maynard, J.E. (1976) Nosocomial viral hepatitis B: A cluster among staff with subsequent transmission to patients. *Ann Intern Med* 85:573.
24. Anonymous (1980) All the collaborators have chosen to remain anonymous to facilitate the reorganization of their colleague's professional life. Report of Collaborative Study by the Communicable Disease Surveillance Center and the Epidemiological Research Laboratory of the Public Health Laboratory Service with a District Control-of-Infection Service: Acute hepatitis B associated with gynecological surgery. *Lancet* i:1.
25. LaBrecque, D.R., Muhs, J.M., Lutwick, L.I., Woolson, R.F. and Hierholzer, W.R. (1986) The risk of hepatitis B transmission from health care workers to patients in a hospital setting. *Hepatology* 6:205.
26. Beasley, R.P, Hwang, L.Y., Lin, C.C. et al. (1981) Hepatitis immunoglobulin efficacy in the interruption of perinatal transmission of hepatitis B carrier state. *Lancet* i:388–93.
27. Harrison, T.J., Chen, J.Y. and Zuckerman, A.J. (1986) Hepatitis B virus and hepatocellular carcinoma. In: *Clinics in Tropical Medicine and Communicable Diseases*, (Zuckerman, A.J., ed). A.R. Liss Inc., New York, pp. 395–410.
28. Bassendine, M.F., Chadwick, R.G., Saberom, J., Shipton, U., Thomas, H.C. and Sherlock, S. (1981) Adenosine arabinosive therapy in HBsAg positive chronic liver disease. *Gastroenterology* 80:1016–22.
29. Scullard, G.H., Smith, C.L., Merigan, T.C., Robinson, W.S. and Gregory, P.B. (1981) Effects of immunosuppressive therapy or viral marker in chronic active hepatitis B. *Gastroenterology* 81:987–91.

30. Weller, I.V.D., Bassendine, M.F., Craxim, A. et al. (1982) Successful treatment of HBs and HBeAg positive chronic liver disease. *Gut* 23:717–23.

31. Thomas, H.C. and Scully, G.J. (1986) Antiviral therapy in chronic hepatitis B virus infection. *Br Med Bul* 41:374–80.

32. Greenberg, H.B., Pollard, R.B., Lutwick, L.L., Gregory, P.B., Robinson, W.S. and Merigan, T.C. (1976) Effect of human leucocyte interferon or hepatitis B virus infection in patients with chronic active hepatitis, *N Engl J Med* 295:517–22.

33. Smith, C.I., Weissberg, J., Bernhardt, L., Gregory, P.B., Robinson, W.S. and Merigan, T.C. (1983) Acute done particle suppression with leucocyte recombinant interferon in chronic HBV infection. *J Infect Dis* 148:907–13.

Chapter 17
Nutrition in Perioperative Care

Graham Neale

All patients with liver disease should be screened for nutritional disorders (Table 17–1), an assessment that is particularly important in those requiring surgery. Sometimes the correction of a single deficiency (e.g., vitamin K, potassium, magnesium) may have a major influence on the recovery from surgical trauma. In other circumstances the deliberate provision of protein and energy may ameliorate the catabolic processes of the perioperative period and so improve the chances of a speedy recovery, free from septic complications.

In the overall care of surgical patients, the relationship of nutrition to the processes of intermediary metabolism, many of which are mediated by the liver, must be considered. Assessment is often made more difficult because major surgery also causes metabolic disturbances. Moreover, a major systemic illness may unmask occult liver pathology that in turn may adversely affect healing processes and the recovery of the patient.

The liver plays a key role in intermediary metabolism, especially in relation to the processing of nutrients, the production of circulating proteins, and the handling of drugs and toxins (Table 17–2). These functions may be modulated by diet or the administration of nutrient solutions. Unfortunately, it is usually impossible to disentangle the adverse effects of malnutrition from those of other variables such as organ underperfusion, bacterial and nonbacterial toxins, drugs, and mediators of the inflammatory response. The clinician must apply general principles and make therapeutic decisions on the basis of the best available, but often incomplete, evidence.

Table 17–1. Important Nutritional Disorders in Patients with Liver Disease

Pathological Process	Nutritional Disorder
Chronic liver parenchymal disease	Weight loss
	Hypoalbuminemia
	Hypoprothrombinemia
	Electrolyte disturbances
Alcoholism	Muscle loss
	Magnesium deficiency
	Phosphate deficiency
	Electrolyte disturbances
	Vitamin deficiencies (B group, Folic acid, Vitamin C)
Cholestasis (several weeks)	Vitamin K deficiency
(several months)	Osteomalacia
	Fat: soluble vitamin deficiency
Malignant disease affecting liver	Usually severe generalized malnutrition
	Electrolyte and mineral disorders

Any patient with chronic liver disease may develop iron deficiency as a result of blood loss from varices or an associated gastropathy.

The Assessment of Hepatic Function

Common causes of liver damage are listed in Table 17–3. Liver function may be impaired by poor blood flow, loss of cell function, or impaired excretion (cholestasis). Hepatic reserve is considerable and thus patients with compensated liver disease may not show overall impairment of intermediary metabolism. Standard biochemical markers are useful for diagnosis but are not useful in predicting the likelihood of liver failure, which is manifested clinically by the development of encephalopathy or coagulopathy.

Liver Failure

Metabolic dysfunction in liver disease may be caused by a decreased number of functioning cells and by the impaired delivery of both nutrients and hormones because of intra- and extra-hepatic shunting of the hepatic circulation. Levels of insulin, glucagon, adrenalin, and cortisol tend to increase, thereby enhancing catabolic processes.[1,2] Gluconeogenesis is normally well maintained but the storage of glycogen is impaired. Thus impaired glucose tolerance is common. The sick liver may be unable to metabolize long-chain fatty acids completely, thereby reducing the availability of ketones for gluconeogenesis.

In severe hepatic dysfunction the liver has increasing difficulty in metabolizing aromatic amino acids (AAA) (tyrosine, phenylalanine, and tryptophan) and other liver-dependent amino acids, especially methionine and glutamine. Plasma concentrations increase. The branched chain amino acids (BCAA) (leucine, isoleucine, and valine) are mainly metabolized in skeletal muscle. In chronic liver disease, circulating concentrations decrease possibly because of the effects of higher concentrations of circulating insulin. The molar ratio of BCAA:AAA has been correlated with hepatic encephalopathy.[3,4] In normal subjects:

$$\frac{\text{Isoleucine} + \text{Valine} + \text{Leucine}}{\text{Phenylalanine} + \text{Tyrosine}} = 3.0 - 3.5$$

In hepatic encephalopathy values decrease to less than 1. Amino acids in cerebrospinal fluid show a similar imbalance, and this may explain the reduction in concentration of brain neurotransmitters (dopamine and noradrenalin) and an increase in serotonin and the false neurotransmitters, octopamine and phenylethyl amines, in response to saturation of the phenylalanine-catecholamine pathway.[5] In addition ammonia, derived from the catabolism of protein and amino acids and from bacterial metabolism in the colon, is poorly cleared from the circulation in patients with liver failure. It also impairs cerebral function.

Table 17–2. Important Functions of the Liver in Relation to Nutrition

Function	Nutritional Component	Clinical Disorder
Storage and interconversion of fuels	Reduced glycogen stores Insulin resistance	Hypoglycemia Hyperglycemia
Deamination of amino acids	Urea produced from excess nitrogen	Urea production falls
Synthesis of export proteins	Need adequate supply of amino acids	Hypoalbuminemia Low transport proteins
Synthesis of coagulation factors	Need vitamin K	Hypoprothrombinemia
Synthesis of lipoproteins	From cholesterol, triglycerides, and protein	Upset lipoprotein profile (e.g., hypercholesterolemia with cholestasis
Enzyme systems for excretory pathways	Many systems inducible by alcohol	Disturbed metabolism of steroids, xenobiotics
Storage of vitamins	Vitamin A, vitamin B_{12}	Usually not clinically significant
Metabolism of vitamins	25-hydroxylation of vitamin D	Predisposition to osteomalacia
	Vitamin K-epoxide	Coagulopathy not responding to vitamin K

Table 17–3. Common Disorders of the Liver

Acute Liver Pathology
Hypoperfusion
   Heart failure
   Circulatory insufficiency
   Shock
Direct hepatocellular damage
   Viral hepatitis
   Drug hepatitis
   Alcohol
Cholestatic liver disease
   Intrahepatic
      Drugs
      Cholestatic hepatitis
   Extrahepatitic
      Stone
      Stricture
      Neoplasm
Chronic Liver Pathology
Chronic hepatitis
   Persistent hepatitis
   Active hepatitis
   Reactive hepatitis
Cirrhosis
   Alcoholic
   Post-hepatitic
   Chronic active hepatitis—cirrhosis
   Primary biliary cirrhosis
   Hemochromatosis
   Wilson's disease
   Anti-trypsin deficiency
   Muscoviscidosis
   Tyrosinosis
Fibrosing conditions causing portal hypertension without
   cirrhosis
   Noncirrhotic portal hypertension
   Schistosomiasis
Chronic extrahepatic cholestasis
   Sclerosing cholangitis
   Extrahepatic biliary atresia
Hepatic venous occlusion
   Budd-Chiari syndrome
   Bush tea disease

Metabolic dysfunction to the point of encephalopathy is not solely a function of liver parenchymal cell mass and its access to the circulation. Encephalopathy may be precipitated by infection, fluid and electrolyte imbalance, gastrointestinal bleeding, or drugs. Correction of all adverse factors is paramount in the management of hepatic failure.

The readily available laboratory tests of liver "function" (Table 17–4) provide markers of the nature of the pathologic process but only a crude index of function.

Table 17–4. Laboratory Tests for Elucidation of Hepatobiliary Dysfunction

Serum Tests	Value
Total bilirubin	Severity of jaundice
Unconjugated bilirubin	Diagnosis of Gilbert's syndrome of hemolysis
Alkaline phosphatase (AP)	Diagnosis of cholestasis, hepatic infiltration
Gammaglutamyl transpeptidase	Marker for liver AP, alcohol abuse
Aspartate transaminase (AST)	Hepatocellular damage
Alanine transaminase (ALT)	More specific, less sensitive than AST
Albumin	Synthetic function of liver (but see Figure 17–1)
Prothrombin time (after vitamin K)	Synthetic function
Urine Tests	**Value**
Bilirubin	Conjugated hyperbilirubinemia
Urobilinogen	Hepatocellular dysfunction Hemolysis

Bilirubin

A modest increase in bilirubin without disturbance in other liver tests and without bile in the urine may be due to hemolysis but usually indicates only the clinically unimportant condition of unconjugated hyperbilirubinemia (Gilbert's syndrome), which occurs in up to 5% of normal people. It is important to remember that in Gilbert's syndrome serum bilirubin is increased in the fasting state and during most illnesses.

Enzymes

The transaminases (especially alanine transferase [ALT]) are useful markers of hepatocellular damage. Minor elevations are of little significance, although they may alert the clinician to episodes of poor hepatic perfusion or to damage by toxins (e.g., bacterial endotoxins). Values of above 100–200 IU/L indicate more serious damage, although conditions causing acute cholestasis (both intra- and extrahepatic) may cause a short-lived elevation of ALT up to 500 IU/L. Values above 500 IU/L are usually due to hepatocellular pathology.

Alkaline phosphatase (AP) the first circulating enzyme to be of clinical use, is usually elevated in patients with serious liver disease. High values indicate cholestasis or malignancy, but it is important to remember that the enzyme may be derived from bone, gut, and malignant tissue (the Regan isoenzyme) as well as from the liver. A high value for gamma-glutamyltranspeptidase (GGT) is helpful in assigning a raised AP to an hepatobiliary cause. As an isolated biochemical finding, a raised GGT may indicate induction of the cytochrome P450 mixed oxidase enzyme system as a result of alcohol or drugs (e.g., anti-convulsants) or hepatocellular regeneration (e.g., as seen in active cirrhosis or during the recovery phase of hepatitis). In contrast, an isolated finding of a high value for alkaline phosphatase frequently indicates bone pathology, especially Paget's disease of bone and osteomalacia which is a diagnosis to be considered in any patient with chronic liver disease, especially if there is a cholestatic element.

Proteins

Serum albumin is an important marker in the assessment of the surgical patient. Unfortunately a reduced serum albumin is nearly always the result of multiple factors (Figure 17–1) and its significance may be difficult to interpret. It is important not to equate hypoalbumimemia with protein–calorie malnutrition. Indeed, in affluent countries a low serum albumin is rarely caused primarily by undernutrition. Starving for a month and losing 5–10 kg weight has little effect on the concentration of circulating albumin. Low values are usually caused by increased tissue catabolism and altered body distribution. In such cases feeding protein or amino-nitrogen have little influence on the size of the albumin pool. In acute liver disease, albumin synthesis is usually well maintained. On the other hand, hypoalbuminemia is an important and serious prog-

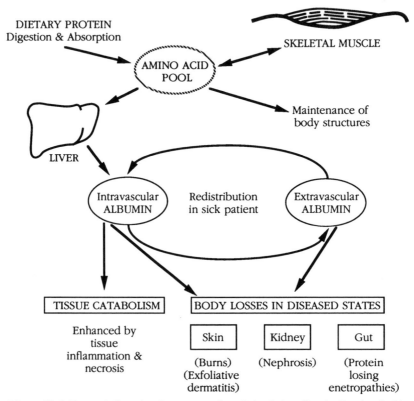

Factors influencing the concentration of circulating albumin

Figure 17–1. Factors influencing the concentration of circulating albumin. Reprinted with permission from Neale, G. *Clinical Nutrition.* London: Heinemann Medical, 1988, p. 60.

nostic marker for chronic liver disease, especially cirrhosis.

Clotting Factors

Liver disease is frequently associated with disturbances of the clotting process. Laboratory assessment of the prothrombin–thrombin complex is necessary. Patients with jaundice of several weeks' duration are likely to develop vitamin K deficiency. All patients with chronic liver disease should be given parenteral vitamin K (IM or IV vitamin K 10 mg/day) to correct potential or actual deficiencies.

Mental State

The mental state of patients with liver dysfunction is assessed clinically using a scale for the level of consciousness (Table 17–5). More objective evi-

Table 17–5. Features of Acute Liver Failure

Encephalopathy
Grade 1   Mild confusion, change in affect, sleep disturbance
Grade 2   Drowsy, inappropriate behavior, tremor
Grade 3   Asleep but rousable, confused, marked tremor
Grade 4   Coma
Cerebral Edema
Occurs in 75–80% of patients with fulminant hepatic failure in grade 4 encephalopathy and is a major cause of death
Hemorrhage
Major coagulation defects often with bleeding into the gut, the bronchial tree, the skin and retroperitoneal space
Respiratory Complications
Hyperventilation (loss of autoregulation)
Hypoxia (often as a result of associated pulmonary edema or pneumonia)
Renal Failure
Prerenal uremia
Acute tubular necrosis
Functional renal failure (7 associated with endotoxemia and/or disseminated intravascular coagulation)
Other Biochemical Disturbances
Metabolic acidoses (especially after paracetamol overdose)
Hypoglycemia (Samson et al., 1987)
Hyponatremia (dilutional, sodium shifts)
Hypokalemia
Hypocalcemia (Parbhoo et al., 1971)
Hypophosphatemia

Table 17–6. Recognition of Encephalopathy

Clinical behavior
  Apathy, slowness, brevity of response
  Personality change: irritable, lack of concern (cf. frontal lobe disorder)
  Hypersomnia (inverted sleep rhythm)
  Intellectual deterioration
  Occasional hypomania (especially in children)
Physical signs
  Asterixis ("flapping tremor")
  Muscle twitching
  Exaggerated deep tendon reflexes (flexor plantar)
  Reflexes lost in deep coma (extensor plantar)
  Grasping and sucking reflexes
Clinical tests
  Reitan trail making
  Constructional praxia
  Psychometric testing
Biochemical tests (little used)
  Blood ammonia and amino acids
  CSF glutamine
Electroencephalopathy
  Slowing of alpha rhythm (normally 8–13 cps)
    (an early change before psychological disturbances but occurs in other metabolic disorders)
Factors complicating diagnosis of hepatic encephalopathy:
1. Electrolyte disorders
  Water intoxication
  Hyponatremia
2. Alcoholism
  Delirium tremens
  Wernicke's encephalopathy
3. Latent psychiatric disturbance unmasked by encephalopathy
  Depression
  Paranoia
4. Hepatolenticular degeneration in Wilson's disease

dence of encephalopathy may be obtained from the use of standardized tests, measurements of circulating ammonia and amino acids, and electroencephalographic assessments (Table 17–6).

The Assessment of Nutritional Status in Patients with Liver Disease

The principles of nutritional assessment of patients with liver disease are the same as for any patient with chronic illness,[6] but certain points require special attention. The main features of assessment are shown in Table 17–7.

A logical sequence for the assessment of an individual patient is as follows:

Table 17–7 Principles of Nutritional Assessment

	Routine Assessment	Readily Available Tests	Special Investigations
Body build	Clinical Impression; Height Weight (compare ideal and previous)		
Body Composition			
Fat	Skinfold thickness		Isotope methods for
Protein	Serum urea, creatinine	Simple nitrogen balance	body water, nitrogen potassium
Active tissue mass			
Skeletal muscle	Clinical assessment	Muscle circumference, cross-sectional area Grip strength	Muscle stimulation tests Histology
Liver	Clinical (e.g., jaundice, edema) LFTS; coagulation factors; Circulating proteins	Isotope breath tests	Tests of intermediary metabolism
Blood	Full blood count Examination of blood film	Iron/IBC Folate/RBC/folate. B12	Ferritin Marrow morphology
Immune system	Lymphocyte count Circulating immunoglobulins	(Delayed hypersensitivity skin tests)	Secretory Immunoglobulins T and B cells
Heart	Clinical assessment	ECG	Measurement cardiac output
CNS	Clinical assessment	EMG; EEG	
Supporting tissues			
Hair, skin, nails, mucous membranes	Clinical assessment		Tests of protein, vitamin trace element, EFA status
Skeleton	Clinical assessment Circulating Ca, P, Alk phos 25-HOCholecalciferol	Radiology; chest, pelvis, hands, spine Isotope scanning	Bone biopsy
Plasma	Clinical assessment of hydration Circulating urea/electrolytes	Direct measurement of CVP for effective plasma volume	Isotope methods
Specific factors			
Vitamins	Clinical assessment Effects on circulating substances e.g., Ca, P, AP (vit D); Prothrombin (vit K)	Response to treatment	Red cell enzymes (vit B) Leucocyte vitamin C Retinol/RBP (vit A)
Minerals	Plasma Ca, Mg, P Radiology skeleton	Tests of neuromuscular excitability	Isotope methods
Trace elements	Clinical assessment	Serum zinc	Serum concentrations of other trace elements

1. Clinical history to define disorders that may be associated with nutritional deficiencies:
   a. Nausea, vomiting, diarrhea, steatorrhea, and jaundice, any of which may cause a reduced food intake and loss of weight
   b. Infective, inflammatory, or neoplastic pathology which is often associated with weight loss
   c. Blood loss causing iron deficiency (as in chronic liver disease)
   d. Associated metabolic disorders (e.g., impaired glucose tolerance)
   e. Symptoms that may be associated with nutritional deficiency (e.g., muscle cramp in magnesium deficiency, weakness and skeletal pain in vitamin D deficiency)
2. Dietary history to identify:
   a. Long continued undernutrition
   b. Possible specific deficiencies (e.g., vitamin C and folic acid deficiency in patients with a poor intake of fruit and vegetables)
   c. Intake of protein, sodium, and fluid which are important determinants of well-being in patients with liver disease.

3. Clinical examination for assessment of:
   a. Body weight (compared with normal weight and ideal weight)
   b Fat stores (skinfold thickness) and skeletal muscle mass (midarm circumference corrected for fat), but remembering that nonnutritional factors such as prolonged bedrest cause muscle wasting
   c. Signs of possible protein, trace element, or vitamin deficiencies (see Table 17–5); the signs are usually nonspecific but may serve to remind the clinician of dietary needs
   d. Body fluids
4. Laboratory tests to provide measures of:
   a. Hematological variables and hematinic status
   b. Fluid and electrolyte balance
   c. Divalent cations—iron, calcium, and magnesium phosphate
   d. Trace elements, especially zinc, copper, selenium
   e. Circulating proteins (albumin, immunoglobulins and acute phase reactants); the values must be assessed in the light of associated pathology
   f. Circulating lipids
   g. Coagulation factors, especially important with respect to vitamin K in the jaundiced patient
5. Nutritional factors in relation to hepatic failure:
   a. Nature of protein in diet
   b. Laboratory measurement of ammonia:amino acid ratio

To confirm a suspected nutritional deficiency, it may be necessary to undertake special tests (see Table 17–7) or to treat the patient and observe results. Sequential observations are invaluable and clinicians should be aware of unusual disorders (e.g., deficiencies of trace elements or of essential fatty acids that may develop in patients with prolonged liver disease).

General Principles of Nutritional Support

The general principles of nutritional support of sick patients are now well established,[6] but there are some special considerations for those with liver dysfunction. Nausea is a common symptom so dietary intake may be poor especially by patients in hospital who may find institutional food unpalatable. It is important to encourage such patients to eat, and ward clinicians, nurses, and dietitians should all try to ensure that an adequate quantity of food is taken. It may be helpful to enlist the help of relatives who can supplement hospital food with delicacies and who can assist in feeding a disabled patient.

Supplementary Feeding

Undernourished patients may benefit from the provision of high-protein, energy-dense liquid feeds offered between meals to boost the normal dietary intake.

Patients with liver disease have fickle appetites. What is acceptable one day may be deemed unappetizing the next. Thus it is as well to have a choice of feeds that are best served direct from the refrigerator. The amount offered should be within the patient's capacity, and half-completed drinks should not be left sitting at the patient's bedside.

Enteral Tube Feeding

A liquid feed may be infused directly into the gastrointestinal tract through a fine-bore tube. Usually the nasogastric route is used but, in some cases, it may be better to position the tube in the small intestine. A percutaneous feeding gastrotomy is only occasionally necessary. Patients with feeding tubes are most conveniently fed by continuous infusion over 24 hours. This convenience must be balanced against the fall in morale that occurs in patients denied the ordinary social contacts of mealtimes.

Standard feeds contain approximately 1 kcal (4.2kJ)/per ML and 4.5–6.0 g nitrogen (28–36 g protein) per liter. Most adults require 1,500–2,500 kcal (6300–10500 kJ) per day and 10–12 g nitrogen. Often modifications must be made for patients with hepatic decompensation.

Parenteral Feeding

Parenteral feeding becomes necessary if the small intestine is unavailable or nonfunctioning. A peripheral line may be adequate for a few days. Water and electrolyte balance is easy to maintain by this route, but the amount of carbohydrate, fat, and amino acids that can be infused is limited. The osmolarity of the nutrient solution should not exceed 500–600 mOsm/l and, even so, phlebitis often appears after less than a week of peripheral venous feeding.

If the small intestine is likely to be unavailable for 10 days or more then feeding through a large central vein is indicated. Ideally a tunneled line should be inserted so that the tip comes to lie in the superior vena cava. The catheter is best inserted via a subclavian vein but, if necessary, a cephalic or jugular vessel may be used. Once established the line should be used for no purpose other than feeding. If carefully placed using a full aseptic technique and subsequently managed by trained staff, such a catheter should remain trouble-free for many months. Infection of the line is the main complication, but a properly inserted, well-maintained feeding line is rarely the cause of a pyrexial illness especially in the first month after insertion. The infection rate for multi-lines is greater than for single lines. Unfortunately multi-lines are most often necessary in very sick patients, and it is these patients who are at the greatest risk of infection.

Nutrition Requirements

Energy

Whatever the route of feeding, sufficient calories should be given to meet energy needs, usually between 1,500 and 2,000 kcals (6300 and 8400 kJ) per day. The appearance of the patient and changes in weight are sufficient to determine the adequacy of caloric intake. In practice it is usual to give rather more than half the nonprotein calories as carbohydrate and the rest as fat. Patients with liver disease are often told to take a low fat diet, but in most cases this does nothing more than reduce the intake of calories without benefiting the patient. Fatty foods may be nauseating, but an ordinary healthy diet containing 70 g fat is usually well tolerated. It may be necessary to modulate the intake of carbohydrate because of glucose intolerance. Complex carbohydrates are useful in slowing the uptake of the products of digestion. Alcohol is an undesirable source of calories in any patient with liver disease.

In long-continued illness, requiring artificial nutritional support, the clinician should carefully consider the most desirable intake of calories.

Sometimes it is possible to help an obese patient lose weight by limiting the intake of calories. This may be especially helpful in the patient with liver disease who has a limited tolerance for carbohydrate.

Protein

The clinician should aim to keep patients in nitrogen balance by providing an optimal intake of amino-nitrogen backed by sufficient calories. Patients with chronic liver disease are often wasted and will lose further muscle when they become bedbound. It is possible to measure nitrogen losses sufficiently accurately for clinical purposes by using the rather crude formula: nitrogen losses (g/24 h) = 2 + (24 h urinary urea in mmol $\times$ 0.028), with modifications if the blood urea is changing consistently or if the patient has abnormal nitrogen losses from the kidney or gut.[6] It is reasonable to try to show that a negative protein balance is not caused by inadequate intake, but it is important to remember that increasing the nitrogen intake of immobilized patients will often do no more than increase the metabolic load on the liver and kidney.

Nitrogen intake becomes critical in patients with encephalopathy. In the severely affected, protein by mouth should be restricted to 20 g in 24 hours and may be best given as a liquid feed (casein-based) through an enteral tube. As encephalopathy improves the intake may be increased in increments of 10–20 g protein per day every second or third day. Protein from milk[7,8] or from vegetables[9-11] is better tolerated than that from a mixed dietary source or from meat. The mechanism for the increased tolerance is uncertain but may be related to the amino acid profile of the protein together with the effect of diet on bowel flora and the effect of different proteins on the clearance of ammonia through intermediate metabolic pathways. Nitrogen balance may also be improved using vegetable diets,[10] but such diets are bulky and often not well tolerated because of abdominal distension, flatulence, and diarrhea.

An artificial diet containing high concentrations of branched chain amino acids (BCAA) has theoretical advantages for the severely encephalopathic patient. An increase in available BCAA should reduce the flux of AAA into the brain and thus the production of false neurotransmitters and improve nitrogen balance by providing an optimal substrate for amino acid metabolism in skeletal muscle. Although BCAA supplements are well tolerated,[8,12,13] there is no evidence that patients benefit from the regular administration of these expensive preparations.[14]

Vitamins and Minerals

Recommended daily intakes of the vitamins are listed in Table 17–8. These recommendations may need to be modified in patients with liver disease. Vitamin A is derived from animal tissues mainly as retinyl palmitate and from vegetables as beta carotene. The absorption of these precursors may be affected by a deficiency of bile acids. Vitamin A is stored in the liver as retinyl ester. This ester is hydrolyzed and the retinol is released as a complex with retinol-binding protein (RBP). In the retina, retinol is converted to its aldehyde (retinal) which is a photoactive chemical. Vitamin A also plays a role in spermatogenesis and general growth and development. In long-standing cholestasis body stores of vitamin A may decrease, and in parenchymal disease release of retinol from stores may be impaired.[15] As a result night blindness may occur, but

Table 17–8. Guide to Baseline Nutritional Requirements for an Adult Requiring Artificial Nutrition

Nitrogen	8–12 g
Energy	1200–2000 kcals (5.0–8.4 MJ)
Electrolytes	
Sodium	70–150 mmol
Potassium	50–100 mmol
Chloride	70–220 mmol
Calcium	5–15 mmol
Magnesium	5–20 mmol
Phosphate	20–60 mmol (very variable)
Trace elements	
Iron	50 μmol
Zinc	100 μmol
(plus traces of chromium, copper, manganese, molybdenum, selenium, vanadium, iodide and fluoride)	
Vitamins	
B group in milligram quantities	
Thiamin 1.5, Riboflavin 2.5, Pyridoxine 2.5, Nicotinamide 15, Pantothenic acid 15, Biotin 0.5)	
B12	3 μg
Folic acid	0.5 mg
Ascorbic acid	20–50 mg
Retinol	1000 IU
Calciferol	5–15 μg
Tocopherol	5–15 μg

the more serious manifestations of vitamin A deficiency have not been described in patients with liver disease. Nevertheless, it is suggested that patients with chronic cholestasis may benefit from regular supplements of vitamin A[16–16a] and possibly additional zinc, which seems to improve the response. Care must be taken because the safe therapeutic range is rather narrow. The regular ingestion of 40,000 IU per day may damage the liver.[17]

In health, vitamin D compounds are derived primarily from irradiation of the skin. There is no absolute requirement for dietary vitamin D, although 400–500 IU (10–12.5 μg) is recommended. Patients with long-standing liver disease (especially if this has a cholestatic element) may become vitamin D deficient and as a result develop osteomalacia with a variable proximal myopathy. The etiology of vitamin D deficiency in chronic liver disease is probably multifactorial, including reduced exposure to sunlight, impaired photolysis by retained bilirubin, reduced absorption, and alterations in intermediary metabolism.[18] In patients at risk (chronic biliary obstruction of greater than one year) it is reasonable to give vitamin D 10,000 IU intramuscularly once a month. Again clinicians must be wary of overdosage.

Hypoprothrombinemia is common in patients with chronic cholestasis. It is readily corrected by giving vitamin K 10 mg IM daily for 3 days. In contrast the hypoprothrombinemia of hepatic failure is part of a more complex coagulopathy in which there is failure of synthesis of clotting factors (not correlated with vitamin K) and increased peripheral consumption. Hemorrhage occurs most commonly when there is an associated thrombocytopenia and can be treated only by infusions of fresh frozen plasma and platelet concentrates.

Clinical vitamin E deficiency has been described in children with biliary atresia and rarely in primary biliary cirrhosis. It may be treated with α-tocopherol acetate orally (up to 1 g/day) or parenterally (up to 100 mg/week).

Water-soluble vitamins are absorbed adequately in patients with liver disease, but significant deficiencies of thiamine and folic acid occur, especially in alcoholics.

Apart from iron, mineral deficiencies are not commonly recognized in patients with liver disease. Nevertheless, there may be specific problems in the management of alcoholics and of patients with acute liver failure. These are discussed in the section on specific disorders.

Nutritional Problems in Acute Liver Disease

The Jaundiced Patient

The acutely jaundiced patient who is being considered for surgical intervention usually presents little difficulty in perioperative care. Nevertheless, accurate diagnosis before operation is essential because the patient with jaundice due to severe hepatocellular damage or intrahepatic cholestasis tolerates anesthesia and major surgery poorly. In the postoperative period they may need prolonged high-dependency care, including nutritional support.

Acute Cholestasis

Patients with extrahepatic biliary obstruction develop steatorrhea and vitamin K deficiency. The prothrombin time may become prolonged, but should respond promptly to treatment with parenteral vitamin K_1 (10 mg daily for 2 or 3 days). Failure to respond indicates severe intrinsic liver pathology that needs to be understood before any major surgical procedure is attempted.

Acute Liver Failure

Acute liver failure is a rare but extremely serious condition for which liver transplantation may be the only effective treatment. It may be defined as severe hepatic dysfunction manifested by either encephalopathy or coagulopathy developing within 6 months of the first symptoms of liver disease and in the absence of long-standing hepatic pathology. Fulminant hepatic failure (FHF) is a subgroup in which encephalopathy intervenes within 1–2 months of the onset of symptoms. If the clinical course is more protracted the condition is sometimes termed *subacute* or *late onset* hepatic *failure*. The causes are listed in Table 17–9 and the major features in Table 17–5.

The prognosis of acute hepatic failure is poor especially if coma becomes deep; if the disorders of coagulation persist despite treatment; and if renal failure supervenes. Outcome is not readily predictable. Nevertheless grade 4 coma carries a mortality rate of 80–90% and grade 3 approximately 50%.

Table 17–9. Causes of Acute Liver Failure

Viral hepatitis	Hepatitis B ($\sim$ 50%)
	Hepatitis A ($\sim$ 20%)
	Hepatitis C
	Cytomegolovirus Herpes simplex, Epstein-Barr virus
Drugs	Paracetamol (large overdose)
	Halothane (rare)
	Antituberculosis drugs (isoniazid, rifampicid)
	Other drugs (monoamineoxidise inhibitors; nonsteroidal anti-inflammatory drug; Gold; sodium valproate; sulphonamides; retoconazole)
Toxins	*Amanita phalloides* (especially in France)
	Aflatoxins
	Carbon tetrachloride (and other halogens)
Other causes (all rare)	Reye's syndrome
	Fatty liver of pregnancy
	Postobesity operations (especially jejunoileal bypass)
	Circulatory failure
	Diffuse metastatic disease

(Wilson's disease may also present as acute liver failure, but such patients have an established cirrhosis at the onset of symptoms.)

Patients with FHF require intensive care. The aim of management is to prevent multisystem failure. Risk factors include persistent hypermetabolism, foci of dead, injured or infected tissue, the presence of the respiratory distress syndrome and poor perfusion leading to tissue hypoxia. The transition from hypermetabolism to multiorgan failure parallels the degree of liver failure. It appears to be mediated by the release of cytokines from macrophages responding to a series of events including tissue necrosis, infection and gut-translocated toxins.[19]

No specific nutritional regimen alters the prognosis of FHF but it is important to maintain the intake of essential nutrients (Table 17–10) to try to prevent organ failure[20] and its associated worsening prognosis, which in turn appears to depend on the arrest or reversal of the primary pathophysiological process. Liver transplantation is indicated before systems fail.

Alcoholic Hepatitis

So far as possible surgery should be deferred in the patient who has a coexisting alcoholic hepatitis. Nevertheless, alcoholics not infrequently develop

Table 17–10. Nutritional Support in Acute Liver Failure

Fluid and Electrolytes	Sodium depletion uncommon despite hyponatraemia
	Potassium depletion common (may need up to 500 mmol per day)
	Calcium and magnesium supplements often necessary
	Phosphate may be needed but levels rise rapidly if renal failure supervenes
Glucose	Continuous intravenous infusion of dextrose (5–15 g per hour) needed to prevent hypoglycemia. Control rate of infusion against blood sugar checked hourly if necessary.
Amino Acids	Amino acid profile enriched with branch chain (BCAA) and deficient in aromatic amino acids and methionine. Improves nitrogen balance but probably no effect on encephalopathy.
Lipid	Use with caution (check daily for clearance of fat from circulation)
Vitamins	Vitamin K status to be maintained
	Vitamin B complex and folic acid may be necessary.

conditions requiring surgical expertise, including bleeding from the upper gastrointestinal tract, pancreatitis, gallstones, and cancer of the bowel. Thus it is necessary to consider the nutritional and metabolic disturbances in some detail.

A high intake of alcohol (which provides 7 kcal (29.6 kJ) energy/g) is often associated with a poor intake of food and hence a degree of malnutrition. Moreover, alcohol interferes with absorption (e.g., of thiamine); may increase requirements for some nutrients (e.g., folic acid) and the turnover of others (e.g., magnesium); and may alter intermediary metabolism (e.g., by predisposing individuals to hyperlipidemia). The increase in hepatic lipids and the increase in the activity of the microsomal cytochrome P450 and ethanol oxidizing systems appear to be due to the effects of alcohol. Experimentally the changes are not modified by a diet supplemented with vitamins and minerals.[21]

Subjects with alcoholic hepatitis presenting with jaundice will have had suboptimal health for weeks or months. This is usually associated with serious nutritional disorders, although there is no clearcut correlation between these and the degree of liver disturbance.[22] Deficiencies of individual nutrients (see Tables 17–7, 17–8) can often be corrected over a period of 2–3 weeks and the patient's condition

may improve sufficiently to allow semi-elective surgery for a serious condition such as gastrointestinal cancer. Restoration to an optimal nutritional state, however, usually takes several months.

It may be difficult to distinguish between the toxic effects of alcohol and the results of malnutrition. For example, alcohol impairs hematopoiesis by a direct effect on the marrow which leads to a macrocytic anemia, but deficiencies of folic acid and pyridoxine may also contribute to the marrow dysfunction. Similarly, in the patient addicted to alcohol the heart may be affected by thiamine deficiency but also damaged by the direct effects of alcohol. Thus the first step in management is not only to wean the patient from alcohol but also to provide a good quality diet. Attempts have been made to determine whether or not such patients benefit from increasing food intake to 50% above demand. In a controlled study it was not possible to demonstrate any positive benefit in terms of recovery of hepatic function or of improvement of nutritional status, although the mortality in the overfed group was somewhat lower.[23]

In the early phases of managing the sick alcoholic patient it is necessary to correct electrolyte and mineral perturbations. At presentation acid–base abnormalities are common, especially ketoacidosis, but hyperchloremic acidosis and metabolic or respiratory alkalosis may also occur.[24] Hyponatremia is usually dilutional because of excessive water intake (as in the beer drinker) or because of an inappropriate secretion of ADH. Hypokalemia may occur especially in those who are receiving diuretics for edema and in those who are magnesium deficient. Phosphate depletion often becomes manifest during the refeeding phase, and it is important to be aware of this complication which may cause muscle weakness by depletion of cellular ATP and tissue anoxia because of the effect on red cell 2,3-diphosphoglycerate. If circulating phosphate levels decrease to less than 0.5 mmol/L supplements should be given.

Magnesium deficiency caused by renal tubular dysfunction is common in the alcoholic. Symptoms include tremors, tetany (with associated hypocalcemia and often hypokalemic alkalosis), and cardiac dysrhythmias. A serum magnesium of less than 0.5 mmol/L indicates depletion (urine values may be difficult to interpret because of associated renal dysfunction). It is difficult to replete body magnesium by oral medication (magnesium salts are poorly absorbed and cause diarrhea) and it may be necessary to give repeated intravenous infusions of 20 mmol magnesium over 12 hours. Values for circulating zinc and selenium are often low in alcoholics, but the significance of such observations is difficult to determine. Experimentally selenium deficiency predisposes to liver injury possibly as a result of accentuated lipo-peroxidation due to decreased activity of the seleno-enzyme, glutathione peroxidase.[25]

Postoperative Liver Dysfunction

Jaundice after major surgery is not uncommon.[26] Usually it is unrelated to nutritional status and the etiology is multifactorial. Infection, blood loss, drugs, (including anesthetic agents), and episodes of hypotension or hypoxia are likely contributory factors (see Table 17–3). Preexisting liver disease[27] and upper abdominal surgery[28] are predisposing causes but not the duration of anesthesia.[29] In the patient with known liver disease care should be taken to correct anemia (and deficiency of hematinic factors), hypoprothrombinemia, hypoproteinemia, and disturbances of water and electrolyte status before surgery. Most cases of postoperative jaundice are self-limiting. Nevertheless, it is important to exclude hemolysis and extrahepatic obstruction by appropriate investigation. It is rarely necessary to modify the mode of nutritional support except perhaps in small infants requiring total parenteral nutrition who are particularly prone to intrahepatic cholestasis (see later).

Jaundice in Association with Parenteral Nutrition

Disturbances of liver function are common in patients on total parenteral nutrition (TPN), and overt jaundice may occur with inappropriate use of large amounts of intravenous lipid or an imbalance in the ratio of carbohydrate to nitrogen in the nutrient solution.[30] It is often difficult, however, to disentangle the effects of intravenous feeding from other causes of postsurgical cholestasis. Experimental studies suggest that TPN is not a direct cause of jaundice, but that it may aggravate the cholestasis of a concurrent liver disorder.[31]

During TPN adults often develop hepatocellular changes (fatty liver or steatonecrosis) but only rarely cholestasis. The changes are usually mild and reversible, although there are occasional reports of progressive liver pathology.[32] In experimental animals the administration of polymyxin B (to decontaminate the bowel and to counteract the effect of bacterial endotoxins) reduced hepatic steatosis during total parenteral nutrition.[33,34] Thus the possible effects of bacterial overgrowth should be considered in any patient on long-term TPN who develops liver dysfunction.

In contrast to adults, infants on TPN are prone to intra-hepatic cholestasis. Carbohydrate overfeeding; infusion of lipid emulsions; carnitine deficiency; and aluminum toxicity have been implicated.[32,35] In these patients there appears to be a reduction in the flow of bile, gallbladder stasis and possibly toxicity from retained bile salts which may contribute to progressive liver failure and death. Without clearcut evidence regarding the pathogenesis of cholestasis treatment is difficult. It seems sensible to provide a balanced intake of nutrients using aluminum-free solutions and to give sufficient stimulus orally to promote contraction of the gallbladder and stimulate the flow of bile. In long-continued TPN-associated cholestasis it may be helpful each month to monitor plasma levels of fat-soluble vitamins and trace elements. In particular manganese levels may increase because this element is excreted mainly via bile. If monitoring is not possible it is suggested that manganese should not be added to TPN fluids being given to infants with severe cholestasis.[36]

Nutritional Problems in Chronic Liver Disease

Patients with chronic liver disease who require surgery should undergo a full nutritional assessment as outlined previously (Table 17–7). Nutritional status will vary with etiology, stage of the disease, and previous care. For example, patients with well-compensated postnecrotic macronodular cirrhosis are usually well-nourished, whereas most long-standing alcoholics show some evidence of malnutrition.

Chronic Cholestasis

In adults, primary biliary cirrhosis and sclerosing cholangitis are the most common causes of chronic cholestasis. Reduction in the flow of bile leads to a reduced concentration of bile salts in the gut and disturbed micelle formation. As a result the absorption of fat is impaired. Although steatorrhea is rarely severe, the fat-soluble vitamins (A, D, E, K) are poorly absorbed and patients with prolonged disease should be given IM supplements (10 mg vitamin K_1, 10,000 units vitamin A, 10,000 units vitamin D) a month. Patients with chronic cholestasis have poor appetites and tend to lose weight. They may benefit from dietary supplements, and medium chain triglycerides may be a useful way of increasing the intake of calories.

In children, growth failure is a complication of chronic cholestasis.[37] The mechanisms are not well understood, but they are resistant to the growth-promoting, diabetogenic, and lipolytic properties of growth hormone.[38,39] Such children are also osteopenic and remain so even if the diet is supplemented with calcium and vitamin D.[45] It is also important to correct vitamin E deficiency in infants because failure to do so may lead to progressive neuromuscular disease. It is usual to give α-tocopherol acetate orally starting with a small oral dose of 25 mg daily, increasing to 1 g per day depending on circulating levels. If this is not effective, it is necessary to give vitamin E parenterally in doses of up to 100 mg once a week.

Portosystemic Encephalopathy (PSE)

Nitrogenous substances absorbed from the gut play a central role in the pathogenesis of PSE. Three steps should be taken in the management of this condition:

1. Correct or eliminate precipitating factors such as infection, electrolyte disturbances (especially hypokalemia), drugs (especially sedatives and narcotics), and blood loss (especially into the gut).
2. Purge the intestine (lactulose is usually used) and administer neomycin (1 g o.d.s. for 1 week) to reduce bacterial proteolysis.
3. Prescribe a low-protein diet. (In view of the characteristic pattern of circulating amino acids in patients with PSE [elevated aromatic amino acids and depressed branch chain amino acids] there have been several trials of IV infusions of BCAA in the treatment of PSE. The overall con-

clusion suggests that BCAA speed the resolution of PSE without altering outcome.[46])

Patients who have had one encephalopathic episode are at risk of recurrence, and much effort has been expended in trying to determine the optimal dietary regimen. Reducing the intake of protein to 40 g or less per day leads to a negative nitrogen balance, wasting of lean body mass, and possible trace element deficiencies.[40] This may be a high price to pay in patients who are often already wasted. The use of a vegetable protein diet may be advantageous for some patients and should be tried in patients who have a tendency to encephalopathy.[11,41]

Ascites

Salt and water retention causing ascites is a common complication of cirrhosis and can usually be managed by a combination of diet and drugs (Table 17-11). A small group of patients become refractory and require large-volume paracenteses[42] or peritoneovenous shunting.[43] Such patients lose lean body mass and become very wasted.

Cirrhosis and Diabetes

Up to 70% of patients with cirrhosis have impaired carbohydrate tolerance and 30% are frankly diabetic. Most of these patients behave as late-onset diabetics with down-regulation of insulin receptors, increased fasting levels of insulin, and hyperinsulinism in response to the administration of glucose. Fasting blood glucose levels are reduced by giving a vegetarian diet: The slower absorption of glucose and amino acids appears to be advantageous.[44] Thus a high-fiber, high vegetable protein diet may improve carbohydrate tolerance and reduce the requirements for insulin as well as lessening the tendency to encephalopathy.

Nutritional Support of Patients Undergoing Liver Transplantation

Liver transplantation is now an accepted treatment for end-stage hepatic failure and certain metabolic disorders (such as type 2 hypercholesterolemia). In

Table 17–11. Management of Ascites

1. Bed rest. Low sodium diet (less than 40 mEq/day reducing to 20 mEq if possible). Maintain potassium intake (100 mEq/day). Restrict fluid intake (1 litre/day). Monitor weight, urine output, serum and urinary electrolytes.

2. If weight loss does not occur within a few days and urinary sodium losses <25 mEq/day, treat with a distal diuretic (e.g., Spironolactone 150 mg; amiloride 10 mg daily) and reduce potassium intake to 50 mEq/day.

3. One week after admission, if weight loss <2.5 kg with satisfactory serum electrolytes and urinary sodium losses <5 mEq/day, add a loop diuretic (e.g., Frusemide 80 mg; bumetamide 1 mg/day).

4. After a further 2–3 days be prepared to double the dose of distal diuretic and more cautiously increase the dose of the loop diuretic.

5. Aim for an average weight loss of 0.5 kg/daily. Discontinue treatment with diuretics if patient develops signs of hepatic pre-coma, hypokalaemia, marked hyponatraemia (<120 mEq/1), uraemia or marked alkalosis. Reduce diuretics if weight loss excessive (>1 kg/day). Patients on a low sodium diet who are losing >25 mEq sodium per day in the urine do not respond to treatment with diuretics.

6. In patients with tense ascites resistant to treatment paracentesis may be necessary (drain 5 l and repeat if necessary).

many cases patients are moderately to severely malnourished before being admitted to a transplant unit,[47] although this seems to be improving as patients are referred earlier in the course of their disease. Even so, all too often there is too little time before surgery to do more than correct anemia, electrolyte disorders, and hypoprothrombinemia. Ideally a patient who has chronic liver disease, that might progress to a requirement for liver transplantation, should be monitored by an hepatologist who is skilled in recognizing and preventing nutritional and metabolic abnormalities.[48]

The management of nutritional abnormalities in patients with chronic liver disease has been described in previous sections of this chapter. If liver transplantation is deemed necessary then the preceding nutrition support regimen has an added degree of urgency. Often artificial supplemental feeding, by either the enteral or the parenteral route, is indicated and the patient's general condition may be strikingly improved.[49]

The patient who recovers smoothly after liver transplantation improves rapidly. Within a week appetite returns and meals are eaten with relish. Nutritional disturbances are quickly corrected and further support becomes unnecessary. In contrast, the patient who requires long-continued intensive care will need artificial feeding usually by the parenteral route and continued attention to the special features outlined in the section on acute liver failure (see Table 17–10).

References

1. Sherwin, R., Joshe, P., Hendler, R., et al. (1974) Hyperglucagonaemia in Laennec's cirrhosis: The role of portal-systemic shunting. *New England Journal of Medicine* 290:239–42.

2. Soeters, P. B. and Fischer, J. E. (1976) Insulin, glucagon, amino acid imbalance and hepatic encephalopathy. *Lancet* 2:880–2.

3. Rikkers L. F., Jenko, P., Rudman, D., Friedes, D. (1978) Subclinical hepatic encephalopathy: detection, prevalence, and relationship to nitrogen metabolism. Gastroenterology 75:462–9.

4. McCullough, A. J., Czaja, A. J., Jones, J. D., Go, V. L. (1981) The nature and prognostic significance of serial amino acid determinations in severe chronic active liver disease. Gastroenterology 81:645–52.

5. Nespoli, A., Bevilacqua, G., Staudacher, C. et al. (1981) Pathogenesis of hepatic encephalopathy and hyperdynamic syndrome in cirrhosis. Role of false neurotransmitters. *Archives of Surgery* 116:1129–38.

6. Neale, G. (1988) *Clinical Nutrition*. London: Heinemann Medical Books.

7. Fenton, J. C. B., Knight, E. J. and Humpherson, P. L. (1966) Milk and cheese diet in portal-systemic encephalopathy. *Lancet* 1:164–5.

8. Christie, M. L., Sack, D. M., Pomposelli, J. and Horst, D. (1985) Enriched branched-chain amino acid formula versus a casein-based supplement in the treatment of cirrhosis. *Journal of Parenteral and Enteral Nutrition* 9:671–8.

9. Greenberger, N. J., Carley, J., Schenker, S., et al. (1977) Effect of vegetable and animal protein diets in chronic encephalopathy. *American Journal of Digestive Diseases* 22:845–55.

10. de Bruijn, K. M., Blendis, L. M., Zilm, D. H., et al. (1983) Effect of dietary protein manipulations in subclinical portal systemic encephalopathy. *Gut* 24:53–60.

11. Weber, F. L., Jr., Minco, D., Fresard, K. M. and Banwell, J. G. (1985) Effects of vegetable diets on nitrogen metabolism in cirrhotic subjects. *Gastroenterology* 89: 538–44.

12. McGhee, A., Henderson, M., Millikan, W. J., et al. (1983) Comparison of the effects of Hepatic-Aid and a casein modular diet on encephalopathy, plasma amino acids and nitrogen balance in cirrhotic patients. *Annals of Surgery* 197:288–93.

13. Horst, D., Grace, N., Conn, H. O. et al. (1981) A double-blind randomised comparison of dietary protein and an oral branched chain amino acid (BCAA) supplement in cirrhotic patients with chronic portalsystemic encephalopathy (PSE). *Hepatology* 1:518.

14. Alexander, W. F., Sandel, E., Harty, R. F. and Cerda, J. J. (1989) The usefulness of branched chain amino acids in patients with acute or chronic hepatic encephalopathy. *American Journal of Gastroenterology* 84: 91–6.

15. Kanai, M., Raz, A., Goodman, D. S. (1968) Retinolbinding protein: the transport protein for vitamin A in human plasma. Journal of Clinical Investigation 47: 2025–44.

16. Herlong, H. F., Russell, R. M. and Maddrey, W. C. (1981) Vitamin A and zinc therapy in primary biliary cirrhosis. *Hepatology* 1:348–51.

16a. Walt, R. D., Kemp, C. M., Lyness L. et al. Vitamin A therapy for night blindness in primary biliary cirrhosis. *British Medical Journal* 1984;288:1030–1.

17. Farrell, G. C., Bhatal, P. S. and Powell, L. W. (1977) Abnormal liver function in chronic hypervitaminosis A. *American Journal of Digestive Diseases* 22:724–8.

18. Krawitt, E. L., Grundman, M. J. and Mawer, E. B. (1977) Absorption, hydroxylation and excretion of vitamin D in primary biliary cirrhosis, *Lancet* 2:1246–9.

19. Cerra, F. B., West, M., Keller, G. et al. (1988) Hypermetabolism/organ failure: The role of the activated macrophage as a metabolic regulator. *Progress in Clinical and Biological Research* (New York) 264:27–42.

20. Latifi, R., Killam, R. W. and Dudrick, S. J. (1991) Nutritional support in liver failure. *Surgical Clinics of North America* 71:567–78.

21. Lieber, C. S. and DeCarli, L. M. (1989) Effects of mineral and vitamin supplementation on the alcohol induced fatty liver and microsomal induction. *Alcoholism: Clinical and Experimental Research* 13:142–3.

22. Mitchell, M. C. and Herlong, H. F. (1986) Alcohol and nutrition: Calorific value, bioenergetics and relationship to liver damage. *Annual Reviews in Nutrition* 6:457–74.

23. Bunout, D., Aicardi, V., Hirsch, S. et al. (1989) Nutritional support in hospitalised patients with alcoholic disease. *European Journal of Clinical Nutrition* 43: 615–21.

24. Wrenn, K. D., Slovis, C. M., Minion, G. E. and Rutkowski, R. (1991) The syndrome of alcoholic ketoacidosis. *American Journal of Medicine* 91: 119–28.

25. Dworkin, B., Rosenthal, W. S., Jankowski, R. H. et al. (1985) Low blood selenium levels in alcoholics with and without advanced liver disease. Correlations with clinical and nutritional status. *Digestive Diseases and Sciences* 30:838–44.

26. La Mont, J. T. and Isselbacher, K. (1985) Post-operative jaundice. *Liver and Biliary Disease* (Wright, R., Millward-Sadler, G. H. and Alberti, K. G. M. M., eds) London: Balliere Tindall, pp. 1367–78.

27. French, A. B., Barss, T. P., Fairlie, C. S. et al. (1952) Metabolic effects of anaesthesia in man. V. A comparison of the effects of ether and cyclopropane on the abnormal liver. *Annals of Surgery* 135:145–63.

28. Clarke, R. S. J., Doggart, J. R. and Lavery, T. (1976) Changes in liver function after different types of surgery. *British Journal of Anaesthesiology* 48:119–27.

29. Fairlie, C. W., Barss, T. P., French, A. B. et al. (1951) Metabolic effects of anesthesia in man. IV. A comparison of the effects of ether and cyclopropane anesthesia on the normal liver. *New England Journal of Medicine* 244:615–22.

30. Allardyce, D. B. (1982) Cholestasis caused by lipid emulsions. *Surgery Gynaecology and Obstetrics* 154: 641–7.

31. Fabri, P. J., Deutsch, S., Gower, W. Jr. et al. (1987) Parenteral nutrition: Short term effects on hepatic clearance of sodium taurocholate and indocyanine green. *Clin Biochem* 20:57–60.

32. Fisher, R. L. (1989) Hepatobiliary abnormalities associated with total parenteral nutrition. *Gastroenterology Clinics of North America* 18:645–6.

33. Capron, J. -P., Ginston, J. -L, Herve, M. -A. and Braillon, A. (1983) Metronidazole in prevention of cholestasis associated with total parenteral nutrition. *Lancet* 1:446–7.

34. Pappo, I., Becovier, H., Berry, E. M. and Freund, H. R. (1991) Polymyxin B reduces cecal flora, TNF production and hepatic steatosis during total parenteral in the rat. Journal of Surg Res 51:106–12.

35. Klein, G. L. (1989) Aluminium in parenteral products. *Journal of Parenteral Science and Technology* 43: 120–4.

36. Hambridge, K. M., Sokol, R. J., Fidanza, S. T. and Goodall, M. A. (1989) Plasma manganese concentrations in infants and children receiving parenteral nutrition. *JPEN* 13:168–71.

37. Novak, D. A. and Balisteri, W. F. (1985) Management of children with chronic cholestasis. *Pediatric Annals* 14:488–92.

38. Bucuvales, J. C., Cutfield, W., Horn, J. et al. (1990) Resistance to the growth promoting and metabolic effects of growth hormone in children with chronic liver disease. *Journal of Pediatrics* 117:397–402.

39. Cywes, C. and Millar, A. J. (1990) Assessment of the nutritional status of infants and children with biliary atresia. *South American Medical Journal* 77:131–5.

40. Quivy, D., Never, J. and Adler, M. (1990) Intake of essential trace elements (selenium, copper, iron) in the nutrition of patients hospitalised with liver cirrhosis. *Acta Gastroenterol Belg* 53:286–91.

41. Uribe, M., Marquez, M. A., Garcia Ramos, G., et al. (1982) Treatment of chronic portal-systemic encephalopathy with vegetable and animal protein diets. A controlled crossover study. Digestive Diseases and Sciences 27:1109–16.

42. Gines, P., Arroyao, V., Quintero, E. et al. (1987) Comparison of paracentesis and diuretics in the treatment of cirrhotics with ascites. *Gastroenterology* 93:234–41.

43. Franco, D., Charra, M., Jeambrun, P. et al. (1983) Nutrition and immunity after peritoneovenous drainage of intractable ascites in cirrhotic patients. *American Journal of Surgery* 146:652–7.

44. Jenkins, D. J. A., Thorne, M. J., Taylor, K. H. et al. (1987) Effect of modifying the rate of digestion of foodstuffs on the blood glucose, amino acid and endocrine responses in patients with cirrhosis. *American Gastroenterology* 3:223–30.

45. Bucuvales, J. C., Heubi, J. E., Specker, B. L. et al. (1990) Calcium absorption in bone disease associated with chronic cholestasis in childhood. *Hepatology* 12:1200–5.

46. Cerra, F. B., Cheung, N. K., Fischer, J. E. et al. (1985) Disease specific amino acid infusion (F080) in hepatic encephalopathy. *Journal of Parenteral and Enteral Nutrition* 9:288–95.

47. Hehir, D. J., Jenkins, R. L., Bistrian, B. R. and Blackburn, G. L. (1985) Nutrition in patients undergoing orthotopic liver transplant. *JPEN* 9:695–700.

48. Hasse, J. M. (1990) Nutritional implications of liver transplantation. *Henry Ford Hospital Medical Journal* 38:235–40.

49. Shronts, E. P., Teasley, K. M., Thoele, S. L. and Cerra, F. B. (1987) Nutrition support of the adult liver transplant candidate. *Journal of American Dietary Association* 87:441–8.

Chapter 18
Drug-Induced Liver Disease

Dagmar Schaps

It is unknown how frequently liver damage caused by drugs occurs, most has a subclinical course. However, up to 25% of all cases of fulminant hepatitis have been attributed to drugs and drugs may be the cause of one-quarter to one-third of chronic liver diseases.[1]

Mechanism

Detoxification of Drugs

In all higher organisms most xenobiotics, including drugs, are metabolized in the liver, where the highest concentrations of enzymes can be found. Most drugs go through two stages of metabolism. Phase I metabolism includes hydroxylation and oxidation. These processes are catalyzed by the mixed-functional oxidase systems (MFO), exemplified by the cytochrome P450s. Phase II metabolism is characterized by conjugation with groups such as glucuronic and sulphonic acids.

These enzymes are not equally distributed throughout the liver lobule. For example sulphate reactions are principally periportal, while glucuronidation occurs pericentrally.[2] An age-related decline in oxidative biotransformation occurs in humans.[2,3] The activity and state of induction of these enzymes are influenced by nutrition.[4]

The detoxification systems can be induced by a variety of substances: polycyclic aromatic hydrocarbons, pesticides, industrial chemicals, and drugs such as barbituric acid and rifampicin. Barbituric acid is bound quickly to the endoplasmic reticulum after uptake into the liver cell. Six hours later a significant increase in MFO and an increase in surface and volume of smooth and rough endoplasmic reticulum can be shown. Here the hyperplasia of the endoplasmic reticulum—which also leads to an expansion of the liver itself—markedly exceeds the increase in enzymic activity.[5] Not all drugs have the same effect. Dexamethasone is a strong inducer of the microsomal enzymes but does not cause an increase in size of the endoplasmic reticulum. The microsomal drug-degrading enzyme system can be inhibited because of complex formation with metabolites, destruction by active metabolites, or interference by different pharmacological agents.

Mechanisms of Damage

Even though enzyme systems are able to convert and degrade a great variety of organic compounds, the number of metabolites that can be made are limited. In some instances they may not only detoxify drugs but also may transform some substances into toxic compounds. The best example of this is the

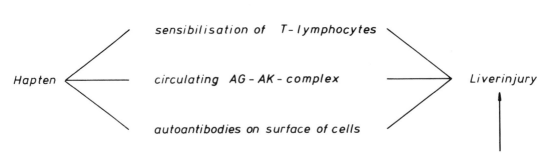

Figure 18-1. Humunologically medicated drug-induced liver damage.

liver damage caused by carbon tetrachloride. Metabolism of carbon tetrachloride by MFO causes the formation of a free trichlormethyl radical. This radical leads to lipid peroxidation of the endoplasmic reticulum with destruction of the membrane's structure and causes direct damage to the cell membrane. Paracetamol is another drug that causes liver damage in overdose, by swamping the normal metabolic pathway.[6] Because of their dose-dependence, paracetamol and carbon tetrachloride cause predictable liver damage. However, some substances cause unpredictable (idiosyncratic) damage, usually by being metabolized by an alternative pathway that produces a toxic metabolite. Alternatively, the metabolites of these drugs may become haptens and damage liver parenchymal cells by an immunologically mediated reaction. This damage might be worsened if the metabolites of the drugs are also cytotoxic (Figure 18-1).[7]

Diagnosis

Laboratory Findings

Large increases in aminotransferases and glutamate dehydrogenase (GLDH) are seen only with acute impairment of blood supply or severe toxic liver damage, for example in intoxication with carbon tetrachloride, halothane, or paracetamol. A hepatitis-like picture with an increase in transaminase activity up to 300–500 U/l, but a smaller increase in GLDH activity is common. The differential diagnosis usually includes viral hepatitis with concomitant cholestasis, intrahepatic obstruc-

tions (because of a space-occupying lesion), chronic inflammation, and extrahepatic obstruction of the biliary ducts.[8] In a small number of cases of liver damage caused by drugs there is a moderate increase in transaminases, a small increase in cholestasis, and a moderate decrease in cholinesterase (CHE).

Immunological Changes

In the serum of patients with a halothane hepatitis an antibody against membrane-neoantigens can be shown. It is specific, acts cytotoxically, and persists for a long time.[9] Using similar methods it is also possible to trace specific antibodies in the serum of patients with liver damage caused by methyldopa[10] and isoniazid.[11] Antibodies against microsome fractions of halothane-treated rabbits were found in the serum of 70% of patients with severe halothane hepatitis. This simple test has been suggested for screening of patients at risk of halothane hepatitis before using halothane.[11,12] An increase in antinuclear and smooth muscle tissue antibody can indicate an immunologically mediated drug reaction. This can be especially useful if clometacine, papaverine, oxyphenisatine, methyldopa, nitrofurantoin, prazosin, or halothane are suspected.[10,11,13]

Histology

Potent inducers of the MFO such as barbiturates, antiepileptics, some psychoactive drugs, etc. may lead to hyperplasia of the smooth endoplasmic reticulum. Strong reactions, viewed with a light microscope, show that the cytoplasm of these cells changes to fine granules, with web-like clearings and an increase in eosinophilia. The cell membrane is wider. According to Klinge this picture can easily be distinguished from the changes of the smooth endoplasmic reticulum occurring in cases of chronic hepatitis B virus (HBV) infections.[14] In addition, cells affected by poisoning are found in the center of the lobule, whereas in viral infections the changes are spread across the entire lobule. Some anti-inflammatory agents, such as phenacetin and acetylsalicylic-acid–containing compounds, may cause lipofuscinosis in the lysosomes. Fatty degeneration may occur with tetracycline. Inflammatory reactions are significantly less with drug-induced damage. With chronic drug damage the morphologic picture often resembles that of chronic-persistent or chronic-progressive viral hepatitis. However, with drug-induced damage more leukocytes, especially eosinophils, are seen in the infiltrated portal fields as well as increased bile deposits. The greater variability of change in the portal tracts also suggests a toxic cause.[14]

Potentially Hepatotoxic Drugs

The rest of this chapter surveys some of the drugs commonly used in the perioperative period that may cause liver damage. Many other drugs may exacerbate poor hepatic function and these can be found in pharmacology textbooks.

Drugs Used during Anesthesia

Volatile Anesthetic Agents

Halothane causes a wide range of liver damage ranging from a subclinical illness with little increase of enzyme activities (type 1) to the rare, severe, and fulminant liver-cell necrosis (type 2).[14a] Changes in enzyme activity can be seen in up to 20% of all patients after repeated exposure to halothane (type 1 damage). The total incidence of liver damage after halothane exposure is estimated to be one in every 9,000 and severe damage occurs with an incidence of one in every 40,000.

Of the halogen-substituted inhalation anesthetics different amounts are metabolized by the liver: 15–25% of halothane, 50% of methoxyflurane, 2.4% of enflurane, and 0.2% of isoflurane.[15] De-

pending on the oxygenation of the liver they are either oxidized into trifluoracetate by a cytochrome P450 or they undergo reduction.[15a] The oxidases taking part in the degradation of halothane can be induced by barbiturates and also by halothane itself.[16] This could explain the increase in damage after repeated exposure. The radicals produced by reduction cause lipid peroxidation leading to damage of cellular membranes. More are produced in the lobule's center, the most hypoxic region.

Only in severe cases are there specific antibodies against liver-cell particles altered by halothane. Presumably, metabolites produced by oxidative conversion become antigens and cause an immunoallergic reaction. These antibodies (IgG) can induce a cytotoxic reaction toward rabbit liver cells pretreated with halothane. To demonstrate these antibodies, which are not found in severe liver damage of a different cause, an enzyme-linked immunosorbent assay (ELISA) has been designed.[12] It showed positive findings in two-thirds of patients with halothane damage.[17] A conspicuous finding, relatively typical for halothane damage, in comparison with an acute virus jaundice, is the small increase of gamma glutamyl transferase (GGT) in relation to the transaminase activities.[18]

Lymphocyte sensitization of patients with halothane damage by metabolite-containing serum of healthy patients with halothane exposure[19] and concomitant clinical phenomena such as fever, eosinophilia, and arthritis, also suggest an immunoreactive cause.[20] Probably, the severe liver damage seen after repeated halothane exposure is a hypersensitive reaction of a genetically predisposed group. Halothane hepatitis can even be caused in these patients by the halothane remaining in the anesthetic apparatus when other volatile agents are being used.[21]

Liver damage after repeated halothane exposure can be seen if it is used within 6 weeks after the first exposure.[22] The intervals grow smaller each time it is used. Women develop halothane hepatitis twice as often as men. It is also seen more often in obese patients.

The histologic picture may be similar to that of a viral jaundice. However, necrosis may be more pronounced towards the center of the lobule.[18] Mallory bodies, a mononuclear infiltration with little fatty degeneration and granulomas, are seldom seen. Changes, similar to those in chronic hepatitis, have also been described.[23]

The mortality of severe halothane hepatitis averages 50%. Therapy is similar to that of necrotizing hepatitis; the use of steroids seems effective,[24] and liver transplantation may be life-saving. It is unknown whether chronic liver damage and cirrhosis may develop as a result of a halothane hepatitis. Cases of recurrent liver damage in anesthetists and nurses exposed to low doses of halothane have been reported.[25,26] The degree of exposure in these health workers may be determined by measuring the concentration of the oxidation product, trifluoroacetate.[27]

Liver damage after exposure to enflurane[15] or methoxyflurane[28] has been reported but is rarer.[29,30] The clinical picture is almost identical to the damage caused by halothane. Because the toxicity of alkylfluranes is caused by their metabolites, liver damage should not follow the use of isoflurane because it is hardly metabolized. Halothane is thus being replaced by enflurane and isoflurane.

Of the other agents diethyl ether causes only a small increase of transaminase activities, but vinyl ether has brought on several cases of massive liver-cell necrosis. The risk is increased with repeated exposure.

Hypnotics, Sedatives, Anxiolytics

There are sporadic descriptions of liver damage after the intravenous injection of thiopental.[31] Nitrous oxide does not cause liver damage. Liver damage caused by phenobarbital is rare; when it occurs it is usually accompanied by a skin eruption (sometimes exfoliative dermatitis), fever, and lymphadenopathy. Barbiturates, however, can also induce an acute hepatic porphyria or a porphyria variegata. The benzodiazepines (alprazolam, clobazam, chlordiazepoxide, chlorazepam, diazepam, flurazepam, thiazolam) cause only a moderate increase in enzyme activity and there are only a few reported cases of liver damage.[32] Chlorazepam and flurazepam have resulted in a cholestatic hepatitis and there has been a death after triazolam. Mild reactions of cholestatic inflammation have been described after chlormezanone[33] and meprobamate. In high doses paraldehyde and chloral hydrate have also caused hepatotoxicity.

Neuroleptics

Chlorpromazine has several effects on hepatocytes. It inhibits the liver-cell membrane Na^+/K^+ ATPase and Mg^{2+} ATPase. There may be a small increase (10–42%) in enzyme activity when these are given. This returns toward normal, even if therapy is continued. More rarely, 0.5–1% of patients becomes icteric because of a cholestatic hepatitis. Eosinophilia is present in 60% of patients and is sometimes accompanied by a skin rash. Rarely hepatic necrosis may occur. In the majority of patients the cholestasis gradually disappears. However, symptoms resembling an icteric and chronically destructive, nonsuppurative cholangitis may develop.[34] Cases of liver parenchymal cell damage with or without marked cholestasis have also been described with other phenothiazines such as fluphenazine, perazine, perphenazine, promazine, thioridazine, and thiofluoperazine.[31] Liver damage caused by the butyrophenones haloperidol and droperidrol does occur, but is rare.[35]

Antiepileptic Drugs

When antiepileptics are given there is a marked, isolated increase in serum-GGT and occasionally an increase in alkaline phosphatase (AP). The increase in GGT represents enzyme induction. Phenytoin may lead to hepatitis-like damage of the liver and, rarely, massive necrosis.[32] The damage manifests itself several weeks after the drug is started. The cause of the liver damage remains unclear. It may be a hypersensitive type of reaction. Indeed, after reexposure a general hypersensitivity reaction can immediately reappear but without derangement of liver function. The parenchymal cell damage is at least partly caused by toxic metabolites formed because of a genetically determined lack of epoxide hydrolase.[36] Patients with severe liver damage have a bad prognosis, especially if they also suffer from exfoliative dermatitis. A transition into a chronic hepatitis has not been seen. Cases of liver damage caused by the antiepileptic agents ethosuximide[37] and trimethadione[31] have been reported.

Carbamazepine may also damage the liver, as well as cause agranulocytosis, aplastic anaemia and thrombocytopenia.[32,37a] Valproic acid may cause two types of damage. First, there may be subclinical damage with a moderate increase in enzyme activities. Second, there may be severe and even lethal liver necrosis.[38] The incidence of the latter is an estimated one in 20,000, occurring mostly in patients under 10 years of age.[39] Although the combination of enzyme-inducing drugs, such as phenobarbital or diphenylhydantoin, in combination with a poor nutritional state (that decreases glucuronidation ability) leads to similar observations.[40] Histology shows a fine drop-like fatty degeneration of liver cells as well as necrosis in the lobule's center. There is a similarity between this and Reye's syndrome. The toxic metabolites of carbamazepine cause mitochondrial damage and a reduction of fatty acid oxidation.[20]

Analgesics

Aspirin causes not only allergic reactions but also liver damage. Histologically, the liver has changes of a nonspecific hepatitis. There is a large increase in enzymes and marked hepato-cellular necrosis.[41] The damage is reversible by dose reduction.[42] Salicylates trigger Reye's syndrome in children being treated for chickenpox or influenza.[43] The syndrome begins with vomiting and an encephalopathy. The bilirubin is moderately increased, while the transaminases increase greatly. Histology shows a fine drop-like fatty degeneration of the liver.[44] In 1980 the mortality rate was 23%; however, of those surviving, 34–36% had long-term neurologic or psychiatric problems.

In therapeutic doses paracetamol has no major side effects. The drug's major route of elimination is by conjugation. A small amount is oxidatively metabolized to N acetyl-*p*-benzoquinone. This metabolite is toxic. It is inactivated mostly by conjugation with glutathione (a small amount is also excreted as the catechol derivative). After ingestion of large amounts of paracetamol there is insufficient glutathione to metabolize the paracetamol to innocuous substances. Severe necrosis of the liver and the kidney occurs if amounts of paracetamol greater than 10 g are taken.[45] After 2–5 days transaminase activities increase up to 50–500 times the normal followed by a decreased activity of clotting factors. At a plasma concentration of 150 μg/mL the risk of hepatic necrosis is low; at a level of over 300 μg/mL it is high. After 12 hours, toxic intermediates have already been formed and bound. *N*-acetylcysteine, part of the glutathione synthesis reaction, can be given before this to prevent toxicity.[45] Another possible treatment is the inhibition of the MFO by cimetidine,[46] but this is rarely done.

In contrast to the relatively uniform type of liver damage caused by many drugs, phenylbutazone shows three different types.[47] There is severe hepa-

tocellular, mainly centrolobular damage with or without bridging necroses. A picture of a "classical" viral hepatitis with cell necrosis and portal infiltration with or without cholestasis may also be seen. Finally, changes similar to primary biliary cirrhosis with a reduction of interlobular biliary ducts and the appearance of granulomas may occur. The various types of damage are based on different causes. Apart from a hypersensitive reaction there is direct, toxic cell damage. This toxic cell damage is estimated to be brought on by the reduction of glutathione in the liver.[48] The changes usually appear during the first 6 weeks after starting the therapy. Severe damage leads to death in 23–28% of patients.[23]

Diclofenac rarely seems to cause severe damage to the liver.[49] Similarly, ibuprofen only causes a small amount of hepatocellular damage,[50] but one case of fulminant hepatitis has been reported.[51] Indomethacin has caused hepatocellular, as well as cholestatic, reactions without signs of hypersensitivity when given for a long time.[52,53]

Antibiotics

Liver damage caused by penicillin is rare, but is being increasingly reported.[54] When it does occur it usually causes a reversible cholestatic jaundice. Granulomatous hepatitis is also possible.[16] Of the derivatives of penicillin, cloxacillin has caused an eosinophilia and an increase in transaminase activities up to 1000 U/L in children.[55] Mild reversible and anicteric hepatitis could be traced back to carbenicillin[56] and oxacillin[57] when patients were re-exposed to the drugs. Changes in enzyme activity caused by flucloxacillin,[8] methicillin, and nafcillin have also been described.[58] Chloramphenicol rarely leads to hepatocellular necrosis with or without cholestasis. Clindamycin showed an increase in transaminases in 15–20% of patients, but jaundice is rare.[59] Cephalosporins increase transaminase activities rarely, but may cause a chronic cholestatic hepatitis.[60] Intolerance to alcohol, after the use of various cephalosporins, is caused by their inhibiting acetaldehyde dehydrogenase.

Tetracyclines can cause dose-dependent damage to the liver, kidney, and pancreas.[8] Histologically the liver shows a fine, drop-like, fatty degeneration pericentrally with little cholestasis and inflammatory reactions. Severe, fatal liver damage may occur.[61] In 1–2% of adults tetracyclines may cause a cholestatic jaundice accompanied by rash, fever, and eosinophilia.[62] Similar signs have been seen after giving erythromycin estolate, ethylsuccinate and lactobionate.[63]

The incidence of hepatitis-like reactions caused by sulfonamides is about 0.6%. The prognosis is generally good, although one case of chronic hepatitis after long-term administration of sulfonamides[64] and reexposure has been described.[29]

Antiarrhythmics, Coronary Dilators, Calcium Antagonists

Amiodarone is a valuable antiarrhythmic agent that has a long half-life and is stored in organs of high fat content. One of its side effects is liver damage. The increase of transaminases correlates with the plasma concentrations of amiodarone and its major metabolite, diethylamiodarone. If the drug is stopped these changes in enzyme activity may disappear, although there is a chance of cirrhosis or even liver failure. Histology shows a picture of an nonspecific reactive hepatitis. Long-term treatment may result in damage resembling that of alcohol-poisoning, with fatty degeneration, Mallory bodies, ballooning of hepatocytes, focal necrosis, and inflammatory infiltrations with collagen in the centrizonal areas of the lobule.[65,66] Hepatocellular damage, with or without cholestasis, is seen after use of aprindine.[67] Histology shows monocellular necrosis, central cholestasis, and portal tract infiltrations. Giving disopyramide, amrinone, and mexiletine may also be followed by toxic liver damage. Procainamide, tocainidine, and verapramil cause only mild damage,[46,68] while propafenone leads to cholestatic hepatitis.[69]

Antihypertensives

A wide range of liver damage is caused by methyldopa. An asymptomatic increase in enzyme activities accompanied by fever and myalgia may be seen. Alternatively there may be an acute fulminant hepatitis or granulomatous hepatitis or chronic liver disease.[70] The severe damage with a transaminase increase of over 1000 U/L is difficult to distinguish from a viral hepatitis. Recovery is possible if the necrosis is not too massive; alternatively, chronic liver dysfunction may develop.

The mechanism causing this is immunological. There is usually a positive Coombs test and lupus erythematosus (LE) cell test. Reexposure may trigger strong, and even lethal, reactions. There may be an immediate allergic–toxic reaction with hydropic parenchymal cell degeneration and focal, confluent, or massive necroses with secondary inflammation. Alternatively, there may be fatty degeneration with the formation of granuloma and fibrosis.[71] Captopril has caused some damage to the liver.[72]

Liver Damage Caused by Drug Abuse

Up to 50–90% of narcotic addicts show change in liver function,[73] although the liver damage is small. Toxic liver damage by cocaine is rare.[74] More than 90% of cocaine is degraded into nontoxic metabolites. However, it can also be oxidatively metabolized by MFO,[75] and the peroxide radicals and cocaine metabolites may then cause liver cell necrosis of lipid peroxidation or the formation of covalent protein bonds.[76] Inhalation of narcotics, solvents, or anesthetics causes damage to the central nervous system or to the heart, rather than to the liver. Halothane sniffers are the exception to the rule. There have been deaths from liver failure among this group. However, even in this group the most frequent causes of death are respiratory depression and cardiac arrhythmias.[77]

Besides these effects there are other reasons for liver damage in drugs addicts. Simultaneous use of a combination of drugs and alcohol may accentuate liver damage. Also in such patients 42% showed toxic cirrhosis and 10% of these showed positive HBV markers.[78–80] The "eking-out" of substances with an impure or dirty substance (usually talcum powder) can cause granulomatous hepatitis as well as talc granuloma.[81]

So long as the immune system is not impaired, liver damage caused by bacterial infections (because of the sharing of injection instruments) is *relatively* rare. However, along with homosexuals,[82,83] drug addicts have the highest risk of an infection with other organisms, especially with HIV. In this group the immune system is depressed and in 12% of drug addicts one can see liver damage caused by histoplasmosis, acid-fast bacilli, and cytomegalovirus (CMV) as well as staphylococcal microabscesses.[76] Many addicts who take their drugs parenterally show markers for hepatitis viruses: of these 90–100% show markers for contact with the hepatitis B virus.[84] About two-thirds end the infection with the production of anti-HBs. The course of the acute viral hepatitis is mostly mild but may be prolonged and about one-third of these patients develop a rather nonactive, chronic hepatitis.[85]

Liver Damage Caused by Chemicals

If chemicals used in industrial processes cause severe acute liver damage then cases are usually published quickly and investigated further. However, little is known about the results of chronic exposure of low-grade hepatotoxins and their interaction with other chemicals, drugs, and nutrition. These are likely to cause less severe liver injury and as such are less likely to be reported and investigated with the same vigor. Patients with a minor degree of hepatic dysfunction from this cause may not have symptoms until after an operation, or as part of another illness or after an accident. In this situation there may be confusion as to the cause of the hepatic dysfunction.

Alcohols

Methanol is eliminated partly by breathing. It is metabolized at a rate of 25 mg/kg/h. This is much slower than ethanol metabolized at a rate of 175 mg/kg/h. An intake of only 15 mL methanol can cause permanent loss of sight, and 30 mL may be lethal in humans. However, there is considerable variability and some patients have survived a dose of 250 mL. The oxidation of methanol into formic acid in the liver causes a metabolic acidosis. It also causes fatty degeneration and focal necrosis. Existing liver damage causes a delay in methanol degradation. Giving ethanol[86] can slow down the acidosis and reduce the toxicity. Animal experiments have shown similar effects for inhibitors of the alcohol dehydrogenase (pyrazol, 4-methylpyrazol).[87]

Halogenated Hydrocarbons

Aliphatic Halogenized Hydrocarbons

It has been known for 50 years that carbon tetrachloride (CCl_4) has a hepatoxic effect. The relatively nontoxic parent compound is converted into the toxic radical CCl_3 by liver enzymes. This, in turn, irreversibly, covalently binds to membrane proteins and lipids and so leads to liver cell necrosis, mostly in the central parts of the liver's lobule.

The damage is greater if the MFO have been induced by alcohol,[88,89] since more toxic radicals are formed. The damage is smaller if the MFO's capacity is reduced by starvation. Heart, lungs, pancreas, and possibly the bone marrow may also be damaged.[90] Hepatic damage after a single acute intoxication is usually reversible, and cirrhosis after a single intoxication is rare. Continuous inhalation of small amounts of CCl_4 can produce this.

The toxic effect of CCl_4 is based on the separation of Cl and the formation of the highly reactive radical CCl_3. Changing $CHCl_3$ (chloroform) into this radical is much more difficult because of its strong C-H bond. The C-F binding of $CFCl_3$ is even stronger, but less energy is needed to split the C-Br bond. Thus the order of ease for activation of the CCl_4 homologues into a toxic radical is: CCl_3 Br > CCl_4 > $CHCl_3$ > $CFCl_3$. This order coincides with that of relative liver toxicity. So, bromtrichlormethane is 10–15 times more hepatotoxic than CCl_4. The toxic effect of $CHCl_3$ is similar to that of CCl_4. However, this is not based on the production of a radical but on an inducible cytochrome P450-dependent oxidation of the molecule into toxic substances. Industrial poisoning by CCl_4 causes fatty degeneration of the liver.[91] Even though both methylene chloride ($CH_2 Cl_2$) and methylchloride ($CH_3 Cl$) form covalent bonds with liver proteins, their acute hepatotoxicity is much smaller. The nonchlorinated homologues of CCl_4, bromomethane and iodo-methane, are less volatile, less stable, and increasingly more reactive than the chloromethane homologues.

Haloethanes

The haloethanes are dehalogenated in the liver and excreted as glutathione conjugates in the urine. There are cases of acute liver damage after chloroethane, bromoethane, and iodoethane, but their main point of action is the central nervous system as well as the cardiovascular system. Animal experiments showed a direct mutagenic effect and also liver damage through the dihaloethanes, 1,2-dichloroethane and 1,2-dibromoethane. Comparative investigation confirmed trichloroethanes to be far less liver toxic than CCl_4.[92] However, inhalation of tetrachloroethane has brought on widespread liver cell necrosis.[93] The anesthetic halothane ($CF_3 CHClBr$) is the most important pentahaloethane in this context.

Three of the haloethylenes have special economic value: trichloroethylene (Cl_2 C=CHCl) is used to degrease metals, perchloroethylene (Cl_2 C=CCl$_2$) is used as a textile detergent, and vinyl chloride (ClHC=CH$_2$) is a source material of plastics. All chlorinated ethylenes are metabolized in the liver, but their relative hepatotoxicity differs from one to the other: 1,1-dichlorethylene > cis-1,2-dichlorethylene > trans-1,2-dichlorethylene > trichloroethylene > vinyl chloride > perchlorethylene. Damage to the liver occurs mainly in the structures of the endoplasmic reticulum of the centrilobule area. It is increased by induction of the MFO 1,1-dichlorethylene, which apparently becomes biotransformed in a different way, is the exception to the rule. Industrial accidents with trichloroethylene resemble those with CCl_4. Acute neurologic symptoms as well as kidney and liver damage are seen.

It is unknown whether or not liver damage in "solvent sniffers"[94] can be solely explained by the effect of trichloroethylene or contamination with CCl_4.[95] Animal experiments showed that trichloethylene strongly increases CCl_4 hepatotoxicity.[96] Repeated severe intoxications with trichloroethylene and later with trichloroethane lead to the development of a cirrhosis,[97] but a long-term exposure with perchloroethylene does not cause liver damage.[98] Vinyl chloride causes a selective reduction in the MFO, including the cytochrome P450 oxidase, and chronic exposure leads to slow but progressive liver damage with marked fibrosis of the perisinusoidal area.

The collective name dioxin includes all polychlorinated dibenzoparadioxins (PCDD). They are closely related to the polychlorinated dibenzofuranes (PCDF). The PCDD are formed as by-products in the production of chlorinated phenols and in the burning of organic material and wood. Both compound groups consist of aromatic ethers. Depending on the number and position of the chlorine atoms the compounds are more or less toxic. The most poisonous of the known dioxins is the one called "Seveso" dioxin. The acute toxicity of this 2,3,7,8-PCDD is markedly species dependent; there have been many accounts of intoxications with dioxins and dibenzofuranes.[99] Usually liver damage is limited to a temporary increase of enzyme activities; rarely it produces the manifestation of chronic hepatic porphyria.[100] Histology showed fatty degeneration, periportal fibrosis, and Kupffer cell activation.[101] Chlorinated hydrocarbons and their derivatives are used as insecticides and herbicides. They may enter the body percutaneously, enterally, or by inhalation and then accumulate in the fat tissue as well as in the liver.[102] The acute poisoning with DDT or lindane, as with other polyhalogenated cyclic hydrocarbons, leads to hyperexcitability of the central and the peripheral motor neurons. Extremely high doses may bring on convulsions and cause necrotic liver damage.[103]

References

1. Wilson, J.H.P. (1984) Drugs and the liver. In: *The Liver Annual 4/1984*, (Arias, I.M., Frenkel, F. and Wilson, J.H.P. eds). Amsterdam: Elsevier Science Publishers, pp. 413–434.
2. James, O.F.W. (1985) Drugs and the ageing liver. *Journal of Hepatology*, 1:431–35.
3. Popper, H. (1985) Coming of age. *Hepatology* 5:1224–26.
4. Walter-Sack, I. (1987) The influence of nutrition on the systemic availability of drugs. Part II: Drug metabolism and renal excretion. *Klinische Welheuschrift*, 65:1062–72.
5. Thurmann, R.G. and Kauffman, F.C. (1985) Sublobular compartmentation of pharmacologic events (SCOPE): Metabolic Fluxes in peri-portal and pericentral regions of the liver lobule. *Hepatology*, 5:144–151.
6. O'Grady, J.G., Alexander, G.J., Hayllar, K.M. and Williams, R. (1989) Early indicators of prognosis in fulminant hepatic failure. *Gastroenterology* 97:439–45.
7. Zimmerman, H.J. and Maddrey, W.C. (1987) Toxic and drug induced hepatitis. In: *Diseases of the Liver*, 6th ed., (Schiff, L. and Schiff, E.R. eds). Philadelphia: Lippincott Co, pp. 591–667. Legends: Drug induced liver damage.
8. Combes, B., Whalley, P.J. and Adams, R.H. (1972) Tetracycline and the liver. In: *Progress in Liver Disease*, (Popper, H. and Schaffner, F. eds). New York: Grune & Stratton, pp. 589–596.
9. Neuberger, J., Gimson, A.E.S., Davies, M. and Williams, R. (1983) Specific serological markers in the diagnosis of fulminant hepatic failure associated with halothane anaesthesia. *British Journal of Anaesthesia* 55:15–18.
10. Neuberger, J., Kenna, J.G., Nouri Aria, K. and Williams, R. (1985) Antibody mediated hepatocyte injury in methyl-dopa induced hepatotoxicity. *Gut* 26:1233–39.
11. Warrington, R.J., Tse, K.S., Gorski, B.E., Schwenk, R. and Sehon, A.H. (1978) Evaluation of isoniazid-associated hepatitis by immunological tests. *Clinical and Experimental Immunology* 32:97–104.
12. Kenna, J.G., Neuberger, J. and Williams, R. (1984) An enzyme linked immunosorbent assay for detection of

antibodies against halothane-altered hepatocyte antigens. *Journal Immunological Methods* 75:3–14.

13. Homberg, J.C., Abruaf, N., Hemly-Khalil, S. et al. (1985) Drug induced hepatitis associated with anticytoplasmic organelle antibodies. *Hepatology* 5:722–27.

14. Klinge, O. (1984) Leber. In: *Pathologie,* vol. 2. (Remmele, W. ed). Berlin, Heidelberg: Springer, pp. 589–740.

14a. Neuberger, J. and Williams, R. (1984) Halothane anaesthesia and liver damage. *British Medical Journal* 289:1136–39.

15. Lewis, J.H., Zimmerman, H.J., Ishak, K.G. and Mullick, F.G. (1983) Enflurane hepatotoxicity: A clinico pathologic study of 24 cases. *Annals of Internal Medicine* 98:984–92.

15a. De Groot, H. and Noll, T. (1983) Halothane hepatotoxicity: Relation between metabolic activation, hypoxia, covalent binding, lipid perioxidation and liver cell damage. *Hepatology* 3:601–06.

16. Goldstein, L.I. and Ishak, K.G. (1974) Hepatic injury associated with penicillin therapy. *Archives of Pathology* 98:114–17.

17. Editorial (1986) Halothane-associated liver damage. *Lancet* i:1251–52.

18. Schmidt, E. and Vido, I. (1976) Exogene toxische Leberschäden. In: *Toxische Leberschäden,* (Wannagat, L. ed). Stuttgart: Thieme, pp. 166–179.

19. Berg, P.A. and Brattig, N. (1981) Role of immune mechanisms in drug-induced diseases. In: *Drug reactions and the Liver,* (Davis, T.H., Tredger, J.M. and Williams, R. eds). London: Pitman Medical, pp. 105–110.

20. Farell, G., Prendergast, D. and Murray, M. (1985) Halothane hepatitis: Detection of a constitutional susceptibility factor. *New England Journal of Medicine* 313:1310–14.

21. Conn, H.O. and Scornicki, J. (1985) Halothane hepatitis sans halothane. *Hepatology* 5:1238–40.

22. Dundee, J.W., McIllroy, P.D.A., Fee, J.P.H. and Black, G.W. (1981) Prospective study of liver function following repeat halothane and enflurane. *Journal of the Royal Society of Medicine* 74:286–91.

23. Benjamin, S.B., Goodman, Z.D., Ishak, K.G., Zimmerman, H.J. and Ireay, N.S. (1985) The morphologic spectrum of halothane-induced hepatic injury: Analysis of 77 cases. *Hepatology* 5:1163–71.

24. Varma, R.R. and Kalbfleisch, J.H. (1984) Beneficial effects of corticosteroid therapy in halothane hepatitis: Results of a prospective controlled study (Abstract). *Gastroenterology* 86:1345.

25. Klatskin, G. and Kimberg, D. (1969) Recurrent hepatitis attributable to halothane sensitization in an anesthesist. *New England Journal of Medicine* 23:515–22.

26. Schmidt, G., Börsch, F., Ricken, D., Müller, K.M. and Neuberger, J. (1985) Zentrolobuläre Leberzellnekrosen nach beruflichem Halothan-Kontakt–Assoziation mit Antikörpern gegen Halothan alte-rierte Leberzellkomponenten. *Z. Gastroent.* 23:192–97.

27. Dallmeier, D. and Heuschler, D. (1981) Halothan-Belastung amAr-beitsplatz im Operationssaal. *Deutsche medizinische Wochenschrift* 106:324–328.

28. Cousins, M.J., Plummer, J.L. and Hall, P.D. (1985) Toxicity of volatile anesthetic agents. *Canadian Anaesthetists Society Journal* 32:52–55.

29. Ransohoff, D.F. and Jacobs, G. (1981) Terminal hepatic failure following a small dose of sulfamethoxazole– Trimethoprim. *Gastroenterology* 80:816–19.

30. Touloukian, J. and Kaplowitz, N. (1981) Halothane-induced hepatic diseases. *Seminars in Liver Disease* 1:134–42.

31. Stricker, B.H.C. and Spoelstra, P. (1985) Drug-induced hepatic injury. In: *Series: Drug-induced Disorders.* (Dukes, M.N.G. ed). Amsterdam: Elsevier Science Publishers.

32. Davion, T., Capron-Chivrac, D., Andrejak, M. and Capron, J.C. (1985) Les hépatites dues aux médicamentes antiépileptiques. *Gastroenterology Clinical Biology* 9:117–26.

33. Pomiersky, C. and Blaich, B. (1985) Arzneimittelbedingte Hepatitis und Cholestase nach Therapie mit Chlormezanone. *Z. Gastroent.* 23:684–86.

34. Ishak, K.G. and Irey, N.S. (1972) Hepatic injury associated with the phenothiazines. Clinicopathologic and follow-up study of 36 patients. *Archives of Pathology* 93:283–304.

35. Dinosoy, H.P. and Saelinger, D.A. (1982) Haloperidol-induced chronic cholestatic liver disease. *Gastroenterology* 83:694–700.

36. Spielberg, S.P., Gordon, G.B., Blake, D.A., Goldstein, D.A. and Herlong, H.F. (1981) Predisposition to phenytoin hepatoxicity assessed in vitro. *New England Journal of Medicine* 305:722–27.

37. Coulter, D.L. (1983) Ethosuximide-induced liver dysfunction. *Archives of Neurology* 40:393–94.

37a. Hadzic, N., Portmann, B., Davies, E.T., Mowat, A.P. and Mieli-Vergani, G. (1990) Acute liver failure induced by carbamazepine. *Archives of Disease in Childhood* 65:315–17.

38. Scott, D.A., Gholson, C.F., Netchvolodoff, C.V., Gonzales, E. and Bacon, B.R. (1991) Incidental microvesicular steatosis due to valporic acid anticonvulsant therapy. *American Journal of Gastroenterology* 86:500–02.

39. Harendra, de Silva, D.G., Keembiyahetty, P., Jayantha, U.K. and Theli-singhe, P.U. (1990) Acute liver failure in a patient with hepatitis A infection on sodium valproate therapy. *Ceylon Medical Journal* 35:76–70.

40. Kesterson, J.W., Granneman, G.R. and Machinist, J.M. (1984) The hepatotoxicity of valproic acid and its metabolites in rats. I. Toxicologic, biochemical and histopathologic studies. *Hepatology* 4:1143–52.

41. Schmidt, E. (1978) Zur Praxis der Enzym-Diagnostik der Leber- und Gallenwegserkrankungen. In: *Stand und Entwicklung der Laboratoriumsdianostik von Leber- und Gallenwegserkrankungen,* (Haschen, R.J. and Nilius, R. eds). Halle: KTB, pp. 6–24.

42. Zimmerman, H.J. (1978) *Hepatotoxicity: The Adverse Effects of Drugs and Other Chemicals on the Liver.* New York: Appleton-Century Crofts, p. 395.

43. Ulschen, M.H. (1986) Salicylates and Reye's syndrome. *Gastroenterology* 91:487–88.

44. Partin, J.S., Daugherty, C.C., McAdams, A.J., Partin, J.C. and Schubert, W.K. (1984) A comparison of liver ultrastructure in salicylate intoxication and Reye's syndrome. *Hepatology* 4:687–90.

45. Black, M. (1984) Acetaminophen hepatotoxicity. *Ann Rev Med* 35:577–93.

46. Negro, F., Pessano, B., Marcolongo, M., Presbitero, P., Brunetto, M.R. and Bonino, F. (1986) Severe liver injury possibly due to verapamil. *Italian Journal of Gastroenterology* 18:332–34.

47. Benjamin, S.B., Ishak, K.G., Zimmerman, H.J. and Gruschka, A. (1981) Phenylbutazone liver injury: A clinical-pathologic survey of 23 cases and review of the literature. *Hepatology* 1:255–63.

48. Bien, E. (1983) Einfluβ von Pyrazolonderivaten auf den Gehalt an reduziertum Glutathion in der Rattenleber. *Biomed Biochem Acta* 42:561–76.

49. Lascar, G., Grippan, P. and Levy, V.-G. (1984) Hépatite aiguë mortelleau cours d'un traitment par le diclofenac (VoltareneR). *Gastroenterology Clinical Biology* 8:881–85.

50. Lewis, J.H. (1984) Hepatic toxicity of nonsteroid anti-inflammatory drugs. *Clinical Pharmacology* 3:128–38.

51. Depla, A.C., Vermeersch, P.H., van Gorp, L.H. and Nadorp, J.H. (1990) Fatal acute liver failure associated with pirprofen. Report of a case and a review of the literature. *Netherlands Journal of Medicine* 37:32–36.

52. Kelsey, W.M. and Scharyi, M. (1967) Fatal hepatitis probably due to indomethacin. *Journal of the American Medical Association* 199:586–87.

53. Mitchell, M.C., Schenker, S. and Speeg Jr., K.V. (1984) Selective inhibition of acetaminophen oxidation and toxicity by cimetidine and other histamine H2-receptor antagonists in vivo and in vitro in the rat and in man. *Journal of Clinical Investigation* 73:383–91.

54. BMJ, 1993.

55. Enat, R., Pollack, S., Ben-Arich, Y., Livini, E. and Barzilai, D. (1980) Cholestatic jaundice caused by cloxacillin: Macrophage inhibition factor rest in preventing rechallenge with hepatotoxic drugs. *British Medical Journal* 280:982–83.

56. Wilson, F.M., Belamaric, J., Lauter, C.B. and Lerner, M. (1975) Anicteric carbenicillin hepatitis. Eight episodes in four patients. *Journal of the American Medical Association* 232:818–21.

57. Tauris, P., Jorgensen, N.F., Petersen, C.M. and Albertson, K. (1985) Prolonged severe cholestasis induced by oxacillin derivates. *Acta Medica Scandinavica* 217:567–69.

58. Kitzing, W., Nelson, J.D. and Mohs, E. (1981) Comparative toxicities of methicillin and nafcillin. *American Journal of Diseases of Children* 135.

59. Zimmerman, H.J. (1981) Effects of aspirin and acetaminophen on the liver. *Archives of Internal Medicine* 141:333–42.

60. Wolf, A., Schomerus, H. and Berg, P. (1985) Schwere Leberschädigung als medikamentös-allergischue Reaktion auf Cefoperazon. *Z. Gastroent.* 23: 198–202.

61. Schenker, S., Breen, K.J. and Heimberg, M. (1975) Pathogenesis of tetracyclin-induced fatty liver. In: Drugs and Liver, (Gerok, W. and Sickinger, K. eds). Stuttgart: Schattauer, pp. 269–280.

62. Funck-Brentano, C., Pressyre, D. and Benhamou, J.P. (1983) Hépatites due a diverses dérivés de l'érythromycine. *Gastroenterology Clinical Biology* 7:362–69.

63. Diehl, A.M., Latham, P., Broitnott, J.K., Mann, J. and Maddrey, W.C. (1984) Cholestatic hepatitis from erythromycin ethylsuccinate. *American Journal of Medicine* 76:931–34.

64. Tonder, M., Nordöv, D. and Elgjo, D. (1974) Sulfonamide-induced chronic liver disease. *Scandinavian Journal of Gastroenterology* 9:93–96.

65. Babany, G., Mallat, A., Zafeani, E.S. et al. (1986) Chronic liver disease after low daily doses of amiodarone. *J Hepatology* 3:228–32.

66. Rigas, B., Rosenfeld, L.E., Barwick, K.W., et al. (1986) Amiodarone hepatotoxicity. *Annals of Internal Medicine* 104:348–51.

67. Brandes, J.W., Schmitz-Moormann, P., Lehmann, F.G. and Martini, G.A. (1976) Gelbsucht nach aprindin. *Deutsches medizinische Wochenschrift* 101:111–113.

68. Levy, M., Goodman, M.W., van Dyne, B.G. and Summer, H.W. (1981) Granulomatous hepatitis secondary to carbamazepine. *Annals of Internal Medicine* 95:64–65.

69. Konz, K.H., Berg, P.A. and Seipel, L. (1984) Cholestase nach antiarrhythmischer Therapie mit Propafenon. *Deutsche medizinische Wochenschrift* 109:1525–27.

70. van Maercke, Y., Colement, L., Pelckmans, P. and Buyssens, N. (1987) Ernster Leberschaden durch Methyldopa bei einem Patienten mit Hypertonie. *Verdauungskrankheiten* 29–30.

71. Arranto, A.J. and Satemiemi, E.S. (1981) Morphological alterations in patients with alpha methyldopa induced liver damage after short- and longterm exposure. *Scand J Gastroent* 16:853–63.

72. Zimran, A., Abraham, A.S. and Hershko, C. (1983) Reversible cholestatic jaundice and hyperamylasaemia associated with captopril treatment. *British Medical Journal* 287:1676.

73. Marks, V. and Capple, P.A.L. (1967) Hepatic dysfunction in heroin and cocaine users. *British Journal of Addiction* 62:189–95.

74. Perino, L.E., Warren, G.H. and Levine J.S. (1987) Cocaine induced hepatotoxicity in humans. *Gastroenterology* 93:176–80.

75. Kloss, M.W., Rosen, G.M. and Ranckman, E.J. (1984) Cocaine mediated hepatotoxicity. A critical review. *Biochem. Pharmacol.* 33:169–73.

76. Evans, M.A. (1983) Role of protein binding in cocaine induced hepatic necrosis. *Journal of Pharmacology and Experimental Therapy* 224:73–79.

77. Yamashita, M., Matsuki, A. and Oyama, T. (1984) Illicit use of modern volatile anaesthetics. *Canadian Anaesthetists Society Journal* 31:76–79.

78. Novick, D.M., Enlow, R.W., Geld, A.M. et al. (1985) Hepatic cirrhosis in young adults: Association with adolescent onset of alcohol and patenteral heroin abuse. *Gut* 26:8–13.

79. Novick, D.M., Gelb, A.M., Stenger, R.J. et al. (1981) Hepatitis B serologic studies in narcotic users with chronic liver disease. *American Journal of Gastroenterology* 75:111–15.

80. Sapira, J.D., Ball, J.C. and Penn, H. (1979) Causes of death among institutionalized narcotic addicts. *Journal of Chronic Diseases* 22:733–42.

81. Min, K., Gyorkey, F. and Cain, G.D. (1974) Talc granulomata in liver disease in narcotic addicts. *Archives of Pathology* 98:331–35.

82. Update (1986) Acquired immuno deficiency syndrome—United States. *Morbidity and Mortality Weekly Report* 35:17–21.

83. Update (1986) Acquired immuno deficiency syndrome—Europe. *Morbidity and Mortality Weekly Report* 35:35–46.

84. Hoofnagle, J.H., Seeff, L.B. and Bales, Z.B. (1987) Serologic responses in Hb. In: *Viral Hepatitis,* (Vyas, G.N., Cohen, S.N. and Schmidt, R. eds). Philadelphia: Franklin Inst. Press, pp. 219–242.

85. May, B., Helmstaedt, D., Kramer, D. et al. (1974) Leberschädigung bei drogenabhängigen Patienten. *Verhandl. Dtsch. Ges. Innere Med.* 80:1554–56.

86. Eckhardt, R.E. (1971) Industrial intoxications which may simulate ethyl alcohol intake. *Industrial Medicine and Surgery* 40:33–35.

87. McMartin, K.E., Makar, A.D., Martin, G., Palese, A.M. and Tephly, T.R. (1975) Methanol poisoning. I. The role of formic acid in the development of metabolic acidosis in the monkey and the reversal by 4-Methalpyrazole. *Biochem. Med.* 13:319–33.

88. Cornish, H.H. and Adefuain, J. (1967) Potentation of carbon tetrachloride toxicity by aliphatic alcohols. *Archives of Environmental Health* 14:447–49.

89. Folland, D.S., Schaffner, W., Ginn, H.E., Crofford, O.B. and Murray, D.R. (1976) Carbon tetrachloride toxicity potentiated by isopropyl alcohol. *Journal of the American Medical Association* 236:1853–56.

90. Schmidt, E. and Schmidt, F.W. (1973) Enzym-Diagnostik bei Leberer-krankungen. In: *Gallenwege–Leber,* (Boekker, W. ed). Stuttgart: Thieme, pp. 32–50.

91. Bomski, H., Sobolewska, A., and Strakowski, A. (1967) Toxische Schädigung der Leber durch Chloroform bei Chemiewerksarbeitern. *Int. Arch. Gewebepath.* 24: 127–34.

92. Stewart, R.D. and Andrews, J.T. (1966) Acute intoxication with methyl chloroform. *Journal of the American Medical Association* 195:904–06.

93. Wilson, R.H. and Brumley, D.R. (1944) Health hazards in the use of tetrachlorethan. *Industrial Medicine* 13:233–34.

94. Baerg, R.D. and Kimberg, D.V. (1970) Centrilobular hepatic necrosis and·acute renal failure in Solvent Sniffers. *Annals of Internal Medicine* 73:713–20.

95. Bouygues, M., Danne, O., Bouvry, M., Luciani, F. and Rabreau, D. (1980) Hépatite au trichloroéthyléne. Action synergique du tétrachlorure de carbone. *Nouv. Presse Méd.* 9:3277–84.

96. Pessayre, D., Cobert, B., Descatoire, V., Degott, C., Delaforge, M. and Larrey, D. (1982) Hepatotoxicity of trichloroethylene-carbon tetrachloride mixtures in rats. *Gastroenterology* 83:761–72.

97. Thiele, D.L., Eigenbrodt, E.H. and Ware, A.J. (1982) Cirrhosis after repeated trichlorethylene and 1,1,1-trichlorethane exposure. *Gastroenterology* 83:926–29.

98. Schimmelpfennig, W., Lun, A., Gutewrort, T. and Dietz, E. (1987) Serum enzyme activities in perchlorethylene (Per-)-exposed workers. *Journal of Hepatology* 5, (suppl 1), 199 (abstract).

99. Lelbach, W.K. (1985) Leber und Umweltgifte. *Klinische Wochenschrift* 63:1139–51.

100. Strik, J.J.T.W.A. and Doss, M. (1978) Chronische hepatische Porphyrie durch polyhalogenisierte aromatische Verbindungen beim Menschen. *Therapiewoche* 28:8466–560.

101. Pazderova-Vejlupková, A., Nemcova, M., Picková, J. and Jirásek, L. (1981) The development and prognosis of chronic intoxication by tetrachlorodibenzo-p-dioxin in man. *Archives of Environmental Health* 36:5–11.

102. Klimmer, O.R. (1961) Vergiftungen durch Insektizide. In: *Handbuch der gesamten Arbeitsmedizin,* vol. 2, (Baader, E.W. ed). Berlin, München: Urban & Schwarzenberg, p. 549.

103. Henschler, D. (1987) Gesundheitsschäden durch Lindan. *Deutsche medizinische Wochenschrift* 112:1921.

Index